RECOGNITION, IDENTIFICATION AND PREVENTION OF ACUTE VIRAL INFECTIONS

RECOGNITION, IDENTIFICATION AND PREVENTION OF ACUTE VIRAL INFECTIONS

"The wise heart will know the proper time and procedure"
Ecclesiastes 8:5b (NIV)

by

DONALD M. McLEAN, MD, FRCP(C)
Professor, Division of Medical Microbiology
University of British Columbia
Vancouver, B.C., Canada

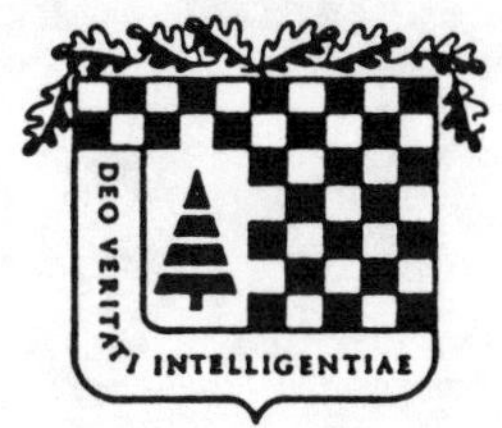

WARREN H. GREEN, INC.
St. Louis, Missouri, U.S.A.

Published by
WARREN H. GREEN, INC.
8356 Olive Boulevard
St. Louis, Missouri 63132, U.S.A.

ISBN No. 87527-480-3

FOREWORD

Virus infections comprise a substantial proportion of illnesses in every community and involve patients in primary, secondary, tertiary and extended care institutions together with medical and allied health professionals who care for patients. Through service as Infection Control Covenor in a University-affiliated Extended Care Unit of 300 beds, since its inception in 1977, the author has collaborated regularly with nursing, physiotherapy, pharmacy, dietary and other allied health professionals. Thus he understands and appreciates the contributions made by each participant in the health care team towards the best standards of patient care. This book provides an historical overview of viruses which cause human illness, followed by a discussion of principles and techniques of recognition, investigation and prevention of virus infections. Succeeding chapters discuss firstly the systematic aspects of each family of viruses associated with human disease, and subsequently the clinical syndromes affecting several systems of the body which are caused by viruses, including approaches to their laboratory investigation and prevention. The concluding chapter demonstrates how allied health professionals are directly involved in the identification, management and prevention of viral illnesses.

Grateful thanks are conveyed to Ms. Julie Nixon and Ms. Rosemary Morgan, Secretaries in the Division of Medical Microbiology, who typed the manuscript.

Electron micrographs were prepared by Ms. Kathleen Wong, Electron Microscopist in the Division of Medical Microbiology, whose collaboration during the past decade is acknowledged gratefully.

Diagrams and artwork were prepared by Mr. Michael Henry and Mr. Bruce Stewart of Biomedical Communications, University of British Columbia, whose endeavours are appreciated keenly.

Donald M. McLean
Vancouver, Canada

TABLE OF CONTENTS

PART III   Clinical categories of viral infections are described as follows:
                       clinical features, incubation period and duration of communicability,
                       specimens and relevant laboratory diagnostic tests, epidemiology,
                       preventive aspects including vaccines and antivirals whenever
                       appropriate.

RECOGNITION, IDENTIFICATION AND PREVENTION OF ACUTE VIRAL INFECTIONS

PART I

CHAPTER 1

VIROLOGY PAST AND PRESENT

SCOPE OF THIS TEXTBOOK

Virology concerns microorganisms with sizes ranging from about 20 to 250 nm which grow or multiply only inside living cells of susceptible hosts (Figure 1-1).

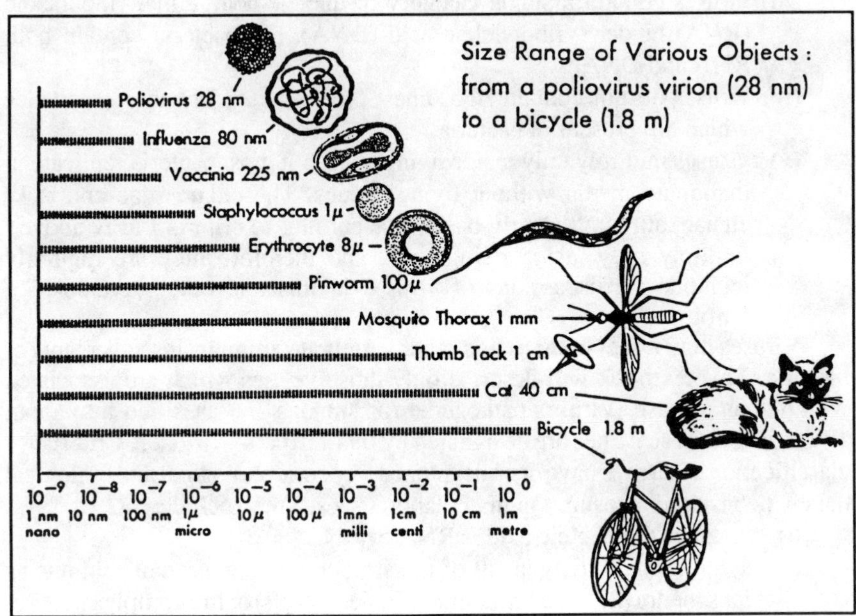

Figure 1-1: Size range of various objects from a poliovirus virion (28nm) to a bicycle (1.8m). Reproduced with permission from McLean DM, 1980. Virology in Health Care, Williams and Wilkins, Baltimore, p2.

Frequently hosts develop disease following growth of viruses within them. Viruses are clearly distinct biologically from bacteria which comprise the other great category of microorganisms which induce disease. The science of virology includes description of viruses as living organisms, the diseases caused by them, laboratory methods for diagnosis of virus infections, and prevention of virus infections either through interruption of virus transmission or administration of virus vaccines and antiviral substances.

Viruses are distinguished from bacteria by several criteria including:

(i)   following virus growth, many daughter virus particles emerge from a cell infected initially by one virus particle, in contrast to bacteria which multiply by binary fission where two daughter bacteria emerge from the initial infecting bacterium.

(ii) rigid cell walls are absent from viruses, but they surround most bacteria.

(iii) viruses contain a single category of nucleic acid, either ribonucleic (RNA) or deoxyribonucleic acid (DNA), but bacteria contain both RNA and DNA.

(iv) viruses do not contain ribosomes, mitochondria or other organelles which are present in bacteria.

(v)   viruses multiply only inside living cells, but most bacteria replicate in inanimate media without living tissues. The chlamydiae and rickettsiae, although clearly bacteria according to criteria i to iv above,[4] multiply only inside living cells, and therefore they are regularly included in discussions of viruses in this and other textbooks of Virology.

Viruses may infect humans and other vertebrate animals, insects, plants or bacteria. This textbook will describe only those viruses which are associated with human disease. Viruses pathogenic for humans are classified into about 19 families, whose names are designated by this suffix "—viridae." Criteria for classification of viruses have been developed from morphological and biological data which can be measured in many laboratories. They include:

(i)   whether the nucleic acid is RNA or DNA,

(ii) symmetrical arrangement of the structural nucleoprotein subunits as icosahedra (20-sided structures), helices (coils) or in a complex pattern.

(iii) whether the nucleic acid is single-stranded or double-stranded.

(iv) presence or absence of an outer viral envelope or coat.

HISTORY OF VIROLOGY IN HEALTH CARE

Modern virology first exerted its impact on health care following Pasteur's

1881 publication[50] of the propagation of rabies virus by intracerebral injection of rabbits (Table 1). This led to the development and effective use of vaccine in prevention of human rabies through the use of brain-passaged rabies virus after inactivation with phenol [51], until superseded in 1975 by vaccine propagated in human diploid cell cultures.

TABLE 1-1

ADVANCES OF SIGNIFICANCE IN MEDICAL VIROLOGY

Year*	Investigator	Technique	Virus
1881	Pasteur et al	rabbits IC	rabies
1886	Buist	light microscopy	vaccinia
1898	Beijerinck	filtration	tobacco mosaic
1902	Reed	mosquito transmission	yellow fever
1909	Landsteiner & Popper	rhesus monkey IC	poliovirus
1928	Maitland	fragment tissue culture	vaccinia
1928	Stokes, Bauer & Hudson	rhesus monkey	yellow fever
1930	Theiler	mice IC	yellow fever
1931	Meyer, Howitt et al	mice IC	western equine encephalitis (WEE)
1931	Woodruff & Goodpasture	chick embryo chorioallantoic membrane	fowlpox
1932	Paul & Bunnell	heterophil hemagglutination	mononucleosis
1933	Andrewes, Laidlaw, & W Smith	ferrets, mice	influenza A (WS)
1934	Francis et al	chick embryo allantoic	influenza A (PR 8)
1937	Trask & Paul	rhesus monkey IC	poliovirus in feces
1937	Theiler & HH Smith	chick embryo tissue cultures	yellow fever 17D vaccine
1939	Ruska et al	electron microscopy	tobacco mosaic
1940	Burnet	chick embryo amniotic	influenza A
1941	Hirst	hemagglutination	influenza
1941	Stanley et al	ultracentrifugation plus electron microscopy	tobacco mosaic
1942	Coons et al	immunofluorescence	influenza, mumps
1948	Dallforf & Sickles	suckling mice	coxsackievirus
1949	Enders, Robbins & Weller	cytopathic effects in primary tissue cultures	poliovirus
1952	Dulbecco et al	plaques in primary tissue cultures	WEE
1953	Scherer, Syverton, & Gey	cytopathic effects in continuous polyploid tissue cultures	poliovirus
1954	Hilleman	continuous polyploid tissue cultures	adenovirus
1954	Casals	hemagglutination at defined pH and temperature	arboviruses
1957	Shelokov	hemadsorption	influenza
1959	Brenner, Horne, Waterson & Wildy	phosphotungstic acid negative stain electron microscopy	adenovirus
1960	Tyrrell et al	tissue cultures at reduced temperature	rhinovirus
1962	Buescher et al	interference in tissue culture	rubella

Continued

TABLE 1-1 (Continued)

Year*	Investigator	Technique	Virus
1962	Kaufman et al	idoxuridine in keratoconjunctivitis	herpesvirus
1967	Henle et al	blastoid transformation plus immunofluorescence	mononucleosis
1967	Krugman et al	institutionalized subjects and serum transaminase levels	hepatitis A and B
1970	Yalow et al	radioimmunoprecipitation	hepatitis B
1972	Ling & Overby	radioimmunoassay	hepatitis B
1973	Feinstone, Kapikian, & Purcell	immunoelectron microscopy	hepatitis A
1973	RF Bishop & Holmes	electron microscopy	rotavirus
1976	Voller et al	enzyme immunoassay	herpesviruses
1977	DHL Bishop	RNA oligonucleotide finger-print analysis	arboviruses
1979	RNP Sutton et al	in situ DNA hybridization	herpesviruses
1982	Nahmias, Roizman, et al	DNA restriction-enzyme analysis	herpesviruses
1983	Brandt et al	monoclonal antibodies (serotype specific)	dengue
1983	Barré-Sinoussi et al Gallo et al	stimulated lymphocyte cultures plus reverse transcriptase assays	retrovirus HTLV-III

*Year of publication of definitive article. Preliminary scientific observations leading to these technical advances were often made 2 to 4 years before publication cited here, and they may already have been published as preliminary communications.

Virus particles were first observed by the Edinburgh physician Buist who described in 1886[8] the 250 nm particles of vaccinia virus in stained preparations using the ordinary light microscopes. Morphological descriptions of other groups of viruses, all of which are smaller than vaccinia within the Poxviridae family, appeared initially from the Ruska group in 1939[36] using an electron microscope, prototypes of which were first developed by the Ruska group in 1932.[37] Electron microscopy paved the way for visualization of objects as small as 0.3 to 1.0 nm due to the substantially shorter wavelength of a beam of electrons that a beam of visible light. Currently human viruses within all families, with diameters as small as 20 nm, have been visualized by electron microscopy and descriptions of their internal architecture have been elucidated following the 1959 publication of the phosphotungstic acid negative stain technique by Horne, Brenner, Waterson and Wildy.[7,34]

Following reports in 1898 that the plant pathogen, tobacco mosaic virus,[2] and the animal agent, foot and mouth disease[44] passed through the pores of porcelain filters which were capable of retaining bacteria, the term "filterable virus" was applied to these infective agents. This term persisted until about 1945, when the current term "virus" came into use generally. Development of collodion membrane filters with graded pore sizes by Elford's group during the 1930's[19] provided a convenient means for determination of the approximate sizes of viruses, until superseded by electron microscopy following technical improvements during the next two decades.

Yellow fever posed a major health barrier against construction of the Panama Canal during the late nineteenth century. Publication in 1902[53] of the Reed commission's findings that:

(i) yellow fever virus circulated in the blood of patients during the initial two days of fever;

(ii) *Aedes aegypti* mosquitoes which fed on blood of febrile patients became infected and transmitted virus by biting humans after 11 days or more of extrinsic incubation at the usual tropical environmental temperature of 28° C, elucidated the urban or domestic component of the natural history of yellow fever.

This knowledge provided the scientific basis for effective control of *Aedes aegypti* in peridomestic situations through adequate drainage of mosquito-breeding sites, and thus rendered possible the completion of the Panama Canal in 1914 through suppression of urban yellow fever. This striking advance in Public Health was achieved without the isolation of the causative yellow fever virus. Isolation of virus was first achieved in Accra, Ghana in 1927[61] through inoculation of the blood of a febrile patient into rhesus monkeys imported from India, where previous attempts had failed through the use of indigenous African monkeys. The adaptation of yellow fever virus to mice was first reported by Theiler in 1930[63] and this paved the way for development of a safe and highly effective live yellow fever vaccine in 1937,[64] after virus attenuation through repeated passage in chick embryo tissue cultures.

During an epidemic of encephalitis affecting humans and horses in the San Joaquin valley of California in 1930, western equine encephalomyelitis (WEE) virus was first isolated from the brains of horses by inoculation of a variety of laboratory animals including weaned mice.[49] This same agent was isolated from the brain of a fatal human case in 1934.[35] Following the successful use of suckling mice aged less than 48 hours for the isolation of coxsackieviruses in 1948,[17] extensive use of suckling mice from about 1950 onwards has resulted in the isolation of over 400 arboviruses (arthropod-borne viruses) from humans with encephalitis, dengue, yellow fever and other tropical fevers, from vertebrate animal reservoirs, and from mosquito, tick or sandfly vectors.[3] During recent years, a variety of tissue cultures have been employed successfully for isolation of dengue and other arboviruses.[3,45] Extensive use of hemagglutination techniques by Casals and associates[11] from 1954 onwards provided a convenient basis for classification of this diverse group of viruses.

Chorioallantoic membranes of chick embryos within fertile hen eggs after incubation at 37° C for 11 days provided a most convenient natural layer of susceptible cells for cultivation of a wide range of viruses,[5] following the 1931 report[72] that localized lesions termed pocks developed following multiplication of fowlpox virus. Strains included fowlpox and vaccinia, *Herpesvirus hominis* and arboviruses such as louping ill and Murray Valley encephalitis. Until the development of the plaque technique in 1952[18] the pock count provided an extraordinarily convenient procedure for titration of virus infectivity.

Influenza A virus was first isolated from the nose and throat secretions of a medical microbiologist, who contracted influenza in 1933,[60] by intranasal inoculation of ferrets, which exhibited fever and sneezing two or more days subsequently. After propagation in the nasal mucosa of ferrets, influenza A strains were adapted to growth in the allantoic cells of chick embryos in 1934.[21] To the present day, allantoic inoculation of fertile eggs provides optimal means of propagation of influenza virus for preparation of diagnostic reagents and vaccines. Application of amniotic inoculation of chick embryos by Burnet in 1940[9] provided a more sensitive technique for isolation of both influenza B strains from patients, but also influenza A strains. This technique was superseded in 1957 following the highly successful use of primary monkey kidney tissue cultures combined with the hemadsorption technique[67] for the isolation of Asian A (H2N2) strains of influenza virus during a pandemic.

Hemagglutination of influenza virus was first reported by Hirst in 1941.[33] Immediately this technique provided a most convenient and simple procedure for titration of virus and determination of influenza antibody titers in patient's sera both for diagnostic tests and epidemiological surveys of influenza prevalence.

The virus causing paralytic poliomyelitis was first isolated in 1909[41] by inoculation of central nervous system tissue from a fatal case intracerebrally into a rhesus monkey which subsequently developed paralysis. Although fecal excretion of poliovirus was initially recorded in 1912, it was not generally recognized until 1937, during investigations of a poliomyelitis epidemic in Connecticut by Paul and associates[65] that poliomyelitis patients excreted virus in the throat and feces. During 1931, Burnet and Macnamara[10] first documented the existence of more than one serotype of poliovirus, but only in 1951[16] was worldwide acceptance achieved regarding the existence of three, and only three, serotypes of poliovirus. By 1949, Enders, Robbins, and Weller showed that all three serotypes of poliovirus multiplied in and caused cytopathic effects to, tissue cultures of human embryonic cells[20] and of rhesus monkey testis and kidney.[54] This provided the current and highly convenient method for isolation of poliovirus from patients and for detection of antibodies by neutralization tests in sera, both from individual patients and from entire populations. This technique also provided the system for propagation of large quantities of poliovirus for production of Salk inactivated vaccine[57] and Sabin live attenuated vaccine.[55]

Numerous hitherto unknown viruses were isolated through the widespread use of tissue culture techniques during the 1950's including the echoviruses,[47] reoviruses,[56] adenoviruses,[31] and rhinoviruses.[66] Demonstration of plaque production by WEE virus in tissue culture monolayers by Dulbecco and associates in 1952[18] provided the present-day technique for accurate titration of virus infectivity, and for determination of antibody titers, interferon activity and antiviral efficacy. Observation of cytopathic effects in monolayer tissue cultures of human polyploid cells by Scherer and associates in 1953[58] increased substantially the range of cell systems for virus and antiviral antibody titrations. Isolation of rubella virus in 1962[48] was achieved initially by demonstration of interference, rather than cytopathic effects, following its growth in African green monkey kidney tissue cultures.

Although the heterophil hemagglutination response in sera of patients convalescent from infectious mononucleosis was described by Paul and Bunnell in 1932,[52] and currently this test is used extensively in presumptive diagnosis of mononucleosis, it was only in 1967 that the causative agent termed Epstein-Barr virus was first isolated from patients with mononucleosis by induction of blastoid transformation in tissue culture cells.[30]

Hepatitis currently remains one of the few virus-induced diseases for which no convenient laboratory techniques have been developed to isolate the causative viruses. Epidemiological observations during the 1930's together with studies on human volunteers[25,26,27] during World War II clearly established that the causative agent of hepatitis A ("catarrhal jaundice" or "infectious hepatitis"), with an incubation period of 30 to 35 days, was transmitted principally by the fecal-oral route, in contrast to hepatitis B ("homologous serum jaundice" or "serum hepatitis"), with an incubation period about 2 months, which was transmitted largely by blood. Through extensive use of serum transaminase determinations as chemical markers of hepatitis, Krugman and associates reported in 1967 the simultaneous prevalence of hepatitis A and hepatitis B among a large population of inmates and staff at Willowbrook State School, New York.[39] Application of the recently developed in vitro techniques of radioimmunoprecipitation[70] and radioimmunoassay[42,43] to hepatitis B provided suitable laboratory tools for diagnosis and epidemiological investigations[40] and paved the way for development of hepatitis B vaccine.[62] Demonstration of 27 nm particles in feces of patients at onset of illness with hepatitis A by immunoelectron microscopy[22] defined the etiological agent, and assisted the development of effective radioimmunoassays for diagnosis and epidemiological surveillance.[23]

Rotaviruses were first described in 1973[6] during electron microscopic examination of biopsy specimens of duodenal mucosa of infants with gastroenteritis in Melbourne, Australia. Within the succeeding 3 years, rotaviruses were observed in feces of 25% or more infants with gastroenteritis world-wide. They continue to comprise the major viral cause of acute gastroenteritis especially in Temperate Zones during winter. However, no convenient tissue culture system has yet been devised for their routine isolation from patients. Currently in 1990, the preferred method of diagnosis of rotavirus gastroenteritis remains electron microscopy of feces,[46] but in the absence of an electron microscope, rotaviruses have been detected conveniently since 1977 by enzyme immunoassay.[74,75]

Widespread application of the enzyme immunoassay (ELISA) technique to many virus systems including the herpesviruses, measles, rubella, coxsackievirus and an arbovirus by Voller and associates 1976[68] provided for the first time a convenient and highly sensitive test system both for detection of antibodies to the complete range of viruses and for detection of virus antigens in specimens from patients,[69] especially rotavirus in feces.[75]

Molecular virology techniques have provided powerful new tools for elucidation of taxonomic relationships, particularly within the large and heterogeneous group of arthropod-borne viruses, following successful application of RNA oligonucleotide fingerprint analysis by D.H.L. Bishop and associates in 1977.[15,24] This procedure complements and extends previous results obtained by serological methods of hemagglutination inhibition, complement fixation and neutralization tests.

Molecular virology techniques have also recently elucidated the pathogenesis of herpesvirus infections of the central nervous system. Detection of *Herpesvirus hominis* type 1 genome in brain tissue from 3 of 6 patients who died with dementia or other psychoses of long duration, by R.N.P. Sutton and associates in 1979,[59] employing the new procedure of in situ DNA hybridization, demonstrated clearly the prolonged persistence of herpesvirus in brain. A 1982 report by Nahmias and associates[71] indicated that strains of *Herpesvirus hominis* were recovered from lip vesicles and brain tissue of 5 patients with herpes encephalitis, using DNA restriction-enzyme analysis.

Development of monoclonal antibody technology in 1967 by Kohler and Milstein[38] provided virologists with a tool of high precision, for demonstration of fine degrees of antigenic similarities or differences between virus strains, which was not available using sera obtained from animals after single injections with high doses of semipurified viruses. Using the indirect immunofluorescence test with monoclonal antibodies against all four dengue serotypes, Brandt and associates in 1983[28] determined the serotypes of dengue virus isolates from humans and mosquitoes, substantially more rapidly and conveniently than by the traditional and cumbersome plaque reduction neutralization test.

Combination of the techniques of culture of lymphocytes, from peripheral blood or lymph nodes of patients with acquired immunodeficiency syndrome (AIDS) and its precursor lymphadenopathy syndrome, with assays for reverse transcriptase in tissue culture supernotant fluids, led to the isolation of the retrovirus HTLV-III* (human T-lymphotropic virus type III) in 1983.[2a,22a]

---

*Termed HIV (human immunodeficiency virus) since 1986.

DIRECT IMPACT OF VIROLOGY ON
HUMAN HEALTH IN THE 1980's

Substantial progress towards complete elimination of certain virus diseases has rewarded the efforts of numerous virus investigators worldwide throughout the past 80 years. Global eradication of smallpox was achieved in October 1977.[29] Developed countries have been virtually free of paralytic poliomyelitis since about 1972,[12] through successful implementation of nationwide vaccination, but poliomyelitis continues to pose a persistent health hazard in underdeveloped nations. Widespread vaccination against measles following licensure of vaccine in 1963, followed by practically universal vaccination of susceptible children and young adults throughout the United States since 1978, has achieved virtual elimination of indigenous measles through 1982.[13] Of 1697 cases during 1982 most were introduced from other countries.* Concerted efforts to administer rubella vaccine to all children aged 12–15 months throughout the United States since licensure of vaccine in 1969 has resulted in virtual disappearance of infants with the congenital rubella syndrome since 1980.[14,32] Urban yellow fever no longer comprises a health hazard throughout much of South America and tropical Africa following routine vaccination of indigenous peoples and travellers, following development of safe and effective yellow fever vaccine in 1937.[64]

Diagnosis of many common virus diseases on the same day that patients seek medical care has become routine in many urban communities through the widespread use of morphological methods such as immunofluorescence[73] and electron microscopy.[46] Short turnaround times of 3–4 hours[45] provide physicians with essential virological criteria to ensure that patients:

(i)   are nursed in appropriate isolation facilities to prevent nosocomial spread of infections,

(ii) do not receive inappropriate antibacterial therapy,

(iii) receive suitable antiviral substances when these are available.

REFERENCES

[1] Aoki FY, Tyrrell DAJ, Hill LE, Turner GS: Immunogenicity and acceptability of human diploid-cell culture rabies vaccine in volunteers. Lancet 1:660, 1975.

[2] Beijerinck NW: Ueber ein Contagium vivum fluidum also Ursache der Fleckenkrankheit der Tabaksblatter. Verh Akad Wetensch Amsterdam II 6 No. 5:1, 1898.

[2a] Barré-Sinoussi F, Chermann JC, Rey F, et al: Isolation of a T-lymphotropic retrovirus from a patient at risk for acquired immune deficiency syndrome (AIDS). Science 220:868, 1983.

---

*Measles cases from 1983 through 1987 showed median 2812 cases annually.

[3]Berge TO (ed): International Catalogue of Arboviruses including certain other Viruses of Vertebrates. 2nd edition US Dept. of Health, Education and Welfare Publ. No. (CSC) 75-8301, 1975 with updatings by the Subcommittee on Information exchange to December 1982.

[4]Bergey's Manual of Determinative Bacteriology, ed. RE Buchanan, NE Gibbons. Williams and Wilkins, Baltimore, 8th Edition, 1974.

[5]Beveridge WIB, Burnet FM: The cultivation of viruses and rickettsiae in the chick embryo. Medical Research Council Special Report Series No. 256, London HMSO, 1946.

[6]Bishop RF, Davidson GP, Holmes IH, Ruck BJ: Virus particles in epithelial cells of duodenal mucosa from children with acute non-bacterial gastroenteritis. Lancet 2:1281, 1973.

[7]Brenner S, Horne RW: A negative staining method for high resolution electron microscopy of viruses. Biochim Biophys Acta 34:103, 1959.

[8]Buist JB: The life history of the micro-organisms associated with variola and vaccinia. Proc. Roy Soc Edinburgh 13:603, 1886.

[9]Burnet FM: Influenza virus infections of the chick embryo by the amniotic route. I. General character of the infections. Australian J. Exp. Biol. Med. Sci. 18:353, 1940.

[10]Burnet FM, Macnamara J: Immunological differences between strains of poliomyelitis virus. Br. J. Exp. Path. 12:57, 1931.

[11]Casals J, Brown LV: Hemagglutination with arthropod-borne viruses. J. Exp. Med. 99:429, 1954.

[12]Center for Disease Control. Poliomyelitis Surveillance Summary 1980–1981. Issued December 1982.

[13]Center for Disease Control. Measles—United States, 1982. MMWR 32:49, 1983.

[14]Center for Disease Control. Rubella—United States, 1974–1982. MMWR 31:568, 1982.

[15]Clewley J, Gentsch J, Bishop DHL: Three unique viral RNA species of snowshoe hare and La Crosse bunyaviruses. J. Virol 22:459, 1977.

[16]Committee on Typing of the National Foundation for Infantile Paralysis. Immunologic classification of poliomyelitis viruses. I. A cooperative program for the typing of one hundred strains. Am. J. Hyg. 54:191, 1951.

[17]Dalldorf G: The coxsackie group of viruses. Science 110:594, 1949.

[18]Dulbecco R: Production of plaques in monolayer tissue cultures by single particles of an animal virus. Proc. Nat. Acad Sc. USA 38:747, 1952.

[19]Elford WJ: A new series of graded collodion membranes suitable for general bacteriological use, especially in filterable virus studies. J. Path. Bact. 34:505, 1931.

[20]Enders JF, Weller TH, Robbins FC: Cultivation of the Lansing strain of poliomyelitis virus in cultures of various human embryonic tissues. Science 109:85, 1949.

[21]Francis T Jr: Transmission of influenza by a filterable virus. Science 80:457, 1934.

[22]Feinstone SM, Kapikian AZ, Purcell RH: Hepatitis A: Detection by immune electron microscopy of a virus-like antigen associated with acute illness. Science 182:1026, 1973.

[22a]Gallo RC, Salahuddin SZ, Popovic M et al: Human T-lymphotropic retrovirus, HTLV-III, isolated from AIDS patients and donors at risk for AIDS. Science 224:500, 1984.

[23]Gust ID, Lehmann HI, Dimitrakakis M: A seroepidemiologic study of infection with HAV and HBV in five Pacific islands. Am. J. Epidemiol. 110:237, 1979.

[24]Hamdy El Said L, Vorndam V, Gentsch JR, Clewley JP, Calisher CH, Klimas RA, Thompson WH, Grayson MA, Trent DW, Bishop DHL: A comparison of La Crosse virus isolates obtained from different ecological niches and an analysis of the structural components of California encephalitis serogroup viruses and other Bunyaviruses. Am. J. Trop. Med. Hyg. 28:364, 1979.

[25]Havens WP Jr: Infectious hepatitis in the Middle East. A clinical review of 200 cases seen in a military hospital. JAMA 126:17, 1944.

[26]Havens WP Jr: The period of infectivity of patients with homologous serum jaundice and routes of infection in this disease. J. Exp. Med. 83:441, 1946.

[27]Havens WP Jr, Ward R, Drill VA, Paul JR: Experimental production of hepatitis by feeding icterogenic materials. Proc. Soc. Exp. Biol. Med. 57:206, 1944.

[28]Henchal EA, McGown JM, Seguin MC, Gentry MK, Brandt WE: Rapid identification of dengue virus isolates by using monoclonal antibodies in an indirect immunofluorescence assay. Am. J. Trop. Med. Hyg. 32:164, 1983.

[29]Henderson DA: The saga of smallpox eradication: An end and a beginning. Can. J. Public Health 70:21, 1979.

[30]Henle G, Henle W, Diehl V: Relation of Burkitt's tumor-associated herpes-type virus to infectious mononucleosis. Proc. Natl. Acad Sci. USA 59:94, 1968.

[31]Hilleman MR, Werner JH: Recovery of a new agent from patients with acute respiratory illness. Proc. Soc. Exp. Biol. Med. 85:183, 1954.

[32]Hinman AR, Bart KJ, Orenstein WA, Preblud SR: Rational strategy for rubella vaccination. Lancet 1:39, 1983.

[33]Hirst GK: The agglutination of red cells by allantoic fluid of chick embryos infected with influenza virus. Science 94:22, 1941.

[34]Horne RW, Brenner S, Waterson AP, Wildy P: The icosahedral form of an adenovirus. J. Molec. Biol. 1:84, 1959.

[35]Howitt BF: Recovery of the virus of equine encephalomyelitis from the brain of a child. Science 88:455, 1938.

[36]Kausche GA, Pfankuch E, Ruska H: Die Sichtbarmachung von pflanzlichern Virus in Ubermikroskop. Naturwissenschaften 27:292, 1939.

[37]Kroll M, Ruska E: Das Electronenmikroskop. Z. Physik 78:318, 1932.

[38]Kohler G, Milstein C: Derivation of specific antibody-producing tissue culture and tumor lines by cell fusion. European J. Immunol. 6:511, 1976.

[39]Krugman S, Giles JP, Hammond J: Infectious hepatitis. Evidence of two distinctive clinical epidemiological and immunological types of infection. JAMA 200:365, 1967.

[40]Krugman S, Overby L, Mushalwar IK, Ling C-M, Frosner GR, Deinhardt F: Viral hepatitis B. Studies on natural history and prevention re-examined. New Eng. J. Med. 300:101, 1979.

[41]Landsteiner K, Popper E: Ubertragung der poliomyelitis acuta auf offen. Z. Immunitatsforsch Orig. 2:377, 1909.

[42]Ling C-M: Radioimmunoassays for hepatitis B virus markers. Chapter 46 in Manual of Clinical Immunology, ed. NR Rose, H Friedman, ASM, Washington, D.C., 2nd edition, 1980.

[43]Ling C-M, Overby L: Prevalence of hepatitis B. Virus antigen as revealed by direct radioimmune assay with ^{125}I-antibody. J. Immunol. 109:834, 1972.

[44]Loeffler F, Frosch P: Berichte der Kommission zur Erforschung der Maul-und Klavenseuche beiu dem Institut fur Infektionskrankheiten in Berlin. Zbl Bakt (1 Abt Orig) 23:371, 1898.

[45]McLean DM: Virology in Health Care. Williams and Wilkins, Baltimore, 1980.

[46]McLean DM, Wong KK: Same-day Diagnosis of Human Virus Infections. CRC Press, Boca Raton, Florida, 1984.

[47]Melnick JL: Tissue culture techniques and their application to original isolation, growth and assay of poliomyelitis and orphan viruses. Ann. N.Y. Acad. Sci. 61:754, 1955.

[48]Parkman PD, Buescher EL, Artenstein MS: Recovery of rubella virus from army recruits. Proc. Soc. Exp. Biol. Med. 111:225, 1962.

[49]Meyer KF, Haring CM, Howitt B: The etiology of epizootic encephalomyelitis in horses in the San Joaquin Valley, 1930. Science 74:227, 1931.

[50]Pasteur L, Chamberland C, Roux E, Thuillier: Sur la rage. Compt Rend Acad. Sci. (Paris) 92:1259, 1881.

[51]Pasteur L: Methods pour prevenir la rage apres morsure. Compt Rend Acad. Sci. (Paris) 101:765, 1885.

[52]Paul JR, Bunnell WW: The presence of heterophile antibodies in infectious mononucleosis. Am. J. Med. Sc. 183:90, 1932.

[53]Reed W: Recent researches concerning the etiology, propagation and prevention of yellow fever, by the United States Army Commission. J. Hyg. 2:101, 1902.

[54]Robbins FC, Enders JF, Weller TH, Florentino GL: Studies on the cultivation of poliomyelitis viruses in tissue culture. V. The direct isolation and serological identification of virus strains in tissue culture from patients with nonparalytic and paralytic poliomyelitis. Am. J. Hyg. 54:286, 1951.

[55]Sabin AB: Present position of immunization against poliomyelitis with live virus vaccines. Br. Med. J. 1:663, 1959.

[56]Sabin AB: Reoviruses. A new group of respiratory and enteric viruses formerly classified as ECHO type 10 is described. Science 130:1387, 1959.

[57]Salk JE, Krech U, Youngner JS, Bennett BL, Lewis LJ, Bazeley PL: Formaldehyde treatment and safety testing of experimental poliomyelitis vaccines. Am. J. Pub. Health 44:563, 1954.

[58]Scherer WF, Syverton JT, Gey GO: Studies on the propagation in vitro of poliomyelitis viruses. IV. Viral multiplication in a stable strain of human malignant epithelial cells (strain HeLa) derived from an epidermoid carcinoma of the cervix. J. Exp. Med. 97:695, 1953.

[59]Sequiera LW, Jennings LC, Carrasco LH, Lord MA, Curry A, Sutton RNP: Detection of herpes-simplex viral genome in brain tissue. Lancet 2:609, 1979.

[60]Smith W, Andrewes CH, Laidlaw PP: Virus [influenza] obtained from patients. Lancet 2:66, 1933.

[61]Stokes A, Bauer JH, Hudson NP: Transmission of yellow fever to *Macacus rhesus*, preliminary note. JAMA 90:253, 1928.

[62]Szmuness W, Stevens CE, Harley EJ, Zong EA, Oleszko WR, William DC, Sodvasky R, Morrison JM, Kellner A: Hepatitis B vaccine. Demonstration of efficacy in a

controlled clinical trial in a high risk population in the United States. New Eng. J. Med. 303:833, 1980.

[63]Theiler M: Studies on action of yellow fever in mice. Ann. Trop. Med. 24:249, 1930.

[64]Theiler M, Smith HH: Use of yellow fever virus modified by in vitro cultivation for human immunization. J. Exp. Med. 65:787, 1937.

[65]Trask JD, Vignec AJ, Paul JR: Poliomyelitis virus in human stools. JAMA 111:6, 1938.

[66]Tyrrell DAJ, Bynoe ML, Hitchcock C, Pereira HG, Andrewes CH: Some virus isolations from common colds. I. Experiments employing human volunteers. Lancet 1:235, 1960.

[67]Vogel J, Shelokov A: Adsorption-hemagglutination test for influenza virus in monkey kidney tissue culture. Science 126:358, 1957.

[68]Voller A, Bidwell DE, Bartlett A: Enzyme immunoassays in diagnostic medicine Theory and Practice. Bull World Health Org. 53:55, 1976.

[69]Voller A, Bidwell DE, Bartlett A: Enzyme-linked immunosorbent assay. Chapter 45 in Manual of Clinical Immunology, ed. NR Rose, H Friedman, ASM, Washington, D.C., 2nd edition, 1980.

[70]Walsh JH, Yalow R, Berson SA: Detection of Australia antigen and antibody by means of radioimmunoassay techniques. J. Infect Dis. 121:550, 1970.

[71]Whitney R, Lakeman AD, Nahmias A, Roizman B: DNA restriction-enzyme analysis of herpes simplex virus isolates obtained from patients with encephalitis. New Eng. J. Med. 307:1060, 1982.

[72]Woodruff AM, Goodpasture EW: The susceptibility of chorioallantoic membrane of chick embryos to infection with the fowl-pox virus. Am. J. Path. 7:209, 1931.

[73]World Health Organization. Rapid laboratory techniques for the diagnosis of viral infection: report of WHO scientific group. WHO Techn. Rep. Ser. No. 661, 1981.

[74]Yolken RH, Kim HW, Clem T, Wyatt RG, Kalica AR, Chanock RM, Kapikian AZ: Enzyme-linked immunosorbent assay (ELISA) for detection of human reovirus-like agent of infantile gastroenteritis. Lancet 2:263, 1977.

[75]Yolken RH, Leister F: Rapid multiple-determinant enzyme immunoassay for the detection of human rotavirus. J. Infect. Dis. 146:43, 1982.

CHAPTER 2

CLASSIFICATION OF VIRUSES AND VIRUS INFECTIONS

PURPOSES OF VIRUS CLASSIFICATION AND NOMENCLATURE

Nomenclature concerns the naming of viruses and virus groupings. Classification signifies the orderly arrangement of clusters of viruses into groupings with similar biological attributes, by which they may be distinguished from other clusters with different biological properties. Virus names should signify the same biological attributes of particular viruses to readers throughout the world. Thus nomenclature provides an essential, succinct and accurate means of communication internationally about particular viruses or virus groups.

Species is the fundamental unit of virus classification. *Strain* is an individual virus isolated from one patient, mammal, bird or mosquito. The concept of a virus species denotes a cluster of virus strains from one or more sources which have in common a set or pattern of correlating stable properties that separates the cluster from other clusters of strains.[19] A species epithet should consist of a simple word, or if essential, a hyphenated word. The word may be followed by numbers or letters.

Genus is a group of species sharing certain common characters.[19] The genus name and species epithet, together with the strain designation, must give an unambiguous identification of the virus. The species epithet must follow the genus name and be placed before the designation of strain, variant or serotype, e.g., *Herpesvirus hominis* type 1. Efforts will be made towards a latinized nomenclature for genus (plural genera) and species. The suffix for the generic name is "....virus." Typically virus names are binomial to include both genus and species.

Virus names are preferably place names which signify the community (city or village), jurisdictional region (county, state or province) or a notable geographic entity such as a river which is close to the site of first isolation of the virus.[1] Care should be taken to avoid the use of disease entities, personal names, or language which may be offensive to virologists of different national origin.

Letters, numerals or combinations thereof may be used to designate a species where these symbols already have wide international acceptance, but usually letters or numerals are used more appropriately to designate individual strains or clusters within a species. Examples of apt virus nomenclature include: (i) coxsackievirus which was first isolated from patients living in Coxsackie N.Y. in 1947[7]; (ii) Powassan virus which was first isolated from a child resident of Powassan, Ontario, Canada in 1958;[15] (iii) Ross River virus which was first isolated from *Aedes vigilax* mosquitoes collected in mangroves along the Ross River near Townsville, Queensland, Australia in 1959.[8]

Family is a group of genera with common characters, and the ending of the name of a viral family is "...viridae," e.g., the family Paramyxoviridae[13] contains three genera with species which are human pathogens: *Paramyxovirus, Morbillivirus* (measles), Pneumovirus (respiratory syncytial virus); and the family Bunyaviridae[5] contains four genera *Bunyavirus, Nairovirus, Phlebovirus, Uukuvirus.*

VIRUS CLASSIFICATION

Viruses which infect humans are classified into 18 families according to the kind, and strandedness, of the nucleic acid making up the viral genome, and the presence or absence of a lipoprotein envelope or outer viral coat[10,18,19] (Table 2-1). Viruses contain either RNA or DNA which may exist in single stranded (SS) or double stranded (DS) forms. There are no known SS-DNA viruses with envelopes.

Retroviridae has been listed as a family containing candidate virus strains as possible human pathogens following the 1983 report[20] of the association of the human T-cell leukemia/lymphoma virus with adult cases of this disease. This agent is now termed human T-cell lymphotropic virus type I (HTLV-I). First reports of the isolation of the antigenically distinct retrovirus HTLV-III* from patients with acquired immunodeficiency syndrome (AIDS) and its antecedent condition lymphadenopathy syndrome also appeared during 1983 and 1984.[3,9]

The arboviruses[4] comprise a functional grouping of more than 400 virus serotypes within more than 60 serogroups which are actually or potentially transmitted biologically through bites of infected arthropods. They are classified within five families; Togaviridae, Flaviviridae, Bunyaviridae, Rhabdoviridae and Reoviridae.

Laboratory detection of the presence of a viral envelope is achieved conveniently in the routine diagnostic laboratory by demonstration of at least one hundredfold decrease of virus infectivity after treatment with sodium deoxycholate 1:1000[21] or overnight exposure to diethyl ether.[2] Determination of the category of nucleic acid is achieved readily by inhibition of replication of

---

*Termed human immunodeficiency virus (HIV) since 1986.

TABLE 2-1

CLASSIFICATION OF KNOWN AND POTENTIAL HUMAN PATHOGENIC VIRUSES INTO FAMILIES AND GENERA ACCORDING TO KIND, AND STRANDEDNESS, OF NUCLEIC ACID, AND PRESENCE OR ABSENCE OF A LIPOPROTEIN ENVELOPE[19]

Nucleic acid	*RNA*					*DNA*		
Strandedness	*SS*				*DS*	*DS*		*SS*
envelope	*non-enveloped*	*enveloped*			*non-enveloped*	*enveloped*	*non-enveloped*	*non-enveloped*
genome strategy	*positive sense genome*	*positive sense genome*	*no DNA step* *negative sense genome*	*DNA step in replication cycle*				
	Picornaviridae Enterovirus Rhinovirus	*Togaviridae* Alphavirus Rubivirus	*Paramyxoviridae* Paramyxovirus Morbillivirus Pneumovirus	*Retroviridae* human T-lymphotropic virus (HTLV)	*Reoviridae* Reovirus Orbivirus Rotavirus	*Poxviridae* Orthopoxvirus	*Adenoviridae* Mastadenovirus	*Parvoviridae* Parvovirus Big
	Calciviridae Calicivirus	*Coronaviridae* Coronavirus *Flaviviridae* Flavivirus	*Orthomyxoviridae* Influenzavirus *Rhabdoviridae* Lyssavirus Vesiculovirus *Bunyaviridae* Bunyavirus Nairovirus Phlebovirus Uukuvirus *Arenaviridae* Arenavirus	Human immuno-deficiency virus (HIV)		*Herpesviridae* Herpesvirus	*Papovaviridae* BK & JC virus	*Hepadnaviridae** hepatitis B

*Hepadnavirus DNA is partly DS and partly SS.

TABLE 2-2
GUIDELINES FOR ASSIGNMENT OF VIRUSES TO FAMILIES AND GENERA USING METHODS AVAILABLE IN ROUTINE DIAGNOSTIC LABORATORIES, INCLUDING NEGATIVE STAIN ELECTRON MICROSCOPY

Virus Family	ICTV Criteria	Capsid		Virion Diameters (nm)				Serological Characterization	
					RNA	surface			
		symmetry	capsomeres	total	helix	projection	test	level	examples
Picornaviridae	SS-RNA non-env	cubic	32	22–30	-	-	NT	serotype	Enterovirus: Poliovirus 1
									Rhinovirus 14
Calciviridae	SS-RNA non-env	cubic	32	35–39	-	cup dep	-	-	-
Togaviridae,	SS-RNA (+) env	cubic	-	40–70	-	-	NT	serotype	WEE
Flaviviridae	SS-RNA (+) env	cubic	-	25–50	-	-	HI, CF	serogroup	Alphavirus: (arbovirus group A)
							NT	serotype	POW, SLE
							HI, CF	serogroup	Flavivirus: (arbovirus group B)
							NT, HI	species	Rubivirus: rubella
Coronaviridae	SS-RNA (+) env	uncertain	-	75–160	11–13	12–24	NT	serotype	Coronavirus OC 43
Orthomyxoviridae	SS-RNA (–) env	helical	-	80–120	9	14 H	HI, NI	serotype	Influenza A (H3N2) A/Philippines/2/82
						8 N	S-CF	species	Influenza A or B
Paramyxoviridae	SS-RNA (–) env	helical	-	150–300	18	10	HI, NI, NT	species	Paramyxovirus: mumps
							HI, NT	serotype	Paramyxovirus: Parainfluenza 1
							HI, NT	species	Morbillivirus: measles
							CF, NT	species	Pneumovirus: Respiratory syncytial
Rhabdoviridae	SS-RNA (–) env	helical (bullet)	-	130–380 x 50–95	50	10	CF, NT	serotype	Lyssavirus: rabies
									Vesiculovirus: VSV
Bunyaviridae	SS-RNA (–) env	helical	-	90–100	1	+	HI, CF	serogroup	Bunyavirus (Bunyamwera supergroup)
							NT	serotype	Snowshoe hare
Arenaviridae	SS-RNA (–) env	uncertain	-	50–300	-	10	CF	complex	Tacaribe complex (Machupo)
							NT, IF	serotype	Lassa

TABLE 2-2 (continued)

| Virus Family | ICTV Criteria | Capsid | | Virion Diameters (nm) | | | Serological Characterization | | |
		symmetry	capsomeres	total	RNA helix	surface projection	test	level	examples
Retroviridae	SS-RNA env (DNA step)	cubic	-	80–100	-	8	NT	serotype	human T-lymphotropic virus (HTLV-III or HIV)
Reoviridae	dS-RNA non-env	cubic (double shelled)	32	60–80	-	spikes	NT, HI NT ELISA	species serotype species	Reovirus I Orbivirus CTF Rotavirus (human)
Poxviridae	dS-DNA env	complex	-	300–450 x 170–260	-	-	NT * HI	species species	vaccinia Orthopoxvirus
Adenoviridae	ds-DNA non-env	cubic	252	70–90	-	fiber	CF HI, NT	genus species	Mastadenovirus Adenovirus 7
Papovaviridae	ds-DNA non-env	cubic	72	45–55	-	-	IF, HI	serotype	Polyomavirus BK
Parvoviridae	SS-DNA non-env	cubic	32	18–26	-	-	IEM IF	genus genus	Parvovirus: Biq Adeno-associated 1

Test abbreviations

CF: complement fixation

ELISA: enzyme immunoassay

HI: hemagglutination inhibition

IEM: immunoelectron microscopy

IF: immunofluorescence

NT: neutralization test (preferably by plaque reduction)

S-CF: complement fixation using the ribonucleoprotein (soluble, S) antigen of influenza virus

Virus abbreviations

POW: Powassan virus

SLE: St. Louis encephalitis virus

WEE: western equine encephalomyelitis virus

DNA-containing viruses by 5-iodo-2'-deoxyuridine[11] or 5-bromo-2'-deoxy-uridine,[12] but the multiplication of RNA-containing viruses is unaffected by these DNA-base analogs. Determination of the strandedness of nucleic acid and the genome strategy require advanced techniques in molecular virology.

When electron microscopy is readily available for diagnostic purposes,[17] the overall size of the virus particle and the internal distribution of nucleoprotein subunits (*capsomere* within the viral body or *capsid*) provide extremely useful data for assigning viruses to families and possibly genera also (Table 2-2).

Immunological reactions are commonly employed in diagnostic laboratories to assign freshly isolated viruses to genera, species and varieties or serotypes within species. Tests frequently used[16] include: (i) neutralization (NT) by plaque reduction or 50 percent endpoint determination—this provides highly specific characterization of the species or serotype within species but it is technically time-consuming and requires large quantities of supplies; (ii) hemagglutination inhibition (HI)—this often provides determination of genus or group but is too broadly reacting for identification of species or serotype, except for the Orthomyxoviridae; (iii) complement fixation (CF)—this may characterize an entire genus, e.g., *Mastadenovirus* or a few serotypes within a serogroup, e.g., the group C arboviruses within the *Bunyavirus* genus. The development of monoclonal antibodies to an ever-increasing range of viruses will augment substantially the specificity of serotyping.

CLINICAL CLASSIFICATION OF VIRUS INFECTIONS

Selection of appropriate laboratory tests to determine the causative virus in the patients' current illness depends on knowledge of the groups (family or genera) of viruses which are regularly associated with particular syndromes. Although a syndrome such as measles is caused by infection with the sole serotype of one single virus species *Morbillivirus* (measles virus) within the family *Paramyxoviridae*, a syndrome such as aseptic meningitis may arise from infection with one of a wide range of serotypes within the genus *Enterovirus* (Picornaviridae family) or a single serotype mumps virus (*Paramyxoviridae* family). Conversely, a particular enterovirus serotype such as coxsackievirus B5 may induce a wide variety of syndromes including pericarditis, pleurodynia, myositis as well as aseptic meningitis in the same patient[14] or one patient may develop pericarditis alone whilst another shows signs of aseptic meningitis without involvement of serous membranes.

From the clinical standpoint, virus families, and individual virus genera, species or serotypes within each family, may be grouped according to the principal target organ or system affected by the virus infection: the central nervous system (Table 2-3), the respiratory tract (Table 2-4), the exanthemata and tropical fevers (Table 2-5), and gastrointestinal infections (Table 2-6).

TABLE 2-3
CENTRAL NERVOUS SYSTEM VIRUS INFECTIONS

Syndrome	Clinical Features	Virus genus or family	Serotypes Commonly Encountered
Aseptic meningitis	headache, vomiting fever, neck stiffness CSF lymphocytosis	Enterovirus Paramyxoviridae	coxsackievirus B5, echovirus 9 mumps
Poliomyelitis	aseptic meningitis plus flaccid paralysis	Enterovirus	poliovirus 1, 2, 3
Encephalitis	headache, high fever, drowsiness to coma CSF lymphocytosis convulsions, spastic paresis	Togaviridae Bunyavirus Rhabdovirus Herpesvirus Paramyxoviridae Flaviviridae	Alphavirus (WEE) LAC rabies Herpesvirus hominis 1, 2 measles Flavivirus (POW, SLE)

LAC: La Crosse virus
POW: Powassan virus
SLE: St. Louis encephalitis
WEE: Western equine encephalomyelitis virus

TABLE 2-4

RESPIRATORY VIRUS INFECTIONS

Syndrome	Clinical Features	Virus genus or family	Serotypes Commonly Encountered
Coryza	running nose, nasal stuffiness, some cough	Picornaviridae	rhinovirus 14
Pharyngoconjunctival fever	reddened eyes, red and sore pharynx, cough	Mastadenovirus	adenovirus 3, 4, 7
Influenza	high fever, malaise headache, myalgia glazed pharynx	Orthomyxoviridae	influenza A Philippines/2/82 (H3N2) influenza B/USSR/100/83
Croup	croupy cough, inspiratory stridor, hoarse voice or cry, respiratory difficulty	Paramyxoviridae	parainfluenza 1, 3 (influenza, measles and chickenpox viruses may occasionally cause croup)
Bronchiolitis bronchopneumonia	cough, mucous secretions, rib retraction plus barrel chest. bronchopn: crepitations and consolidation on X-ray	Paramyxoviridae	respiratory syncytial (RS) (Influenza, parainfluenza, measles and chickenpox viruses may occasionally cause bronchopneumonia)
Pleurodynia	pain in chest on deep inspiration, plural friction rub	Enterovirus	coxsackievirus B1–B5
Pericarditis	pain over precordium, pericardial friction rub	Enterovirus	coxsackievirus B1–B5

TABLE 2-5
VIRAL EXANTHEMATA (RASHES)

Syndromes	Clinical Features	Incubation period (days)	Duration of Infectivity (days)	Virus genus or family	Serotypes Commonly Encountered
Measles	blotchy maculopapular rash, fever, running nose, and eyes, brown staining subsequently	14 (catarrh 2 days earlier)	−2 to +2	Paramyxoviridae	measles
Rubella	peachbloom blush, slight fever, postauricular lymphadenopathy	18	−2 to +7	Togaviridae	rubella
Herpes 1 oral	crops of pinpoint vesicles over face, lips, buccal mucosa	2–4	0 to +4	Herpesviridae	Herpesvirus hominis 1 (herpes simplex type 1)
2 genital	painful pinpoint vesicles on external genitalia	2–4	0 to +4	Herpesviridae	Herpesvirus hominis 2 (herpes simplex type 2)
Varicella-zoster	(a) chickenpox (varicella) crops of vesicles over face and trunk, all have scabbed within 7 days	18	−2 to +4	Herpesviridae	Herpesvirus varicellae (varicella-zoster, varicella or chickenpox virus)
	(b) herpes zoster (shingles) vesicles over cutaneous distribution of sensory nerves			Herpesviridae	Herpesvirus varicellae
Mumps	painful swelling of parotid glands, fever	14	−6 to +4	Paramyxoviridae	mumps
Dengue	'break-bone' fever, retro-orbital pain, headache, maculopapular rash, leukopenia	5–10	0 to +3	Flaviviridae	Flavivirus (dengue 1–4)

TABLE 2-5 (continued)

Syndromes	Clinical Features	Incubation period (days)	Duration of Infectivity (days)	Virus genus or family	Serotypes Commonly Encountered
Hemorrhagic fevers	fever, thrombocytopenic purpura, epistasis, hematuria, gastrointestinal hemorrhage	5–10	0 to +3	Flaviviridae Togaviridae Bunyaviridae	Flavivirus (dengue, Kyasanur Forest disease) Alphavirus (chikungunya) Nairovirus (Congo)
Undifferentiated tropical fevers	fever, headache, arthralgia sometimes	5–10	0 to +3	Togaviridae Bunyaviridae	Alphavirus (Ross River) Oropouche

TABLE 2-6
GASTROINTESTINAL VIRAL INFECTIONS

Syndrome	Clinical Features	Incubation period (days)	Duration of Infectivity (days)	Virus genus or family	Serotypes commonly encountered
Gastroenteritis	watery green stools dehydration	2	0 to +4	Reoviridae Adenoviridae	Rotavirus 1,2 Adenovirus 40,41
Hepatitis A	anorexia, nausea, fever, jaundice	15–40	−15 to +10	Picornaviridae	Enterovirus 72
Hepatitis B	"	50–160	−15 to +60	Hepadnaviridae*	Hepadnavirus 1

*Hepadnaviridae: candidate new virus family containing the single genus Hepadnavirus (hepatitis B virus) which is a double-shelled non-enveloped virus containing double-stranded DNA (Melnick, JL: Intervirology 18:105, 1982).

CENTRAL NERVOUS SYSTEM INFECTIONS induced by viruses comprise the syndromes aseptic meningitis, poliomyelitis, encephalitis (Table 2-3).

Aseptic meningitis consists of headache, vomiting, fever, neck stiffness and leukocytosis of CSF in which more than 50% cells are lymphocytes and the sugar and protein contents are normal. Enteroviruses (many serotypes of coxsackievirus and echovirus) and mumps virus are the principal causative agents.

Poliomyelitis exhibits all the features of aseptic meningitis, accompanied by flaccid paralysis of some component of the skeletal musculature, and concomitant pain and spasm in the affected muscle groups. Characteristically the cerebral functions remain clear. Causative agents are almost exclusively one of the three serotypes of poliovirus, but occasional cases of flaccid paralysis have been attributed to several non-polio enteroviruses.

Encephalitis comprises the syndrome of severe headache, high fever, drowsiness and disorientation which may progress to stupor or coma, along with twitching and spastic paresis of portions of the skeletal musculature. The case fatality rate may be as high as 5–10%. Causative viruses include arthropod-borne viruses within the Togaviridae and Bunyaviridae, together with non-arthropod-borne agents such as rabies virus, herpesviruses and measles virus.

RESPIRATORY TRACT INFECTIONS include coryza (common cold), pharyngoconjunctival fever, influenza and croup which affect mainly the upper respiratory tract, and bronchiolitis and bronchopneumonia which involve largely the lower respiratory tract. However this classification is somewhat arbitrary because croup involves the vocal cords of the larynx, at the division point between upper and lower respiratory tracts. Pleurodynia and pericarditis, where symptoms arise from viral infections of serous membranes, are discussed conveniently with the respiratory infections.

Coryza (common cold) presents with profuse watery nasal discharge accompanied by sneezing and nasal stuffiness, some cough and slight malaise with little or no fever. Symptoms arise from acute catarrhal inflammation of the nasal and pharyngeal mucosa. More than 100 serotypes of rhinovirus have been associated with common colds.

Pharyngoconjunctival fever usually occurs during summertime, especially among users of swimming pools where chlorination is inadequate. Patients exhibit acute reddening of the conjunctivae accompanied by a gritty sensation in the eyes, together with an acutely reddened and sore pharynx, cough and nasal discharge. Common etiological agents are adenovirus types 3, 4, 7.

Influenza is characterized by high fever, severe malaise accompanied by headache, plus aches and pains in the back and limbs, together with reddened, glazed pharyngeal and nasal mucous membranes and a cough. Symptoms arise from acute inflammation of the nasal and pharyngeal mucosa and also the bronchi and bronchioles; viral proliferation is limited to these mucous membranes. Serotypes within the species influenza A and influenza B commonly cause influenza; infections due to influenza C virus are extremely rare. During influenza epidemics, the proportion of deaths attributed to influenza and pneumonia regularly exceed the threshold proportion of 6.5%.[6]

Croup (acute laryngotracheobronchitis) commonly affects children aged less than 3 years, particularly during the cooler months in temperate zones. Characteristic clinical features are croupy cough, inspiratory stridor, hoarse voice or cry, and respiratory difficulty on inspiration, accompanied by indrawing of the chest wall in the subcostal, intercostal or subclavicular areas. Diminished air entry into the lungs is noted both clinically and radiologically. Bronchopneumonia is uncommon. Usually parainfluenza viruses types 1 and 3 are implicated in croup, but occasionally croup may arise during infections with influenza, respiratory syncytial, measles or varicella viruses.

Bronchiolitis characteristically affects infants aged less than 2 years who develop cough and runny nose followed by an abrupt increase in the mucous secretions 1–2 days later. This is accompanied by wheezing, increased coughing and difficulty with respirations resulting in rib-cage retraction, plus a barrel-shaped chest indicating obstruction to outflow of air. Fever is minimal. Over-inflated lungs are observed radiologically. Bronchoscopic suction may be required to remove excessive mucus.

Viral bronchopneumonia effects all age groups. Patients develop fever, severe cough, difficulty with respiration, and rales are heard over portions of the lung fields. Patchy consolidation throughout the lung fields is observed radiologically.

Respiratory syncytial (RS) virus is the principal causative agent in bronchiolitis and bronchopneumonia. Occasionally these syndromes may be associated with parainfluenza, influenza or measles virus infections.

Bacterial bronchopneumonia may follow shortly after virus infections, especially in adults, from overgrowth of bacteria such as *Haemophilus influenzae* or *Streptococcus pneumoniae*, which may be part of the "normal" flora of portions of the lower respiratory tract.

Pleurodynia is characterized by sharp pain over one side of the chest on deep inspiration, usually accompanied by a pleural friction rub over the painful site and a mild fever.

Pericarditis is characterized by severe precordial pain accompanied by a pericardial friction rub and typical electrocardiographic findings of flattening and inversion of T waves in leads V_3 through V_5.

Coxsackievirus B1 through B6 have all been associated with pleurodynia and pericarditis. Less commonly, group B coxsackieviruses have caused serous peritonitis which is manifested by severe generalized abdominal pain and tenderness with fever but normal leukocyte counts. Furthermore serous peritonitis may be accompanied by pleurodynia, pericarditis or acute tenderness of the skeletal musculature (myositis).

EXANTHEMATA comprise febrile illnesses accompanied by the simultaneous appearance of either maculopapular or vesicular rashes. Although rash is not a feature of mumps virus infection, mumps is traditionally discussed with the exanthemata.

Measles exhibits a blotchy maculopapular rash involving principally the face and trunk, accompanied by moderate fever and running nose and eyes which first appear 1 to 2 days before the rash. The incubation period is about 14 days to the onset of rash. Fever subsides 1 to 3 days after onset of rash, which then develops brown staining, and the rash usually disappears after 7 days. Measles virus is the sole causative agent.

Rubella exhibits a pinpoint blush resembling peachbloom over the face and trunk, but scant involvement of the extremities, accompanied by a mild fever and characteristic enlargement of the postauricular or postcervical lymph nodes. The incubation period is about 18 days. Fever subsides after 1 to 2 days and the rash fades after 3 to 4 days. Rubella virus is the sole causative agent.

Herpes affects two main portions of the body surface:
1. the face, lips and buccal mucosa (oral) where crops of vesicles 1–3 mm diameter arise from infection with *Herpesvirus hominis* type 1 usually,
2. the external genitalia (penis or labia-vaginal junction) where painful vesicles 1 mm diameter are induced by infection with *Herpesvirus hominis* type 2.

Varicella (chickenpox) and herpes zoster (shingles) are both caused by infections with *Herpesvirus varicellae*. Chickenpox vesicles, 1–3 mm diameter usually involve the face and trunk with successive crops during a period of 3 to 4 days following an incubation period of 18 days. All vesicles have dried and developed scabs within 7 days. Herpes zoster vesicles involve the cutaneous distribution of one or more sensory nerves.

Mumps usually presents with fever and painful swelling of one or both parotid or submandibular glands after an incubation period of about 14 days. Fever persists 1 to 2 days and salivary gland swelling usually subsides after 3 to 5 days. Mumps virus is the sole etiological agent.

Dengue is manifested by sudden onset of fever and severe frontal headache, accompanied by retro-ocular pain, severe pain in the back and limbs ('breakbone fever'), perversion of taste, and lymphadenopathy, in the absence of persisting respiratory symptoms. A maculopapular rash lasting for 2 to 7 days may affect two-thirds of the patients, and pruritus about half the patients. The incubation period is 5 to 10 days. Fever may persist 3 to 5 days, and it may show a remission followed by a relapse ("saddleback fever") in about half the patients.

Leukopenia with relative lymphocytosis is a constant finding. Complete recovery is the rule after typical dengue. Although clinically typical dengue usually is induced by infection with one of the four serotypes of dengue virus (Flavivirus), chikungunya virus (Alphavirus) has also induced dengue-like disease.

Hemorrhagic fevers have affected many inhabitants of Southeast Asia and the Indian Subcontinent since 1958, and islands of the Southwest Pacific since 1971. Clinical manifestations include purpura, epistaxis, hematuria and gastrointestinal hemorrhage which are accompanied by varying degrees of shock, in addition to dengue-like symptoms. Causative agents include dengue and Kyasanur Forest disease viruses (Flavivirus), chikungunya (Alphavirus) and Congo virus (Nairovirus).

Undifferentiated tropical fevers may arise from infection with a wide variety of arthropod-borne viruses including Ross River (Alphavirus), West Nile (Flavivirus), Oropouche (Bunyavirus), Rift Valley (Phlebovirus). Ross River virus infections are frequently associated with polyarthritis, whilst Rift Valley fever virus may induce exudative lesions and retinal hemorrhages in the eyes.

GASTROINTESTINAL INFECTIONS due to viruses include those involving the intestine only, causing gastroenteritis, and those affecting a major accessory organ, the liver, inducing hepatitis (Table 2-6).

Viral gastroenteritis patients suddenly develop profuse diarrhoea, often passing 10 or more loose watery yellow or green stools during the initial 24 hours. Severely affected patients rapidly become dehydrated with dry flaccid skin, dry glazed mucous membranes of the mouth and nose, sunken eyeballs and the abdomen feels doughy. Diarrhoea may persist 4 to 7 days in untreated patients, but it usually ceases within 1 to 2 days after commencement of intravenous infusion of fluids and electrolytes accompanied by discontinuance of oral feedings. Causative viruses are Rotavirus, Adenovirus, Calicivirus including Norwalk virus, Astrovirus, picornavirus-like agents, and Coronavirus, in decreasing order of frequency, but none of these agents are propagated conveniently in the laboratory.

Hepatitis is manifested clinically by anorexia and nausea, followed shortly by jaundice, dark urine and pale stools, and the liver is frequently enlarged or tender. Elevated levels of serum transaminases are found regularly. Two principal categories arise from infections with completely different viruses, neither of which is cultivated readily in the diagnostic laboratory. (i) Hepatitis A, due to enterovirus 72 (Picornaviridae), has an incubation period 15 to 40 days and is communicable by the fecal-oral route for about 15 days before to 10 days after onset of jaundice. (ii) Hepatitis B, due to Hepadnavirus 1 (Hepadnaviridae) has an incubation period about 60 days (range 50 to 160 days) and is communicable by blood or through mucous membranes for about 2 weeks before to 8 weeks after onset of jaundice. (iii) An additional category, non-A non-B hepatitis, may arise after transfusion of blood from commercial sources, but it is not attributed to agents causing hepatitis A or hepatitis B.

REFERENCES

[1] American Committee on Arthropod-Borne Viruses: Arbovirus names. Am J Trop Med Hyg 18:731, 1969.

[2] Andrewes CH, Horstmann DM: The susceptibility of viruses to ethyl ether. J Gen Microbiol 3:290, 1949.

[3] Barré-Sinoussi F, Chermann JC, Rey F, et al: Isolation of a T-lymphotropic retrovirus from a patient at risk for acquired immune deficiency syndrome (AIDS). Science 220:868, 1983.

[4] Berge TO (comp): International Catalogue of Arboviruses including certain other Viruses of Vertebrates. 2nd ed U.S. Dept. of Health Education and Welfare Publ No (CDC) 75-8301, 1975, with updatings by Subcommittee on Information Exchange to Dec 1982.

[5] Bishop DHL, Calisher CH, Casals J, Chumakov MP, Gaidamovich SYA, Hannoun C, Lvov DK, Marshall ID, Oker-Blom N, Pettersson RF, Porterfield JS, Russell PK, Shope RE, Westaway EG: Bunyaviridae. Intervirology 14:125, 1980.

[6] Choi K, Thacker SB: An evaluation of influenza mortality surveillance, 1962–1979. I. Time series forecasts of expected pneumonia and influenza deaths. Am J Epidemiol 113:215, 1981.

[7] Dalldorf G, Sickles GM: An unidentified, filtrable agent isolated from the feces of children with paralysis. Science 108:61, 1948.

[8] Doherty RL, Whitehead RH, Gorman BM, O'Gower AR: The isolation of a third group A arbovirus in Australia with preliminary observations on its relationship to epidemic polyarthritis. Australian J Sci 26:183, 1963.

[9] Gallo RC, Salahuddin SZ, Popovic M et al: Human T-lymphotropic retrovirus, HTLV-III, isolated from AIDS patients and donors at risk for AIDS. Science 224:500, 1984.

[10] International Committee on Taxonomy of Viruses: Classification and nomenclature of viruses. Intervirology 12:129, 1979.

[11] Kaufman HE, Martola EL, Dohlman C: Use of 5-iodo-2'-deoxyuridine (IDU) in treatment of herpes simplex keratitis. Arch Ophthal 68:235, 1962.

[12] Kaufman HE: Treatment of herpes simplex and vaccinia keratitis with 5-iodo and 5-bromo-2'-deoxyuridine. In M Pollard ed. Perspectives in Virology III pp 90–107, Hoeber, New York, 1963.

[13] Kingsbury DW, Bratt MA, Choppin PW, Hanson RP, Hosaka Y, Ter Meulen V, Norrby E, Plowright W, Roth R, Wunner WH: Paramyxoviridae. Intervirology 10:137, 1978.

[14] McLean DM: Patterns of infections with enteroviruses. J Pediat 54:823, 1959.

[15] McLean DM, Donohue WL: Powassan virus: isolation of virus from a fatal case of encephalitis. Canad Med Ass J 80:708, 1959.

[16] McLean DM: Immunological Investigation of Human Virus Diseases. Vol 5, Practical

Methods in Clinical Immunology, ed. RC Nairn. Churchill Livingstone, Edinburgh, 1982, pp 1–99.

[17]McLean DM, Wong KK: Same-day Diagnosis of Human Virus Infections. CRC Press, Boca Raton FL, 1984, pp 66–67.

[18]Matthews REF: The classification of nomenclature of viruses: summary of results of meetings of the International Committee on Taxonomy of Viruses in Strasbourg, August 1981. Intervirology 16:53, 1981.

[19]Matthews REF: Classification and Nomenclature of Viruses. Fourth Report of the International Committee on Taxonomy of Viruses. Intervirology 17:1, 1982.

[20]Reitz MS, Kalyanaramon VS, Robert-Guroff M, Popovic M, Sarngadharan NG, Sarin PS, Gallo RC: Human T-cell leukemia/lymphoma virus: the retrovirus of adult T-cell leukemia/lymphoma. J Infect Dis 147:399, 1983.

[21]Theiler M: Action of sodium deoxycholate on arthropod-borne viruses. Proc Soc Exp Biol Med 96:380, 1957.

CHAPTER 3

VIROLOGICAL AND IMMUNOLOGICAL TECHNIQUES

REPLICATION OF VIRUSES IN CELLS

Viruses can multiply or replicate only inside living cells. When most of the medically important viruses enter susceptible cells, the viruses multiply and induce destruction (lysis) of cells which is observed microscopically as the cytopathic effect (the lytic interaction). When a few viruses including Epstein Barr virus and the retroviruses enter cells, the viral genome (genetic markers within the nucleoprotein) integrates with the host genome and induces permanent transformation of the host cell morphology, growth characteristics and manner of interaction with adjacent cells (the transforming virus-cell interaction).

Stages in the lytic virus-cell interaction are summarized herein.[3] Most observations have been derived from studies of one-step growth cycles in which all cells are infected synchronously after exposure to virus suspensions containing substantially more than one infectious virus does per cell. The first stage is adsorption of the virus to the cell surface initially by ionic attraction, subsequently interaction with specific receptors. The second stage involves penetration of the virus into the cytoplasm, followed by the third stage of uncoating of virus protein from the nucleic acid which comprises the genome. The actual details vary within the different virus families. Uncoating of virus results in loss of infectivity during the first few hours after exposure of virus to cell (the eclipse phase). The fourth stage of synthesis of daughter virus now commences. This viral genome replicates either in the nucleus, as in the herpesviruses and adenoviruses, or in the cytoplasm for most other virus groups. However viral protein is regularly synthesized in the cytoplasm. The fifth stage comprises assembly of newly formed viral genomes with viral capsid proteins into daughter virus particles. The sixth stage of release of daughter virus from cells is accomplished either: (i) by mechanical release from disrupted cells as in the poxviruses and groups with naked virions such as enteroviruses; or (ii) by budding of the nucleocapsids (genome plus capsid protein) through the outer cell membranes and walls of intracytoplasmic vesicles, so that they acquire viral envelopes which contain both virus-coded proteins and host-cell proteins, as in groups with enveloped virions such as paramyxoviruses and togaviruses. Single cells infected by one virus particle per cell may each liberate 100 or more daughter virus particles.[6] Typically in infections with naked viruses and poxviruses, most of the recently synthesized virus remains cell-bound, so that the concentration of virus released into the supernatant fluid surrounding the cell remains lower than the cell-bound virus concentration until complete disruption of the cell upon conclusion of viral replication. However in infections with enveloped virions, which mature only during the release process, the virus concentration extracellularly regularly exceeds the cell bound virus concentration substantially.

Immunological responses normally occur in humans and other warm-blood vertebrates after infection with all viruses. Responses are mediated by the reticulo-endothelial system through: (i) B-lymphocytes which produce antiviral antibodies of several classes specifically directed towards each virus serotype; (ii) T-lymphocytes with induction of cell-mediated immunity. Resistance to subsequent infections with the same virus serotype normally depends upon inactivation by the specific antibody. In many situations, cell-mediated immunity accelerates the removal of virus with subsequent decrease in severity of symptoms, but in some instances cell-mediated immunity aggravates the disease process.

VIRUS TITRATIONS

The amount of infectious virus in a suspension of ground-up tissue or in a body fluid is measured by a titration procedure involving living cells in tissue cultures. Detection of virus growth depends upon the observation of characteristic changes in the cells (cytopathic effects) upon microscopic examination of tissue cultures after several days incubation. Monolayer cultures of primary cells (e.g., rhesus monkey kidney) or continuous diploid (e.g., human foreskin fibroblast) or polyploid (e.g., HEp-2) cells have been used extensively for titration of a vast range of viruses. Cytopathic effects after growth of poliovirus are illustrated in Figure 3-1.

TITRATIONS OF 50% TISSUE CULTURE INFECTIVITY DOSES (TCD_{50}) are performed conveniently in flat bottomed cups in plastic plates containing either 24 cups 1.5cm diameter x 1.5cm deep (NUNC 1-43982) or 96 cups 8mm

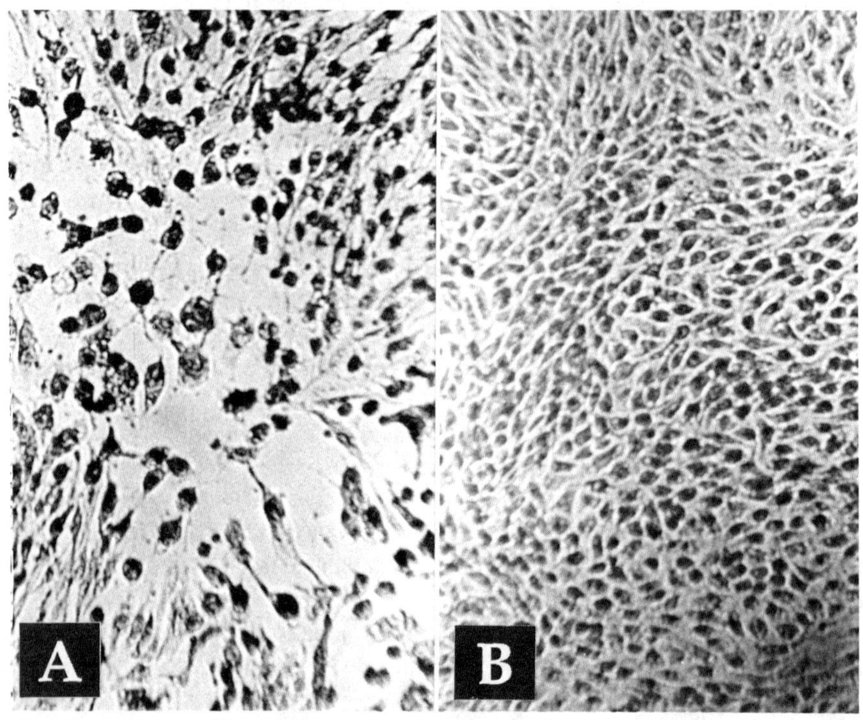

3-1: (A) Cytopathic effects after growth of poliovirus 1 in primary monkey kidney tissue cultures. (B) Uninfected monkey kidney tissue cultures. Crystal violet stain (x21). Reproduced with permission from McLean DM, 1980. Virology in Health Care, Williams and Wilkins, Baltimore, p. 64.

diameter x 10mm deep (NUNC 1-67008) which are incubated in a humidified atmosphere containing 5% CO_2. Serial tenfold dilutions of virus are added to each of 2, 3 or 4 cups per dilution, the plastic plates are incubated at 35 to 37° C for 3 to 4 days, by which time cytopathic effects comprising rounding, shrinkage and detachment will be partial or complete in all cups which received one or more infectious doses of virus such as coxsackievirus B5 or poliovirus 1. Since infection of each cup is an all-or-none effect, it is necessary to express the virus concentration in terms of the dilution required to infect 50% of the cups. This 50% endpoint is calculated conveniently by the Reed and Muench formula[9] as in the following example.

Virus dilution		Observed CPE			Cumulative CPE		
Power	Log	ratio	pos.	neg.	pos.	neg.	percent
10^{-5}	5.0	4/4	4	0	9	0	100
10^{-6}	6.0	4/4	4	0	5	0	100
10^{-7}	7.0	1/4	1	3	1	3	25
10^{-8}	8.0	0/4	0	4	0	7	0

Proportionate distance between 10^{-6} and 10^{-7} (volume of inoculum = 1.0 ml)

$$\frac{50 - \text{next below}}{\text{next above} - \text{next below}} = \frac{50 - 25}{100 - 25} = \frac{25}{75} = 0.3 \text{ approx.}$$

Thus $\log TCD_{50} = 7.0 - 0.3 = 6.7$
i.e., the original preparation contains 6.7 log TCD_{50} per ml.
CPE: cytopathic effect

Actual technical details for the conduct of this and subsequent laboratory tests are described fully by this author in a handbook of techniques.[7]

TITRATIONS OF PLAQUE FORMING UNITS (PFU) are performed either in plastic plates containing 24 cups 1.5 cm x 1.5 (NUNC 1-43982) or in petri dishes 35mm diameter (NUNC 1-50318). Serial tenfold dilutions of virus are added to each of 2 cups per dilution. After holding for 1 hour at 35 to 37° C to permit adsorption of virus tissue culture cells, the supernatant fluids are removed by aspiration. Cell sheets are overlaid with maintenance medium containing 1% agrose which is allowed to gel at bench temperature (23° C) for 1/2 hour. Plates or petri dishes are incubated at 37° C in an atmosphere of 5% CO_2 for 2 to 7 days. The gels are then removed by aspiration, and the cell sheets are stained with 0.1% crystal violet, which is removed 1 minute later. Plaques appear as clear unstained areas against the sheet of unaffected cells which stain violet (Figure 3-2). Since one plaque arises following the growth of one living virus particle (infectious dose), it is straight forward to calculate the amount of infectious virus particles in the original preparation thus:

Virus dilution		Observed plaques		
Power	Log	cup #1	cup #2	mean
10^{-5}	5.0	30	30	30
10^{-6}	6.0	30	30	30
10^{-7}	7.0	7	5	6
10^{-8}	8.0	0	0	0 end point

Since 6 plaques (mean) appeared at dilution 7.0 log (volume of inoculum = 0.1ml), then 1 plaques (mean) would appear at dilution 7.8 log ($\log_{10} 6 = 0.8$ approx.). Thus the original preparation contains 7.8 log PFU per 0.1 ml or 8.8 log PFU per ml.

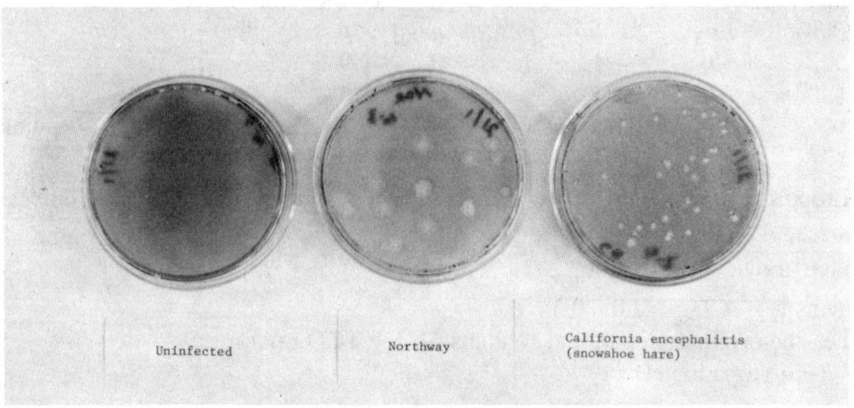

Figure 3-2: Plaques induced by snowshoe hare virus (California encephalitis serogroup) (x2).

ANTIBODY TITRATIONS

NEUTRALIZATION TESTS usually require the addition of a standard amount of infectious virus (100 TCD_{50} or 100 PFU) to serial fourfold or fivefold dilutions of antibody (sera from patients or laboratory animals), followed by incubation of serum-virus mixtures at bench temperature for 30 to 60 minutes in order to permit coupling of antibody to virus. The mixtures are then assayed for residual virus infectivity by inoculation of pairs of tissue culture tubes which are incubated for several days at 37° C, then examined for evidence of cytopathic effects, or for plaque formation if cell sheets received agarose overlays shortly after inoculation. Controls containing serial tenfold dilutions of the estimated 100 TCD_{50} or PFU are always tested simultaneously.

The antibody titre is expressed as the reciprocal of the highest serum dilution which inhibits cytopathic effects in cups which received 100 TCD_{50} (Figure 3-3) or which reduces the plaque count by 90% (Figure 3-4).

HEMAGGLUTINATION INHIBITION (HI) tests depend on the ability of antibody to bind to virus particles and thus render them incapable of attaching to erythrocytes in the proportion of one virus particle to two erythrocytes. Titrations of hemagglutination (HA) and HI are performed conveniently in disposable plastic plates containing 96 U-shaped cups (Dynatech 1-220-24A) employing 0.025 ml volumes of each reagent.

Hemagglutination reactions of some viruses such as influenza, parainfluenza and mumps occur in unbuffered 0.15M (0.85%) saline at pH 7.0 and bench temperature 23° C. Other viruses such as measles, rubella, and some arboviruses

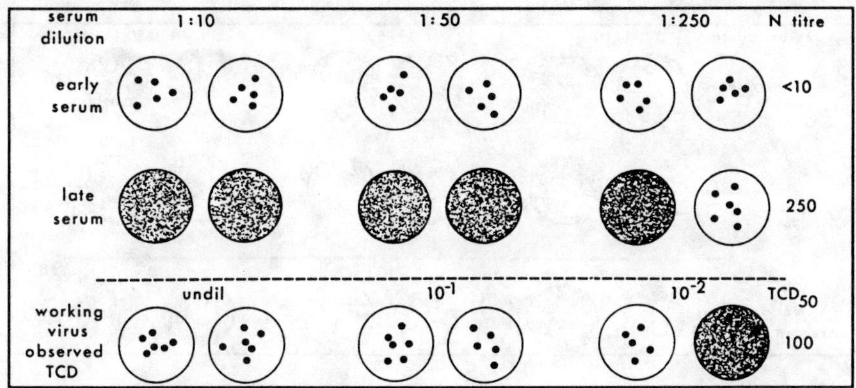

Figure 3-3: Diagrammatic representation of virus neutralization in tissue culture using cytopathic effects. Serial dilutions of patient's sera receive equal volumes of working dilutions of stock virus. Estimated 100 TCD$_{50}$. Reproduced with permission from McLean DM, 1982. Immunological Investigation of Human Virus Diseases, Churchill Livingstone, Edinburgh, p. 6.10^{-1} and 10^{-2}. Plaque reduction of 90% was shown by serum diluted 1:250.

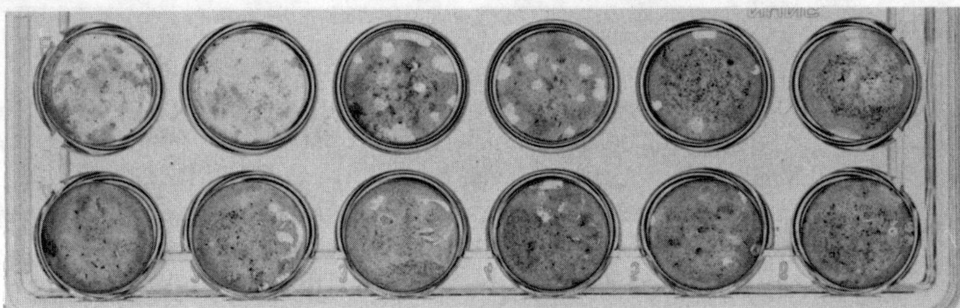

Figure 3-4 A: Plaque reduction neutralization test. Serum dilutions 1:10, 1:50, 1:250 were mixed with 200 PFU snowshoe hare virus and added to pairs of cups in the lower row. The same working dilution of virus was added to pairs of cups in the upper row undiluted at 10^{-1} 10^{-2}. Plaque reduction of 90% was shown by serum diluted 1:250.

agglutinate erythrocytes only in buffered saline at a specific pH, e.g., Powassan virus at pH 6.4 and a particular temperature (4, 23, 37° C).

Certain viruses agglutinate erythrocytes of a particular species of laboratory animal optimally, whilst erythrocytes from other animal species are not agglutinated, e.g., laboratory-passaged strains of influenza virus agglutinate mammalian (human or guineapig) and avian (goose or chicken) erythrocytes to the same titer, but measles virus agglutinates only monkey erythrocytes and Powassan virus agglutinates only erythrocytes from geese or newly hatched chickens.

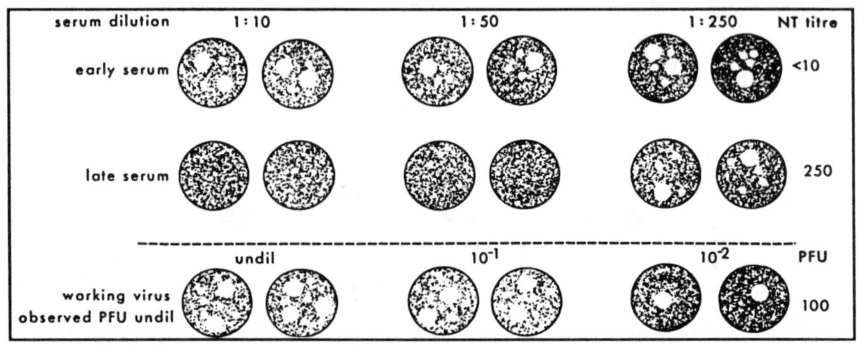

Figure 3-4 B: Diagrammatic representation of virus neutralization in tissue culture using plaque reduction. Serial dilutions of patient's sera receive equal volumes of working dilutions of stock virus. Estimated 100 PFU. Reproduced with permission from McLean DM, 1982. Immunological Investigation of Human Virus Disease, Churchill Livingstone, Edinburgh, p. 7.

Sera from patients or animals usually contain one or more categories of non-specific inhibitors of hemagglutination in addition to antibody. Removal of these inhibitors is essential before conduct of the HI test. In the influenza system, heat-labile (Chu) inhibitors are removed by heating at 56° C for 30 minutes. Thereafter, heat-stable mucoprotein (Francis) inhibitors are removed by treatment either with 0.01 M potassium periodate or with receptor-destroying enzyme (neuraminidase). In the measles and rubella systems, the inhibitors are removed by adsorption with kaolin; in arbovirus systems, acetone extraction effects removal of inhibitors from unheated serum.

Hemagglutination inhibition tests for influenza antibodies in a pair of sera collected early in the course of illness and several days to weeks later are performed as follows. Serial twofold dilutions of the early and late sera, after pretreatment with heat and periodate, are performed in cups of a disposable plastic plate by serial transfer of 0.025ml amounts into equal volumes of saline. Similar quantities of influenza virus, diluted to contain 4 agglutinating doses (AD) per 0.025ml are added to each serum dilution, and in a third row this stock virus is diluted serially in saline. After holding at bench temperature (23° C) for 1/2 hour, 0.025ml drops of 0.5% goose erythrocyte suspension in saline are added to all cups. The plates are incubated at bench temperature for 1/2 to 1 hour, and the pattern of setting of erythrocytes is observed in each cup. Hemagglutination appears as discrete points of erythrocytes distributed over the surface of the cup, as though they were shaken from a table-salt container, but inhibition or lack of hemagglutination appears as red buttons at the bottom of each tube (Figure 3-5, 3-6). The HI titre is expressed as a reciprocal of the highest serum dilution which inhibits hemagglutination by 4AD virus.

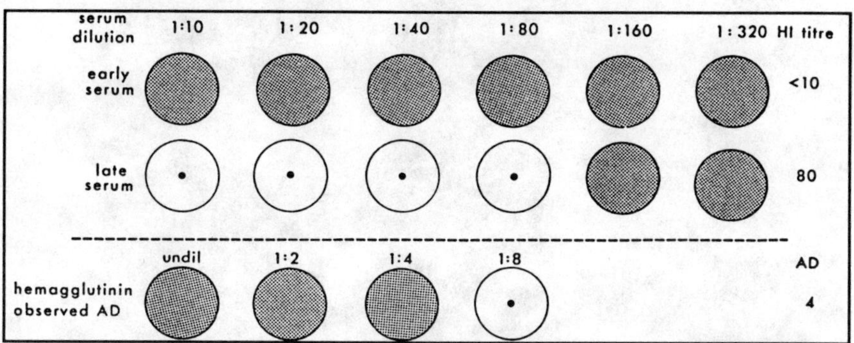

Figure 3-5: Diagrammatic representation of hemagglutination inhibition tests. Serial dilutions of patient's sera receive equal volumes of working dilutions of hemagglutinin (estimated 4 AD). Add washed erythrocyte suspension to each cup of serum-hemagglutinin mixture. Reproduced with permission from McLean DM, 1982. Immunological Investigation of Human Virus Diseases, Churchill Livingstone, Edinburgh, p. 10.

Hemagglutination inhibition tests for arboviruses, e.g., Powassan (POW) virus require buffers. Serial twofold dilutions of acetone-extracted patient's sera (0.025ml) are prepared in borate-saline buffer pH9 which contains 0.4% bovalbumin to stabilize virus during the reaction process. Equal quantities of virus diluted in the borate buffer to contain 8AD per 0.025ml are added to each serum dilution. After holding for 1/2 hour at 4° C, two volumes (0.05ml) 0.25% goose erythrocyte suspension in a phosphate buffer (virus adjusting diluent, VAD) are added to each cup of serum-virus mixture. This immediately changes the pH from 9.0, which is required to maintain virus stability during its interaction with antibody, to a predetermined pH from 6.2 to 7.0 at which the HA reaction occurs. The plate is incubated for one hour on the bench (23° C), or in the refrigerator (4° C) or incubator (37° C) to promote reaction between free virus and erythrocytes at the optimal temperature for the particular virus system (Powassan virus reacts optimally at pH 6.4 and 23° C).

COMPLEMENT FIXATION (CF) TESTS depend on the following principle. Complement (C') is a complex of about a dozen euglobulins which are present

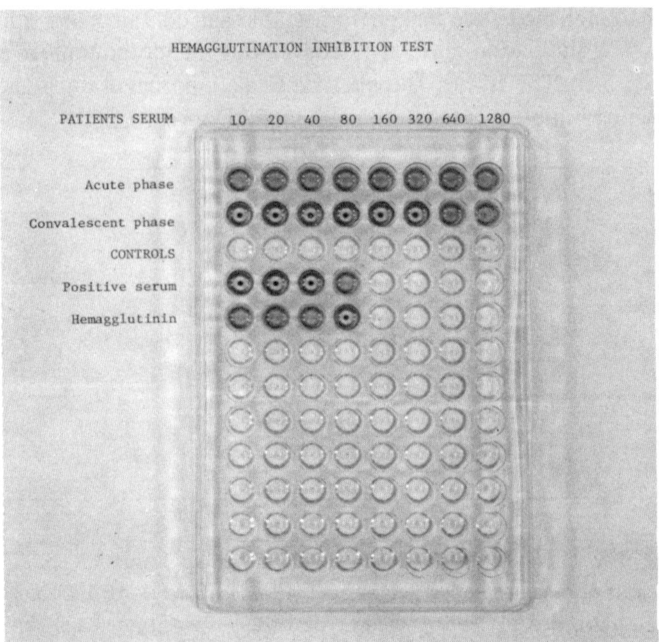

Figure 3-6: Hemagglutination inhibition tests on paired human sera using influenza A (H3N2) virus.

in sera from humans and other mammals. Whenever C' is added to a complex of antigen (e.g., virus) and its homologous antibody in saline, C' is "fixed" (bound) to this complex. Complement is detected by its ability to induce hemolysis through increased permeability of outer membranes of erythrocytes which have been coated previously ("sensitized") by anti-erythrocyte antibody ("hemolysin"). In most situations involving patient's the CF test is employed to assay patient's sera for antiviral antibodies. Usually CF tests are performed in disposable plastic plates with 96 U-shaped cups per plate (Dynatech 220-24A), employing 0.025ml volumes of each reagent.

Actual details of the preparation of reagents such as sensitized erythrocytes and the working dilution of the virus antigen and complement are described in a textbook of techniques.[7] Diagrammatic representation of the result of an antibody titration involving sera collected from a patient both early and late in the course of illness is shown in Figure 3-7, where the antibody titer has increased from an undetectable level of <5, as shown by hemolysis in all cups, to a titre of 80 in the late serum, where erythrocytes remained intact in cups containing dilutions of patient's serum as high as 1:80. An actual test on paired sera from a patient is shown in Figure 3-8.

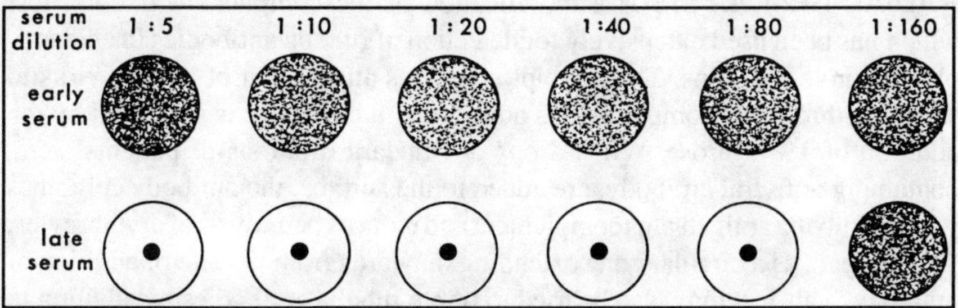

Figure 3-7: Diagrammatic representation of complement fixation test. Serial dilutions of patient's sera receive equal volumes of virus antigen (optimum dilution) and complement. Incubate overnight at 4° C. Add sensitized erythrocytes, incubate at 37° C. Reproduced with permission from McLean DM, 1982. Immunological Investigation of Human Virus Diseases, Churchill Livingstone, Edinburgh, p. 14.

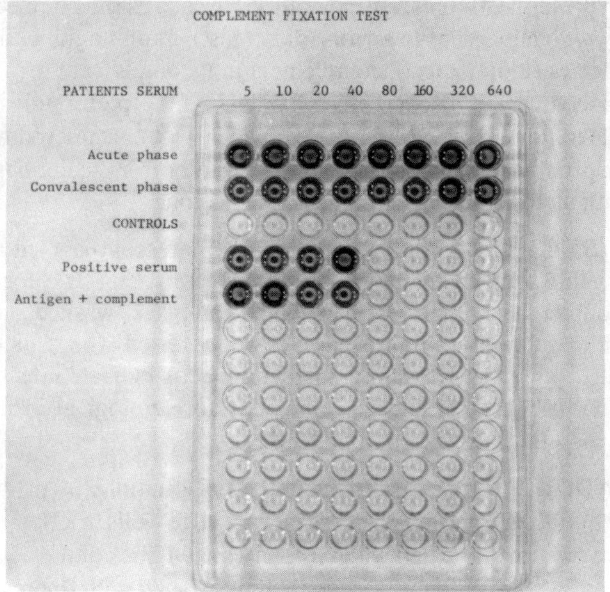

Figure 3-8: Complement fixation test on paired human sera using adenovirus group antigen.

RADIAL HEMOLYSIS is a modification of the complement fixation test which has been used extensively for detection of rubella antibodies in epidemiological investigations. The principle involves attachment of rubella virus to sheep erythrocytes, complement is added, and the mixture is solidified by the addition of 1% agarose. When drops of standard dilutions of patients' sera, containing antiviral antibody, are added to the surface, the antibody combines with the rubella antigen plus complement and induces hemolysis of erythrocytes. This appears as a circular zone extending outwards from the site of addition of antibody. This test may also be used to titrate rubella antibodies by addition to the agar surface a series of two-fold dilutions of patients' sera, as in the illustration.

IMMUNOFLUORESCENCE. The indirect or anticomplement techniques are employed for detection of antibodies in patients' sera; either of these or the direct techniques is used for identification of virus antigen in specimens from patients. In principle, fluorescein or another dye such as rhodamine is combined chemically with antibodies to a virus (direct test), immunoglobulin of a human or other species (indirect test), complement (anticomplement test).

Teflon-coated microscope slides containing 12 perforations each 6mm diameter (Hendley, Essex SM-014 or equivalent) receive microdrops (0.01ml) of virus suspension in infected tissue culture cells or from secretions of patients. After drying at 40° C, the slides are fixed in acetone.

For the **DIRECT** test, a suitable dilution of fluorescein-labeled antiserum is added, the slide is incubated in a humidified chamber at 37° C for 30 minutes, washed, counterstained with 0.01% naphthalene black, washed, and examined under incident ultraviolet light in a microscope fitted with a dichroic prism. Bright yellow-green fluorescent points within cells indicate infection with the particular virus. This test is used principally for serological identification of viruses in secretions or tissues of patients.

For the **INDIRECT** test, microdrops of serial dilutions of patients' sera in phosphate buffered saline (PBS) pH 7.0 are added to wells in teflon-coated slides which were previously coated with virus-infected tissue culture cells. Slides are incubated at 37° C for 30 minutes, washed, incubated with fluorescein-labeled antihuman immunoglobulin (IgG or IgM), washed, counterstained with naphthalene black, washed, and examined by fluorescence microscopy. Wells in which fluorescent foci are seen intracellularly denote the presence of antibody (Figure 3-9).

For the **ANTICOMPLEMENT IMMUNOFLUORESCENCE** (ACIF) test, serial dilutions of patients' sera are applied to wells in teflon-coated slides which

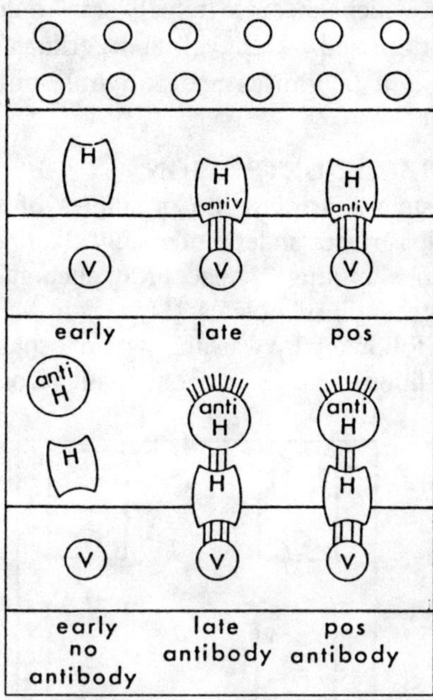

Figure 3-9: Diagrammatic representation of indirect immunofluorescence test for antibodies in paired sera from patient. To virus antigen on slide, add patient's sera, incubate 30 min. Add fluorescein-conjugated anti-human Ig, incubate 30 min, wash, counterstain with naphthalene black and examine by fluorescence microscopy. Reproduced by permission from McLean DM, 1982. Immunological Investigation of Human Virus Diseases, Churchill Livingstone, Edinburgh, p. 20.

were previously coated with virus-infected tissue culture cells. Complement is also added as guineapig serum diluted 1:10. Slides are incubated and washed as above, then a suitable dilution of fluorescein-labeled antiserum to the C'3 component of guineapig complement is added, the slides are again incubated, washed, counterstained with naphthalene black, washed and examined by fluorescence microscopy. Cells in antibody-positive wells exhibit fluorescent staining. This system is used particularly in cytomegalovirus and varicellazoster systems in order to circumvent non-specific binding of the Fc fragment of human IgG to receptors which are produced in tissue culture cells after replication of these viruses.

ENZYME IMMUNOASSAY (enzyme-linked immunosorbent assay, ELISA).

Principles of this test which detects extremely small quantities of antigens and antibodies were first devised by Engvall and Perlman[2] in 1972 and adapted extensively to detection of viruses and antiviral antibodies by Voller and associates[14,15] in 1976.

ANTIVIRAL ANTIBODY DETECTION

The rubella system illustrates the principles of the ELISA test. Proteins adsorb to plastic surfaces under moderately alkaline conditions at pH 9.6. Thus semipurified rubella virus (V) becomes "anchored" to surfaces of cups in 96-cup flat-bottomed plastic plates (Dynatech M129A) after overnight incubation at 40° C, following by washing with phosphate buffer pH 7.4 (Figure 3-10, step 1). Addition of late serum from a patient convalescent from rubella

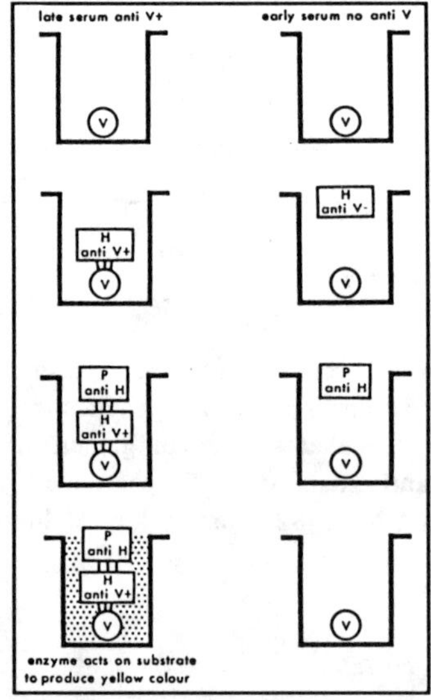

Figure 3-10: Diagrammatic representation of enzyme immunoassay (ELISA) test for detection of antiviral antibody. Step 1: adsorb virus (V) to plastic surfaces of 96-cup plates; step 2: add patient's sera (anti V+), incubate 30 min at 23° C, wash; step 3: add enzyme-labeled anti-human antibody (P anti H), incubate 30 min, wash; step 4: add substrate, read color reaction by spectrophotometer.

permits attachment of anti-rubella antibody (anti V+) to the anchored rubella virus (V) after incubation at 23° C for 1 hour, and this complex remains bound to the plastic surface after washing (step 2). However early serum collected within 2 days after onset of rash and fever does not contain antiviral antibody and therefore it is washed away from the plastic surface. Anti-human Ig antibody (anti H) (prepared in goats or rabbits) which is labeled with alkaline phosphatase (P) or another enzyme (E) such as horseradish peroxidase is added, and the plate is incubated and washed. The anti-human Ig binds to the human species-specific component of the patient's serum which contains antiviral antibody (step 3). Addition of a substrate (P-nitrophenyl phosphate, Sigma 104) in diethanolamine buffer pH 9.8 is followed by development of a yellow color due to enzymic action, and the color intensity is read by a spectrophotometer (step 4). (Figure 3-11).

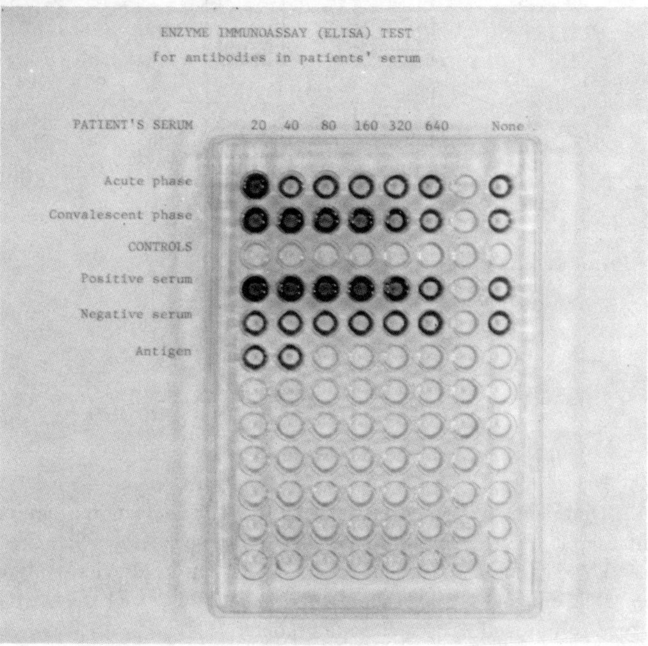

Figure 3-11: ELISA test for antiviral antibodies in paired sera.

The antiviral antibody titer within the IgM component of the patient's serum is determined by the following modification (Figure 3-12). Antibody to human IgM (prepared in goats) is adsorbed to the plastic surface (step 1). After addition of patient's serum, antiviral antibody within the IgM component binds to the attached anti IgM (step 2). Addition of virus (V) permits attachment to antiviral antibody within the IgG component (step 3). Antiviral antibody, prepared in rabbits and labeled with alkaline phosphatase binds to the virus (step 4). Phosphatase bound to the virus-antibody complex acts on the Sigma 104 substrate to produce a yellow color which is read spectrophotometrically (step

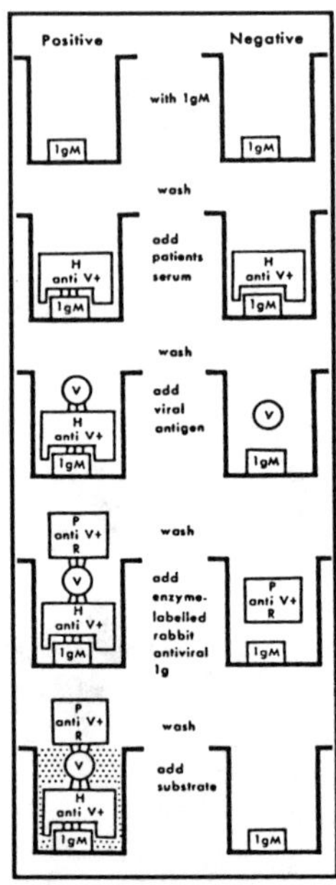

Figure 3-12: Diagrammatic representation of ELISA for detection of antibody in IgM component. Step 1: adsorb goat antihuman IgM to plastic surfaces; Step 2: add patient's serum (H anti V+), incubate 30 min at 23° C, wash; Step 3: add viral antigen, incubate, wash; Step 4: add enzyme-labeled rabbit antiviral antibody, incubate, wash; Step 5: add substrate, read color reaction by spectrophotometer.

5). The difference in antiviral antibody titers between patient's serum added directly to virus attached to wells (Figure 3-10), and after adsorption to anti IgM (Figure 3-12), represents the antiviral antibody titer within the IgM fraction.

Competitive method. Add serial dilutions of patients' serum to virus-coated cups. Antiviral antibody combines with the anchored virus. Add enzyme-labeled antiviral antibody—this cannot combine with the antibody-coated virus. When antiviral antibodies are absent from patients' sera, the enzyme-labeled antiviral antibody attaches to the anchored virus, and a color reaction develops after addition of an appropriate substrate.

VIRUS ANTIGEN DETECTION

The rotavirus system illustrates the principle of detection of virus antigen in

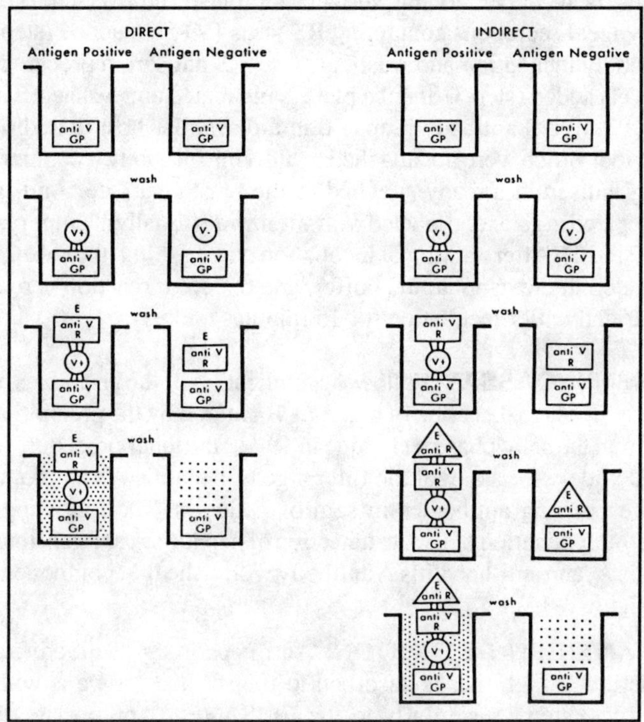

Figure 3-13: Diagrammatic representation of detection of viral antigen by ELISA using direct (enzyme-labeled antiviral antibody in a species different from that adsorbed initially to the plastic surface) and indirect (enzyme-labeled anti-species antiserum) techniques.

feces of gastroenteritis patient's by the *direct* test (Figure 3-13). Anti-rotavirus antiserum (anti V, GP) prepared in guineapigs is adsorbed to plastic cups using carbonate buffer pH 9.6 (step 1). Clarified fecal suspension containing rotavirus (V+) is added next (step 2). After incubation and washing, anti-rotavirus antiserum prepared in rabbits (anti V, R, E) which is labeled with an enzyme (usually alkaline phosphatase) is added (step 3). Finally after additional incubation followed by washing, the substrate (Sigma 104) is added in diethanolamine buffer, and the color reaction is read spectrophotometrically after incubation for 15 minutes (step 4).

The *indirect* test has been employed to detect respiratory syncytial (RS) virus antigen in nasopharyngeal secretions of patients with acute respiratory infections (Figure 3-13). Anti-RS antiserum prepared in guineapigs (anti V, GP) or bovines is adsorbed to the surfaces of plastic cups (step 1). Clarified nasopharyngeal secretions containing RS virus (V+) are added (step 2), which is followed by incubation and washing. Anti-RS antiserum prepared in rabbits (anti V, R) is added (step 3) and the plate is incubated and washed. This permits binding of antiviral antibody prepared in a dissimilar host to additional virus antigenic loci which were not attached to antiviral antibody receptors within the guineapig antiserum already attached to the plastic surface. Anti-rabbit antiserum, prepared in goats and labeled with an enzyme (usually alkaline phosphatase) is added (step 4). After additional incubation and washing, the substrate (Sigma 104) is added in diethanolamine buffer, and the color reaction is read spectrophotometrically after incubation for 15 minutes (step 5).

RADIOIMMUNOASSAY. Following application of the principles of radioimmunoassay (RIA) to detection of hepatitis B antigen by the precipitin technique in 1970[16] and the solid phase technique in 1972,[5] the latter procedure is currently employed widely for assay of the full range of hepatitis A and B antigens plus their corresponding antibodies in sera of patient's. The following examples illustrate the application of RIA to detection of hepatitis A antigen, total antibody to hepatitis A, and anti-hepatitis A antibody within the IgM component of human serum (Figure 3-14).

VIRAL ANTIGEN DETECTION. Anti-hepatitis A antibody (anti V) in human serum at high titer is adsorbed to the surfaces of wells within 96 cup plastic plates (step 1), similarly to the ELISA test. Appropriate dilutions of patient's serum containing hepatitis A virus antigen (V+) are added (step 2) and the cups are incubated, then washed. This permits binding of virus to the plastic surface through the antibody already attached to the cup. Anti-hepatitis A antibody prepared in rabbits and labeled with radioactive iodine[125] I (anti V, R) is added (step 3) to permit binding of this antibody to additional antigen receptor sites on the virus and the mixture is incubated, then washed. The individual cups are cut away from the plate, and the counts per minute of gamma emissions from each cup is measured individually in a scintillation counter (step 4). The sample from the patient is considered positive for hepatitis A antigen when the ratio of radioactive counts per minute in the virus-containing (V+) sample to the counts per minute in the virus-negative (V–) control samples exceeds 2.1. (V+/V– > 2.1).

TOTAL ANTIVIRAL ANTIBODY ASSAY. Patient's serum containing antiviral antibody (anti V+) is adsorbed to the surface of plastic cups (step 1). Addition of a standard amount of hepatitis A virus permits binding of virus to the plastic surface through antibody already attached (step 2) and the mixture is incubated, then washed. Radio-labeled anti-hepatitis A antibody prepared in

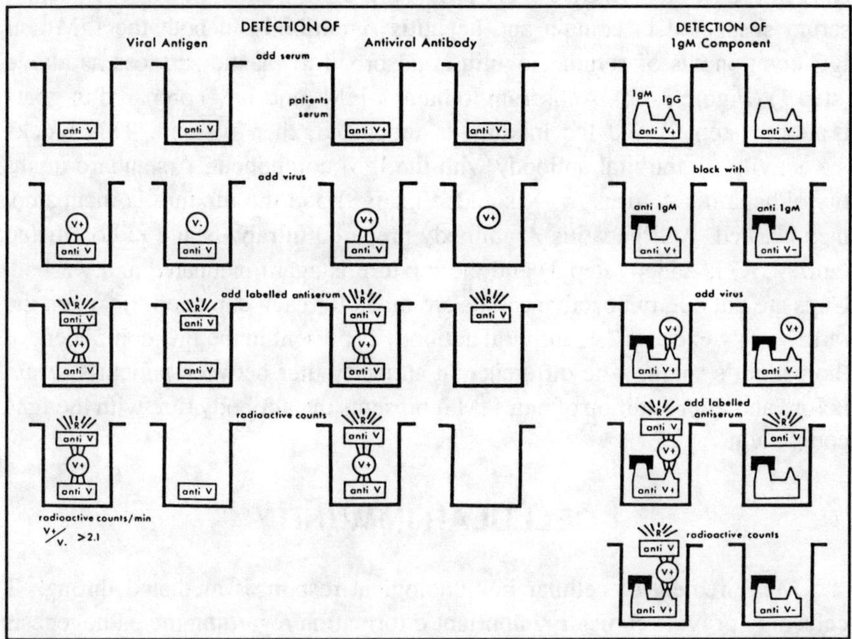

Figure 3-14: Diagrammatic representation of detection viral antigen and total antiviral antibody by solid-phase radioimmunoassay RIA.

Antigen detection: Step 1: adsorb known human antiviral antibody to plastic surface; Step 2: add test viral antigen, incubate, wash; Step 3: add radio-labeled rabbit antiviral antibody, incubate, wash; Step 4: count gamma emissions.

Antiviral antibody (total) in: Step 1: adsorb test antiviral antibody in patient's serum to plastic surface; Step 2: add known viral antigen, incubate, wash; Step 3: add radio-labeled rabbit antiviral antibody, incubate, wash; Step 4: count gamma emissions.

Antiviral antibody (IgM): Step 1: adsorb test antiviral antibody IgM and IgG in patient's serum to plastic surface; Step 2: add goat anti IgM, incubate, wash; Step 3: add known viral antigen; Step 4: add radio-labeled rabbit antiviral antibody, incubate, wash; Step 5: count gamma emissions.

rabbits (anti V, R) is added (step 3) and the mixture is incubated, then washed. This permits attachment of the antiviral antibody to additional antigenic loci on the virus, thus binding the radioactive reagent to the plastic surface. Individual cups are cut away from the plastic plate, then assayed for radioactive counts as above (step 4). Antiviral antibody is present in patient's serum when the ratio V+/V− exceeds 2.1.

ANTIVIRAL ANTIBODY WITHIN THE IgM COMPONENT. Patient's serum suspected to contain anti-hepatitis A antibody in both the IgM and IgG components of serum globulin is adsorbed to plastic surfaces as above (step 1) (Figure 3-14). Antiserum to human IgM (anti IgM) prepared in goats is added (step 2) and the mixture is incubated, then washed. This blocks the activity of antiviral antibody with the IgM component. A standard quantity of hepatitis A virus (V+) is added (step 3) and the mixture is incubated, then washed. Anti hepatitis A antibody prepared in rabbits and radio-labeled (anti V, R) is added (step 4) and the mixture is again incubated and washed. Cups are cut out, radioactive counts are made for each cup (step 5). When the ratio V+/V− exceeds 2.1, antiviral antibody is present in the IgG component of the patient's serum. The difference in antibody titer between patient's serum before and after addition of anti IgM represents the antibody titre with the IgM component.

CELLULAR IMMUNITY

Measurement of cellular immunological responses mediated through T cells may provide clinically important information regarding the pathogenesis and prognosis of some virus diseases. Assays of cellular immunity which are currently employed in virus laboratories include lymphocyte transformation, lymphocyte toxicity and macrophage migration inhibitory factor.

LYMPHOCYTE TRANSFORMATION

This test depends upon stimulation of increased biological activity (transformation of lymphocytes to lymphoblastoid forms), as revealed by increased synthesis of deoxyribonucleic acid (DNA), following exposure of the patient's lymphocytes to heat-inactivated viral antigen. This activity is measured by demonstration of greater uptake of thymidine (a constituent base of DNA) labeled with radioactive carbon ^{14}C[8,10] or tritium ^{3}H[12,13] in virus-treated lymphocytes than in uninfected controls.

Mononuclear cell suspensions are obtained by centrifugation of freshly collected heparinized blood from patient's through a Ficoll-Hypaque gradient.[1] After washing 3 times, cells are suspended at a concentration of 5×10^5 cells/ml in tissue culture maintenance medium RPMI 1640 containing 20% human plasma, gentamicin (50 µg/ml) and L-glutamine (2 mM/ml). Cell suspensions in 0.2ml amounts are placed in groups of 9 wells for each patient within 96-well disposable flat-bottom tissue culture microplates (Figure 3-15).

(i) Clusters of 3 wells for patient receive 10 µl virus antigen, another 3

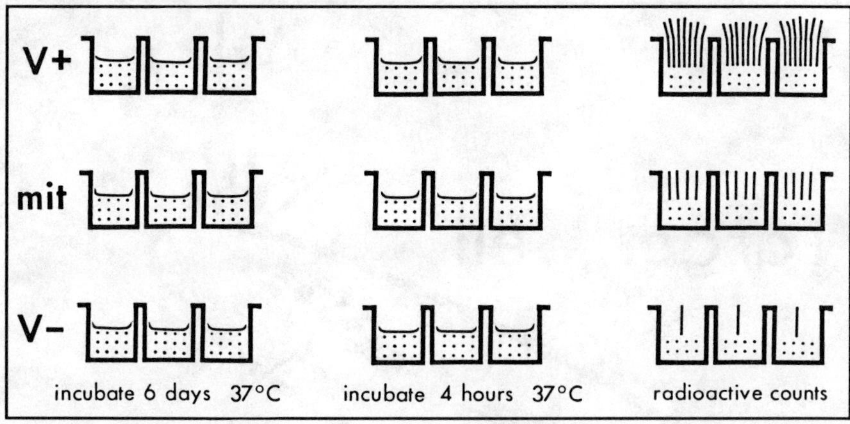

Figure 3-15: Diagrammatic representation of lymphocyte transformation assay. Step 1: place lymphocyte suspensions in groups of 9 wells; to each group of 3 wells add virus antigen, mitogen and control antigen, incubate for 6 days; Step 2: add tritiated thymidine to each well, incubate 4 hours; Step 3: measure radioactive counts.

receive mitogen (phytohemagglutinin M) and the remaining 3 receive uninfected control antigen. The plates are incubated humidified in 5% CO_2 at 37° C for 6 days. (ii) Each well then receives 10 ul quantities containing 0.1μCi (^{3}H) thymidine in tissue culture medium and the plates are incubated for 4 hours at 37° C. (iii) The radioactive counts in each cup are measured in a liquid scintillation counter.

Results of the lymphocyte transformation assay are expressed as the stimulation induces. These represent the quotient of the mean counts per minute in the virus-treated or mitogen-treated cultures and the mean counts in the control preparations thus:

$$\text{stimulation index} = \frac{\text{cpm virus-treated cultures}}{\text{cpm control cultures}}$$

LYMPHOCYTE TOXICITY

This test depends upon the enhanced release of radio-labeled chromium ^{51}Cr from tissue culture cells (target cells) infected persistently with a virus which develop cytopathic effects after incubation with lymphocytes from patients infected with the same virus serotype. Measurement of cell-mediated immunity (CMI) to measles virus will be used as an example.[4] (Figure 3-16).

Target cells such as continuous diploid human fibroblasts (WI-38) persistently infected with measles virus are washed then dispersed in tissue culture

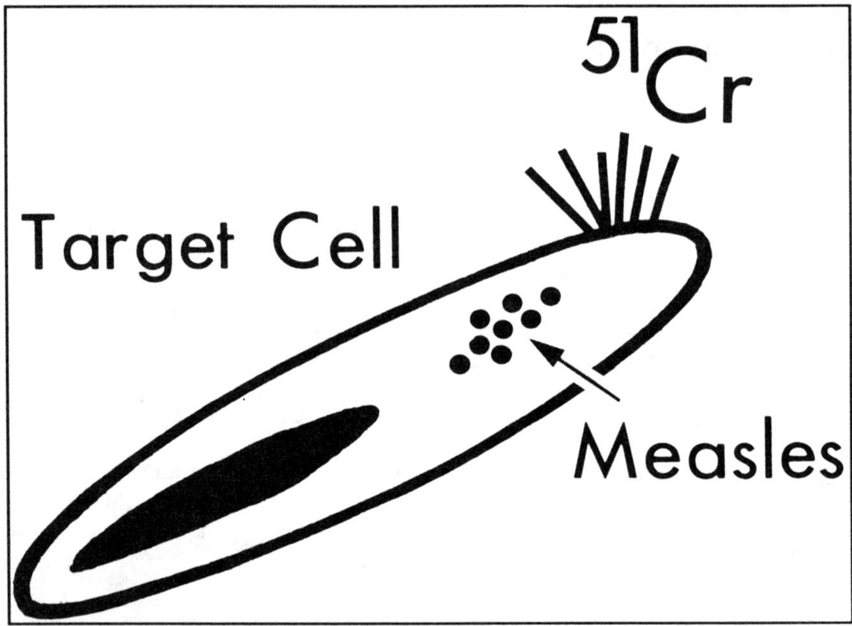

Figure 3-16: Principle of lymphocyte toxicity assay of cell-mediated immunity.

medium containing 10% fetal calf serum to a concentration of 10^7 cells/ml. Cells are incubated with 0.15m Ci ^{51}Cr (sodium chromate) for 30 minutes at 37° C in 5% CO_2 with periodic agitation. The reaction is stopped by the addition of 50 ml medium at 4° C, labeled cells are washed twice with this medium, then diluted to give 5×10^4 cells/ml cold medium which is dispensed in 0.1 ml aliquots to each of 6 wells of a 96-well tissue culture microplate. Uninfected tissue culture cells labeled similarly are placed in another 6 wells as controls (Figure 3-17).

Lymphocyte suspensions from patient's are prepared by centrifugation through Ficoll-Hypaque gradients and diluted to contain 5×10^6 cells/ml maintenance medium. Aliquots of 0.1ml are added to each of 3 wells containing infected labeled target cells and uninfected labeled controls. The lymphocyte: target cell ratio is 100:1. The mixtures are incubated in 5% CO_2 at 37° C for 18 hours, then supernatants are aspirated and radioactive counts are made on them.

The results are expressed as the specific immune release, and they are calculated by subtracting the percentage ^{51}Cr release in the control target cells from the infected target cells thus:

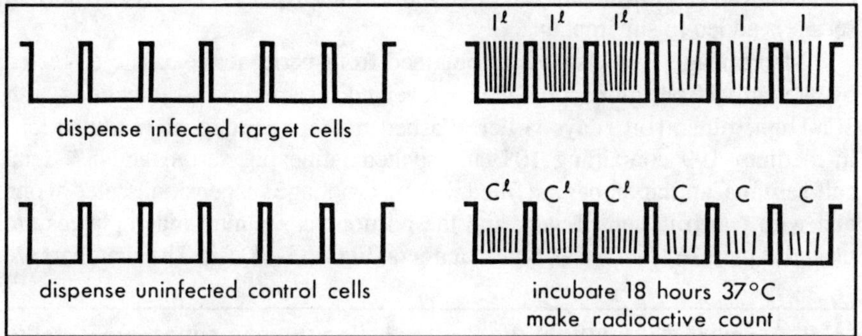

Figure 3-17: Diagrammatic representation of lymphocyte toxicity test. Step 1: incubate persistently virus infected and uninfected control tissue cultures with radio-labeled sodium chromate for 30 min. at 37° C, then add chilled medium at 4° C. Dispense infected and uninfected cultures into each of 6 cups; Step 2: add lymphocyte suspensions from patients to 3 infected cultures and 3 uninfected cultures, incubate for 18 hours at 37° C; Step 3: remove supernatants and make radioactive counts on them.

$$\frac{I^1 - I}{Ti - \text{zero time i}} - \frac{C^1 - C}{Tc - \text{zero time C}} \quad x \quad 100$$

I^1	counts in infected target cells + lymphocytes.	C^1	counts in control target cells + lymphocytes.
I	counts in infected target cells alone.	C	counts in control target cells.
Ti	Total amount of radioactivity in infected cells.	Tc	total amount of radioactivity in control cells.
zero time I	release at zero time infected cells	zero time C	release at zero time control cells

MACROPHAGE MIGRATION INHIBITORY FACTOR

This test depends upon the inhibition of macrophage migration out of a capillary tube containing a suspension of macrophage and T lymphocytes from an immunized subject, when exposed to the immunizing antigen.

Lymphocyte suspensions containing 5×10^6 cells/ml suspended in medium 199 containing 10% antibody-positive serum are obtained from venous blood of patients after centrifugation through a Ficoll-Hypaque gradient.[11] Tubes containing leukocytes are incubated for 3 days at 37° C in 5% CO_2 with appropriate dilutions of virus antigens, for example *Herpesvirus hominis type 1*.[17] (i) Supernatant fluids are removed daily and replaced by fresh medium 199, holding each daily collection at 4° C until all fluids from the same antigen series are pooled and stored at –20° C until tested. For testing, 15% inactivated normal serum is added to supernatants.

Macrophage suspensions are obtained from peritoneal exudate collected by aspiration from guineapigs which received intraperitoneal injections with 30ml light mineral oil 3 days earlier. Washed macrophage deposit is diluted 1:10 in medium 199 containing 10% inactivated guineapig serum and 5% fetal calf serum. Capillary tubes are filled with macrophage suspension, sealed at one end with paraffin, centrifuged, and the portions containing macrophages are placed in pairs in Mackaness-type chambers (Figure 3-18) (ii). The chambers are

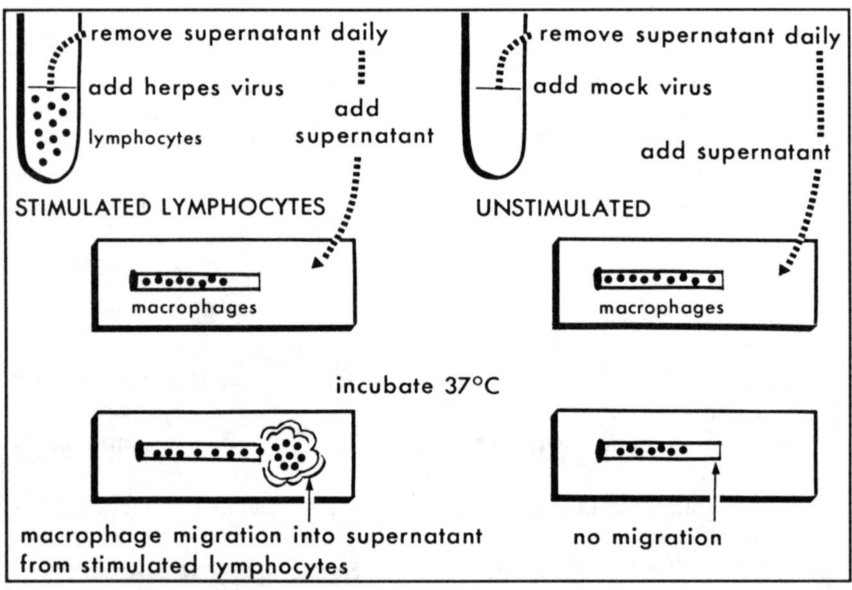

Figure 3-18: Diagrammatic representation of macrophage migration inhibitory factor test. Step 1: incubate lymphocyte cultures with herpesvirus, remove supernatants daily; Step 2: fill capillary tubes with guineapig peritoneal macrophage suspensions and place on glass surfaces in Mackaness-type chambers; Step 3: add supernatant from lymphocyte cultures, incubate 24 hours, then measure extent of migration of macrophages.

filled with 0.8ml supernatant from the leukocyte preparations which were incubated with the virus, and incubated at 37° C for 24 hours. The area of migration of macrophages away from the capillaries is measured by planimetry (iii). Controls comprise antigen in tissue culture medium and tissue culture medium alone.

The migration index is calculated thus:

$$\frac{\text{Macrophage migration in antigen} - \text{stimulated supernatant}}{\text{Macrophage migration in antigen} - \text{reconstituted medium}} \times 100$$

An index of less than 80% is considered significant.

REFERENCES

[1] Boyum A: Isolation of mononuclear cells and granulocytes from human blood. Scandinavian Journal of Clinical Laboratory Investigation *21* (Supplement) 97, 77, 1968.

[2] Engvall E, Perlman P: ELISA III. Quantification of specific antibodies by enzyme-labeled anti-immunoglobulin in antigen coated tubes. J. Immunol. 109:129, 1972.

[3] Joklik WK, ed: Principles of Animal Virology, Appleton-Century-Crofts, New York, 1980, p. 76.

[4] Labowskie RJ, Edelman R, Rustigan R, Bellanti JA: Studies of cell-mediated immunity to measles virus by in vitro lymphocyte-mediated cytotoxicity. J. Infect. Dis. 129:233, 1974.

[5] Ling C-M, Overby LR: Prevalence of hepatitis B virus antigen as revealed by direct radioimmune assay with ^{125}I antibody. J. Immunol. 109:834, 1972.

[6] Lwoff A, Dulbecco R, Vogt M, Lwoff M: Kinetics of the release of poliomyelitis virus from single cells. Virology 1:128, 1955.

[7] McLean DM: Immunological Investigation of Human Virus Diseases. Vol. 5, Practical Methods in Clinical Immunology, Series editor: RC Nairn, Churchill Livingstone, Edinburgh, 1982, p. 3.

[8] Pass RE, Stagno S, Britt WJ, Alford CA: Specific cell-mediated immunity and the natural history of congenital infection with cytomegalovirus. J. Infect. Dis. 148:953, 1983.

[9] Reed LJ, Muench H: Simple method of estimating fifty percent endpoints. Am. J. Hyg. 27:493, 1938.

[10] Reynolds DW, Dean PH, Pass RF, Alford CA: Specific cell-mediated immunity in children with congenital and neonatal cytomegalovirus infection and their mothers. J. Infect. Dis. 140:493, 1979.

[11] Rocklin RE: Production and assay of macrophage migration inhibitory factor. In Rose NH and Friedman H (eds) Manual of Clinical Immunology, 2nd ed. American Society for Microbiology, Washington, D.C. 1980, p. 246.

[12] Scott R, Kaul A, Scott M, Chiba Y, Ogra PL: Development of in vitro correlates of cell–mediated immunity of respiratory syncytial virus infection in humans. J. Infect. Dis. 137:810, 1978.

[13] Starr SE, Toplin MD, Friedman HM, Paucker K, Plotkin SA: Impaired cellular immunity to cytomegalovirus in congenitally infected children and their mothers. J. Infect. Dis. 140:500, 1979.

[14] Voller A, Bidwell DE, Bartlett A: Enzyme immunoassays in diagnostic medicine. Theory and practice. Bull WHO 53:55, 1976.

[15]Voller A, Bidwell DE, Bartlett A: Enzyme-linked immunosorbent assay. Chapter 46 in Manual of Clinical Immunology, ed. NR Rose and H Friedman, American Society for Microbiology, 2nd ed., 1980, p. 359.

[16]Walsh JH, Yalow R, Berson SA: Detection of Australia antigen and antibody by means of radioimmunoassay techniques. J. Infect. Dis. 130:383, 1970.

[17]Wilton JMA, Ivanyi L, Lehrer T: Cell-mediated immunity in Herpesvirus hominis infections. Brit. Med. J. 1:723, 1972.

CHAPTER 4

PATHOGENESIS OF VIRAL INFECTIONS

Pathogenesis concerns the multiplication and movement of virus throughout the body. Studies of pathogenesis include; (i) the entry of viruses; (ii) routes of their transfer within the body to target organs in which they multiply and induce disease; (iii) their means of egress from the body where they are transmitted to other susceptible hosts. Symptoms arise after three typical patterns of interaction between viruses and their human hosts.

PATTERNS OF VIRUS-HOST INTERACTION

SURFACE INFECTION

Influenza provides a typical example of a surface viral infection. Virus enters the body by inhalation of virus-laden droplet nuclei. These traverse the vocal cords and lodge on ciliated columnar epithelial cells of bronchioles or respiratory bronchioles (Figure 4-1). After multiplication within these epithelial cells, virus is expelled into the bronchiolar lumen, where adjacent cells become infected by contact. Cellular damage evokes an acute catarrhal inflammation of the bronchioles with dilatation of bronchiolar capillaries and resultant outpouring of fluid, accompanied by excessive production of mucus by goblet cells plus slowing or cessation of ciliary movements. The latter effect permits accumulation of serous exudate and mucus within the bronchioles, thus restricting the flow of air to the pulmonary alveoli; this occasionally results in atelectasis or bronchopneumonic consolidation. Some exudate reaches the bifurcation of the trachea and stimulates the cough reflex, thus causing dissemination of virus-laden droplet nuclei into the air within a radius of about 2 meters surrounding the patient.

The incubation period is 2 days or less, and virus is excreted via the nasopharynx for 2 to 4 days after onset of illness. Antibodies to the ribonucleoprotein (soluble or S-antigen) first appear in the serum about 1 week after onset, and antibodies to the viral envelope (V), hemagglutinin (H) and neuraminidase (N), appear within 2 to 3 weeks after onset. Anti-S antibodies persist about 3 to 6 months, but antibodies to other viral components may persist at reduced titers for several years.

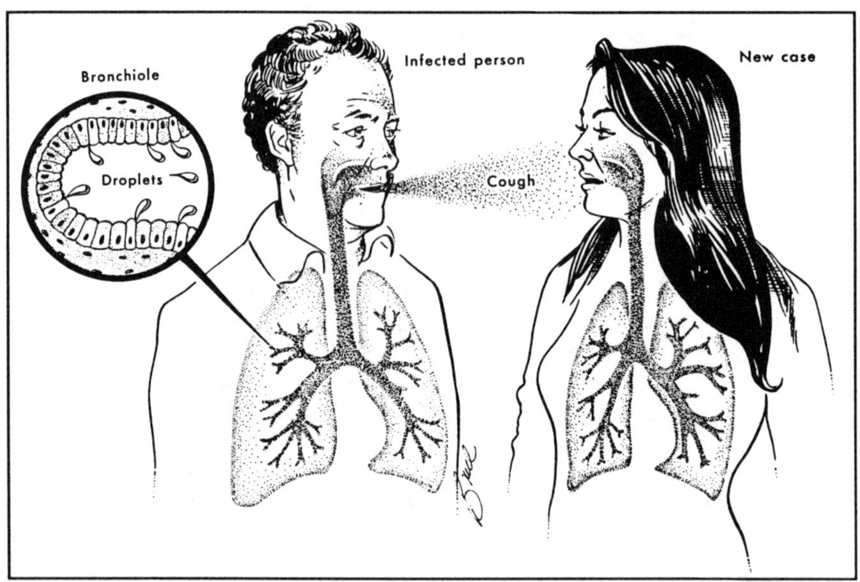

Figure 4-1: Pathogenesis of influenza (surface infection of respiratory tract).

SURFACE AND BLOOD INFECTION

Poliomyelitis provides an important example of a surface infection followed by dissemination by the blood stream. Virus enters the body by ingestion of virus-laden food or water. Some virus particles may lodge and replicate in the pharyngeal mucosa, especially over the tonsils and subsequently it may enter the blood stream. Most of the ingested virus traverses the stomach and lodges on the columnar epithelial cells of the jejunum. Virus replicates in mucosal cells and in the submucosal collections of lymphoid tissue (Peyer's patches). Newly formed virus is released in substantial quantities into the intestinal lumen, and eventually it is discharged into the environment through the feces (Figure 4-2). After replication in the jejunal mucosa, some virus may enter the blood stream by which it is conveyed throughout the body, to reach susceptible target organs such as the central nervous system. Highly susceptible areas within the central system include particularly the motor neurones of the anterior horn of the spinal cord grey matter, plus some foci of neurones in the base of the brain and the cerebral cortex. Destruction of neurones following viral replication within them induces flaccid paralysis of skeletal muscles supplied by their respective nerve axons. Concomitantly virus replicates in the meninges inducing the outpouring of lymphocytes, and the patient exhibits the clinical features of aseptic meningitis including headache and neck stiffness.

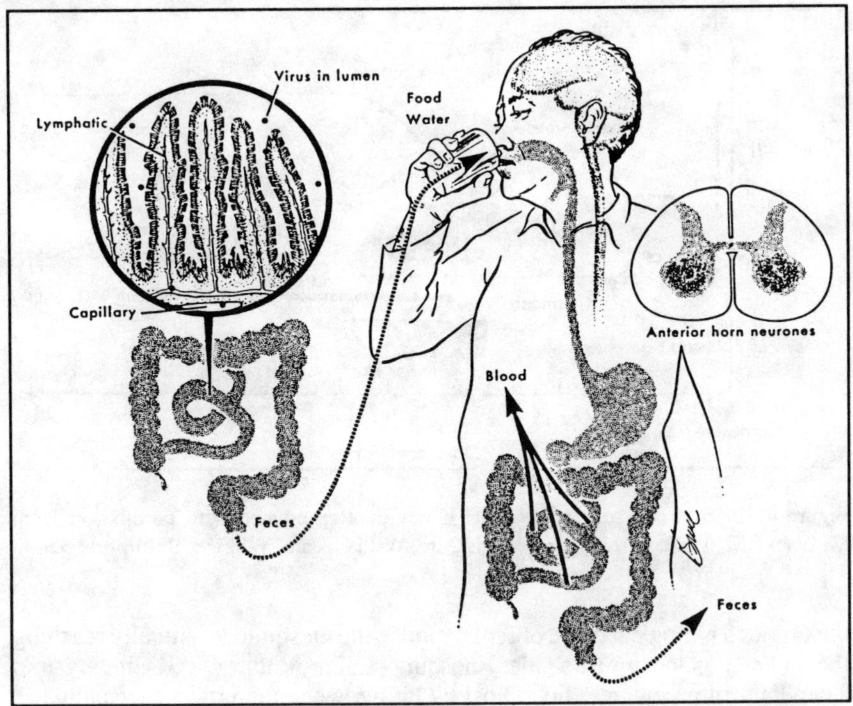

Figure 4-2: Pathogenesis of poliomyelitis (surface infection with spread by blood to target organ).

The incubation period of poliomyelitis is 4 to 8 days. Virus is excreted in the pharyngeal secretions for about one week or less after onset of illness and in the feces for 2 weeks or more after onset. Onset of illness is defined as the moment the patient experiences major symptoms of severe headache and neck stiffness (meningitis), but paralysis characteristically begins one or more days after meningitis. Neutralizing antibodies first appear within one week after onset (often after 2 to 4 days), peak titers are attained about one month after onset, and they persist indefinitely (Figure 4-3).

BLOOD INFECTION

Arbovirus encephalitis caused by western equine encephalomyelitis (WEE) virus exemplifies a blood infection. Typically the virus is maintained in a natural cycle between birds (vertebrate reservoirs) and culicine mosquitoes (arthropod vectors). After the mosquito has fed on a viremic bird, the virus

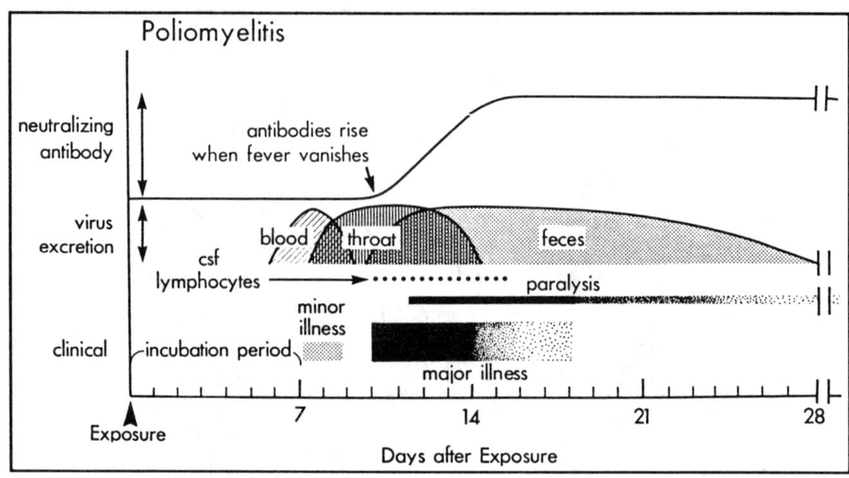

Figure 4-3: Time course of poliovirus infection. Reproduced with permission from McLean DM, 1980. Virology in Health Care, Williams and Wilkins, Baltimore, p. 68.

undergoes a biological cycle of replication in the mosquito, eventually reaching the salivary glands. Virus-laden mosquito saliva is introduced directly into a capillary of a new vertebrate host by biting, when the proboscis cannulates a capillary. Thus virus enters the blood stream directly and it multiplies extensively in reticulo-endothelial cells, so that a high titer of viremia (virus in blood) develops rapidly (Figure 4-4). Virus is conveyed to target organs such as the meninges and cortical neurones of the brain. Viral replication induces extensive inflammation of meninges (meningitis) and damage to cortical neurones (encephalitis) which may terminate fatally.

The incubation period is 4 to 10 days. Virus detected in the blood 2–4 days before to 2–4 days after onset of meningoencephalitis. Antibodies are detected by neutralization and hemagglutination inhibition tests as soon as fever abates, within one week after onset, and they persist in sera indefinitely. Complement fixation antibodies first appear 2 to 3 weeks after onset and persist no longer than 1 to 3 years (Figure 4-5).

ENTRY AND EGRESS OF VIRUS

ENTRY INTO BODY

Portals of entry by which viruses gain access to new human hosts vary according to the particular virus group and the mode of transmission in nature

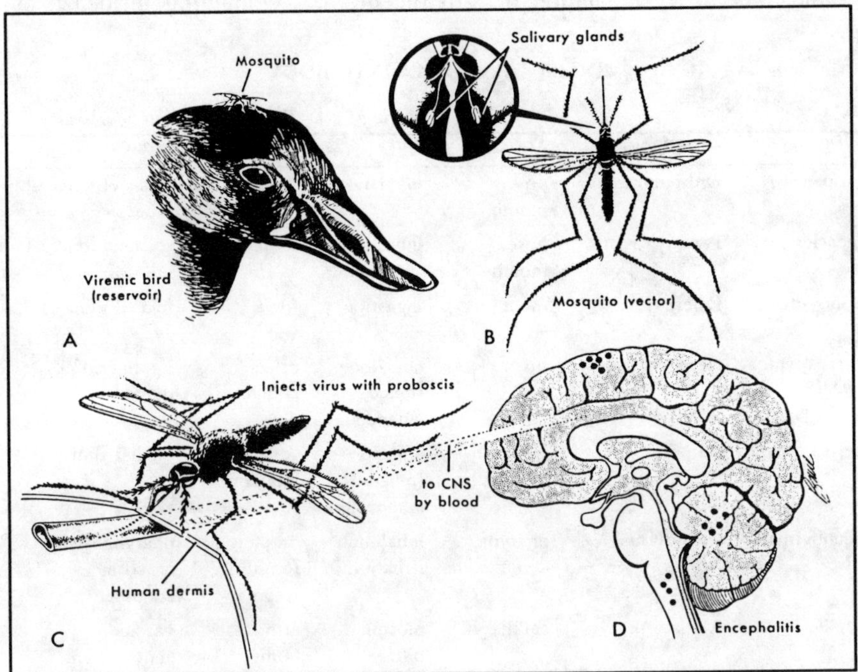

Figure 4-4: Pathogenesis of arbovirus infection (vector-borne blood infection with localization in target organ).

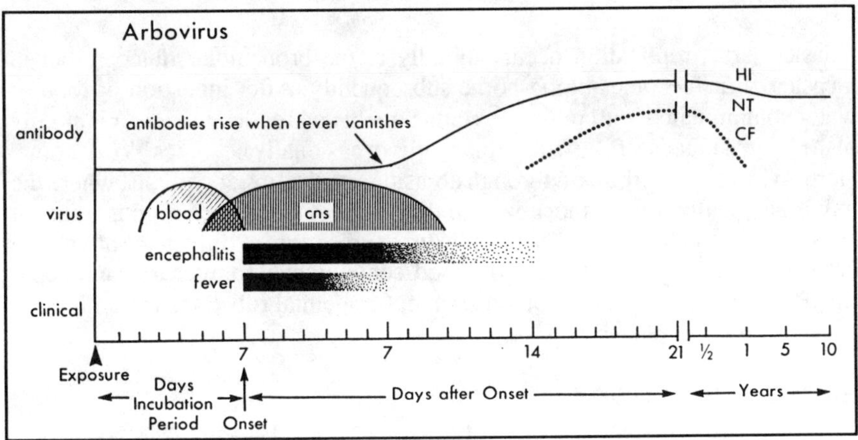

Figure 4-5: Time course of arbovirus infection. Reproduced with permission from McLean DM, 1980. Virology in Health Care, Williams and Wilkins, Baltimore, p. 167.

(Table 4-1). After inhalation of airborne droplets containing influenza or

TABLE 4-1
ENTRY OF VIRUSES INTO BODY

Virus	Group	Portal	Mode of entry	Trans-mission	Site of primary replication
influenza A	Orthomyxovirus	nose, mouth	inhalation	droplets	tracheobronchial mucosa
measles	Paramyxovirus	nose, mouth	inhalation	droplets	tracheobronchial mucosa
poliovirus	Enterovirus	mouth	ingestion	food, water	jejunal mucosa
herpes type 1	Herpesvirus	lip	abrasion (muco-cutaneous)	direct contact	lip, buccal mucosa
herpes type 2	Herpesvirus	genital introtus	abrasion (muco-cutaneous)	sexual intercourse	genital skin
adenovirus	Adenovirus	pharynx conjunctiva	inhalation irritation	droplets fomites, water	pharyngeal-mucosa conjunctiva
WEE	Alphavirus	capillary	mosquito bite	arthropod-borne	vascular endothelium
hepatitis B	Hepadnavirus	Blood vessel	injection	blood	liver cells
rubella (congenital)	Togavirus	placenta	growing through	transpla-cental	developing fetal organs

measles virus, replication occurs initially in the bronchiolar mucosa, but in measles, virus becomes blood-borne subsequently. After ingestion of food or water contaminated with poliovirus, attachment and replication occurs initially in the jejunal mucosa, following which virus occasionally becomes blood-borne. Herpesviruses enter the skin through abrasions on the lips or genitals, where the infection usually remains localized to the portal of entry. Arthropods transmit alphaviruses such as WEE virus by direct injection of infected saliva into capillaries during bites; syringes or blood-contaminated fomites transmit hepatitis B virus directly into the blood stream. Congenital rubella is transmitted to offspring by transplacental passage.

EGRESS FROM BODY

Viruses are expelled into the environment by: (i) airborne droplets during speaking, splitting, coughing, sneezing; (ii) feces which may contaminate (a) the hands of the patient which in turn contaminate food or fomites, or (b) drinking water through improper sewage disposal; (iii) direct contact or discharges from weeping vesicles may contaminate fomites or abraded skin or mucous membranes of other subjects; (iv) imbibing of viremic blood by biting arthropods (mosquitoes, ticks, sandflies); (v) contamination by blood of abraded skin or actual injection of virus-laden blood or its products (Table 4-2).

TABLE 4-2
EGRESS OF VIRUSES FROM THE BODY

Virus	Group	Site of egress	Mode of egress	Dissemination
influenza A	Orthomyxovirus	pharynx	droplets	air
measles	Paramyxovirus	pharynx	droplets	air
poliovirus	Enterovirus	anus	feces	water, food
herpes type 1	Herpesvirus	lip vesicle	surface exudate	direct contact, fomites
herpes type 2	Herpesvirus	genital vesicle	surface exudate	sexual intercourse
adenovirus	Adenovirus	pharynx, eye	droplets, tears	air, water, fomites
WEE	Alphavirus	capillary	mosquito bite	arthropod-borne
hepatitis B	Hepadnavirus	blood vessel	blood	blood contamination, injection
rubella (congenital)	Togavirus	pharynx (infant) placenta	droplets, blood	air; maternal to fetal circulation

METHODS OF SPREAD OF VIRUSES

Virus infections are spread from an infected host to a new susceptible host by contact or blood. However there are several important mechanisms by which each category of infection is transmitted. Contact infections include those transmitted by: (i) direct physical contact of skin or mucous membranes; (ii) contamination of fomites by virus-laden excretions; (iii) ingestion of food or water; (iv) airborne droplets. Blood infections include those transmitted by: (v) intravenous infusion of blood or its fractions; (vi) contamination of equipment such as dental instruments or syringes by blood; (vii) transplacental transfer; (viii) bites by arthropods (Table 4-3).

DIRECT CONTACT: ORAL. Herpesvirus hominis-1 induces vesicular lesions involving especially the lips and face, but vesicles may also appear over the buccal mucosa and the tongue. Vesicles burst within a day or more after their first

TABLE 4-3
MECHANISM OF TRANSMISSION OF SELECTED VIRUS INFECTIONS

Category	Mechanism	Example of virus	
Contact	direct contact:	abraded surfaces	
		oral	Herpesvirus hominis-1
		genital	Herpesvirus hominis-2
	fomites:	contamination	
		salivary	Herpesvirus hominis-1
		fecal	Rotavirus
		urinary	Lassa
	fecal-oral:	inbibing	Poliovirus
		water	Hepatitis A
		food	
	airborne droplets:	inhalation	Influenza
			Parainfluenza-1
blood	intravenous infusion	injection	Hepatitis B
	contamination of equipment	injection	Hepatitis B
			Ebola
	transplacental transfer	congenital	Rubella
	arthropods: biological	bite	WEE, SSH
	- ticks,	bite	POW
	- sandflies	bite	Sandfly fever

appearance, spreading virus over the facial skin and into the saliva during the next 2 to 4 days. Scabs may cover burst vesicles, but virus shedding may persist until epithelium has covered the raw surfaces, thereby completing the healing process about one week later. Direct contact with another person whose lips or face have minute abrasions, for example during the kissing of a baby by an infected mother or guardian, usually results in transmission of herpesvirus to the second person who will develop vesicles 2 to 3 days subsequently, at the site of viral implantation.

In immunocompromised subjects, such as leukemic children who develop herpesvirus infections relatively frequently, virus excretion from herpetic vesicles may persist for several weeks.

The above example illustrates two important attributes of the time course of virus infections: (i) *incubation period* which is the time elapsed between the implantation of an infectious dose of herpesvirus at the time of kissing the baby and the onset of vesicles over the baby's lips and face (2 to 3 days); (ii) *duration of infectivity* which is the number of days (or weeks) during which the patient excretes virus into the environment (2 to 4 days for most who are otherwise healthy).

DIRECT CONTACT: GENITAL. Painful pinpoint vesicles develop around the vaginal introitus or perineum of females with genital herpes due usually to Herpesvirus hominis-2. Within 2 to 3 days after sexual intercourse, similar vesicles may appear on the penile shaft of the male consort. Virus is thus transmitted venerally by direct contact between the skin of the genital areas of the two partners.

FOMITES: SALIVARY. Herpesvirus hominis-1 in saliva of babies with oral or facial herpetic eruptions may contaminate any toy or other object which is placed in the mouth. In a nursery, other babies promptly insert these contaminated objects into their own mouths. Since minute abrasions of the lips or tongue occur frequently, virus on the contaminated object readily penetrates the epithelium of the recipient's lips, and initiates an infection.

FOMITES: FECAL. Rotavirus is excreted in feces of children with acute gastroenteritis for 2 to 7 days after onset of loose watery greenish-yellow stools, thus contaminating the child's diapers and bed linen. Virus transmission to other children may occur either (a) if another child is placed on the contaminated linen, portions of which are promptly placed in the child's mouth; or (b) if an attendant contaminates food delivered to another child by hands which were contaminated fecally by soiled linen from the first child, or if the attendant merely touches the second child's hands which are then placed in the mouth.

FOMITES: URINARY. Arenaviruses of tropical countries, such as Lassa virus in Nigeria, are excreted in the urine for several days or weeks by rodents which are their natural vertebrate reservoirs. Contact of objects contaminated by rodent urine with abraded skin may transmit infection.

FECAL-ORAL ROUTE. After infection with poliovirus-1, virus is excreted in feces for about 2 to 4 weeks, but other enteroviruses such as echovirus-9 are usually excreted for less than 2 weeks. Feces may gain access to drinking water supplies through insanitary sewage disposal practices. Ingestion of water which is not chlorinated adequately may deliver a sufficient dose of virus to infect the recipient. Furthermore, vegetables which are irrigated with sewage may become contaminated with an infectious dose of poliovirus when they are consumed raw. Also, the feet of flies may become contaminated with feces containing poliovirus. When the flies alight on foodstuffs such as ice cream which are consumed without additional preparation, virus may be transferred to these foods.

Hepatitis A virus is excreted in feces from 7 to 14 days before onset of jaundice to about 7 days after onset, thus providing ample opportunity for virus dissemination into the environment long before onset of malaise. Several outbreaks of hepatitis A disease have been attributed to consumption of food or water contaminated fecally by virus excreted before onset of jaundice or by asymptomatic carriers.

AIRBORNE DROPLETS. Influenza and parainfluenza viruses proliferate in the epithelium of the tracheobronchial tree inducing catarrhal inflammation and excretion of virus into mucous secretions which are produced copiously. Virus infection also slows the beat of cilia within the respiratory epithelium, thus promoting accumulation of secretions. Eventually the excess secretions reach the carina at the bifurcation of the trachea, thus stimulating the cough reflex. Virus-laden mucous droplets, 2 to 20/µ diameter are therefore expelled into the atmosphere as far as 2 meters from the virus excretes. Virus-laden droplets are inhaled by persons closer than 2 meters. Particles with diameters 5µ or less pass directly through the larynx and trachea to lodge on epithelium of the bronchioles, thus initiating infection of the recipient. Employing air sampling devices which measure particle diameters, it has been found that the majority of parainfluenza-1 virus excreted by croupy children is contained within mucous particles 3 to 10µ diameter.

BLOOD: INTRAVENOUS INFUSION. Hepatitis B virus may circulate in the blood of chronic carriers over periods of months to years, sometimes in the absence of obvious liver disease. If their blood or plasma, or native plasma fractions such as antihemophilic globulin is administered inadvertently, by intravenous infusion or intramuscular injection, as in passive prophylaxis against measles using pooled human plasma, hepatitis may develop in susceptible recipients.

CONTAMINATION OF EQUIPMENT BY BLOOD. Due to high concentrations (often exceeding 10^6 virus particles per ml) of hepatitis B in peripheral blood of carriers, and on account of resistance to viricidal action of some disinfectants, hepatitis B virus infections have been transmitted by equipment contaminated with blood such as dental instruments, ear-piercing equipment and syringes plus needles treated with ineffective disinfectants such as alcohol or quaternary ammonium compounds. The only procedures to ensure complete inactivation of hepatitis B virus are either prolonged boiling or autoclaving. An epidemic of hemorrhagic fever due to EBOLA virus was transmitted in Zaire through indiscriminate use of syringes plus needles which were not decontaminated adequately between each patient.

BLOOD: TRANSPLACENTAL TRANSFER. Women who contract rubella during the first trimester of pregnancy circulate rubella virus in the blood a few days before the onset of rash. Virus readily enters the fetal circulation after crossing the placental vascular barrier. Virus may localize and multiply in one or more developing fetal organs according to the gestational age, with predilection for heart valves and/or cornea during the initial 4 to 6 weeks, or the cochlea of the ear between 8 and 12 weeks. Tissue damage may occur in these organs, causing the appearance of malformations characteristic of the congenital rubella syndrome at the time of birth of the child.

ARTHROPOD TRANSMISSION. Certain virus infections are transmitted in nature by bites of arthropods, including culicine mosquitoes, ixodid ticks and phlebotomine sandflies. The World Health Organization (1967) defined arboviruses (ARthropod-BORNE animal viruses) as ..."viruses transmitted in nature principally, or to an important extent, through biological transmission between susceptible vertebrate hosts by hematophagous[*] arthropods[+++]; they multiply and produce viremia[+] in the vertebrates, multiply in the tissues of arthropods, and are passed on to new vertebrates by the bites of arthropods after a period of extrinsic incubation[++]. Currently (1989) more than 500 virus serotypes within 5 virus families are definitely or probably transmitted by arthropods. North American examples of mosquito-borne arboviruses include western equine encephalomyelitis (WEE) with *Cultex tarsalis* mosquitoes as principal vectors and various water birds as reservoirs, plus snowshoe hare (SSH) virus (California serogroup) with *Aedes communis* mosquitoes as important vectors and snowshoe hares plus ground squirrels as reservoirs. Powassan (POW) virus is transmitted in nature by *Ixodes cookei* ticks and tree squirrels are important reservoirs. Sandfly fever is a febrile disease affecting human residents of the Mediterranean littoral, with *Phlebotomus papatasi* (sandflies) as vectors and humans as the sole vertebrate reservoir.

---

[*]Hematophagous: Blood-feeding
[+]Viremia: virus circulating in the blood
[++]Extrinsic incubation period: duration between feeding on infective blood and ability to transmit virus by biting a new host.
[+++]Modified by WHO (1985) to include the phrase "or through transovarian and possibly veneral transmission in arthropods."

CHAPTER 5

IMMUNITY TO VIRAL INFECTIONS

Immunity denotes absence of detectable illness following exposure to a virus which induced a clinically manifested or an inapparent infection in a subject after an earlier infection by the same virus. Lifelong immunity characteristically follows symptomatic infections by viruses such as measles, mumps and rubella, all of which exhibit viremia during their incubation periods. Transient immunity for a few months only is characteristic of rhinovirus infections which induce common colds; these viruses involve epithelial surfaces exclusively.

ROLE OF B CELLS AND T CELLS

In most virus infections, immunity is mediated principally through the production of humoral antibodies which are elaborated by antigenic (viral) stimulation of B cells. These B lymphocytes are derived from bone marrow stem cells through a process of antigen-independent maturation, part of which takes place in the bone marrow.[1] B cells migrate to and localize principally in the superficial cortex of lymph nodes, where there are closely packed collections of lymphocytes which form follicles. These follicles develop germinal centers containing large clear proliferating lymphocytes following antigenic stimulation. Viral antigens appear to be taken up by macrophages which are trapped in sinusoids of lymph nodes. Virus-laden macrophages stimulate B cells to proliferate and differentiate principally into plasma cells which secrete antibodies, but some progeny cells acquire immunological memory. Upon subsequent exposure to the same virus serotype, antibodies are produced rapidly (secondary or anamnestic response). These responses usually require cooperative interactions with T cells which abound in the deep cortex of lymph nodes.

Delayed immunological responses may occur after some virus infections. For example, natural infection with measles virus 1 to 5 years after injection of killed measles vaccine has induced "atypical measles" comprising broncho-pneumonia and petechiae in addition to rash and fever.[4] These complications arise from cellular reactions which are mediated principally through T cells.

These T lymphocytes are derived from stem cells within the thymus, and they localize in the deep cortex of lymph nodes and in the spleen.[1] Biological activities of T cells include: (i) regulatory action on B cells and other T cells, either to promote (helper T4 cells) or suppress (suppressor T8 cells) their immunological function; (ii) cellular immunity reactions through elaboration of lymphokines which affect the inflammatory response or the behavior of macrophages; (iii) transplantation immunity reactions such as allograft rejection and graft-versus-host reactions; (iv) cytotoxic responses (killer T cells) especially in immune responses against tumors.

Differentiation between B cells and T cells in the laboratory is shown by proliferation of B cells after addition of bacterial lipopolysaccharide, and stimulation of T cells by addition of phytohemagglutinin or concanavalin A. Also incubation of sheep erythrocytes with T cells permits non-immunological binding of erythrocytes to the T cell surface where they appear as rosettes.

ANTIBODIES

Antibodies are protein molecules which combine specifically with antigens.[1] Antigens are chemical substances capable of inducing a specific immune response. Usually antigens stimulate both the production of antibodies (humoral immunity) and cellular types of immune response. Antigens are usually proteins or polysaccharides with chemical structures different from host constituents. They are recognized as foreign to the host by B and T cells which then respond by production of antibody (B cells) or increased macrophage activity and inflammatory reactions (T cells). In some instances a simple compound (hapten) with a low molecular weight which is attached to a protein of high molecular weight (carrier) may stimulate production of antibodies specifically to: (i) the hapten; (ii) the carrier protein; (iii) occasionally to the hapten plus carrier protein. Viruses behave as antigens upon entry into the human body.

Antibodies are proteins, collectively termed immunoglobulins (Ig), which migrate electrophoretically with the gamma-globulin fraction of human serum proteins. All immunoglobulins contain four polypeptide chains, two large (heavy chain, H) and two small (light chain, L). Disulfide bonds cross-link the two H chains and also bind the L chains to the H chains, as in the diagram. Treatment with the enzyme papain breaks the H chains and liberates 2 Fab fragments plus one Fc fragment. Treatment with pepsin liberates one bivalent Fab' fragment and one Fc fragment; further treatment of the Fab' component with 2-mercaptoethanol breaks the disulfide bonds and liberates 2 Fab fragments.

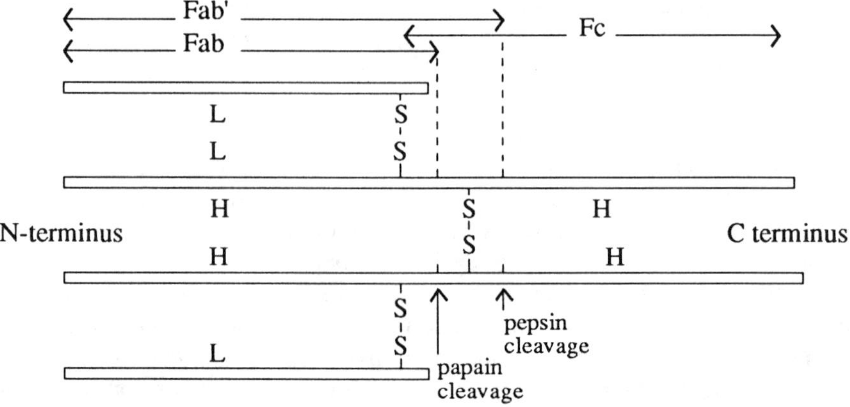

Human immunoglobulins occur in five classes according to the structures of their respective heavy chains IgG, IgA, IgM, IgD, IgE. The heavy chains are termed respectively, gamma, alpha, mu, delta, epsilon. In human serum, about 65% of IgG molecules contain two κ (kappa) light chains and 35% contain two lambda light chains.

Molecules of IgG have a molecular weight of about 150,000 and a sedimentation coefficient of 7 S. Molecules of IgM have a molecular weight of about 900,000, they consist of 5 identical subunits each with molecular weights of about 180,000, together with an additional joining (J) chain. Molecules of secretory IgA, with molecular weight about 71,000 are found mainly in secretions such as saliva, tears, tracheobronchial secretions, etc. IgD is found mainly as a constituent of multiple myeloma protein and plays little part in antiviral immunological reactions. IgE is important in hypersensitivity and anaphylactic responses but plays little or no role in responses to virus infections.

TIME COURSE OF ANTIBODY PRODUCTION AND CELL-MEDIATED IMMUNITY

Three patterns of antibody responses may occur after exposure to viruses or their antigens (Figure 5-1). Although the ensuing description represents the average sequence of events common to all virus infections, actual times of initial appearance of antibodies after exposure to virus may vary by several days, according to the incubation period of the virus. Measles is a typical example of the general principles currently under discussion.

PRIMARY RESPONSE. After exposure to virus (day zero), virus

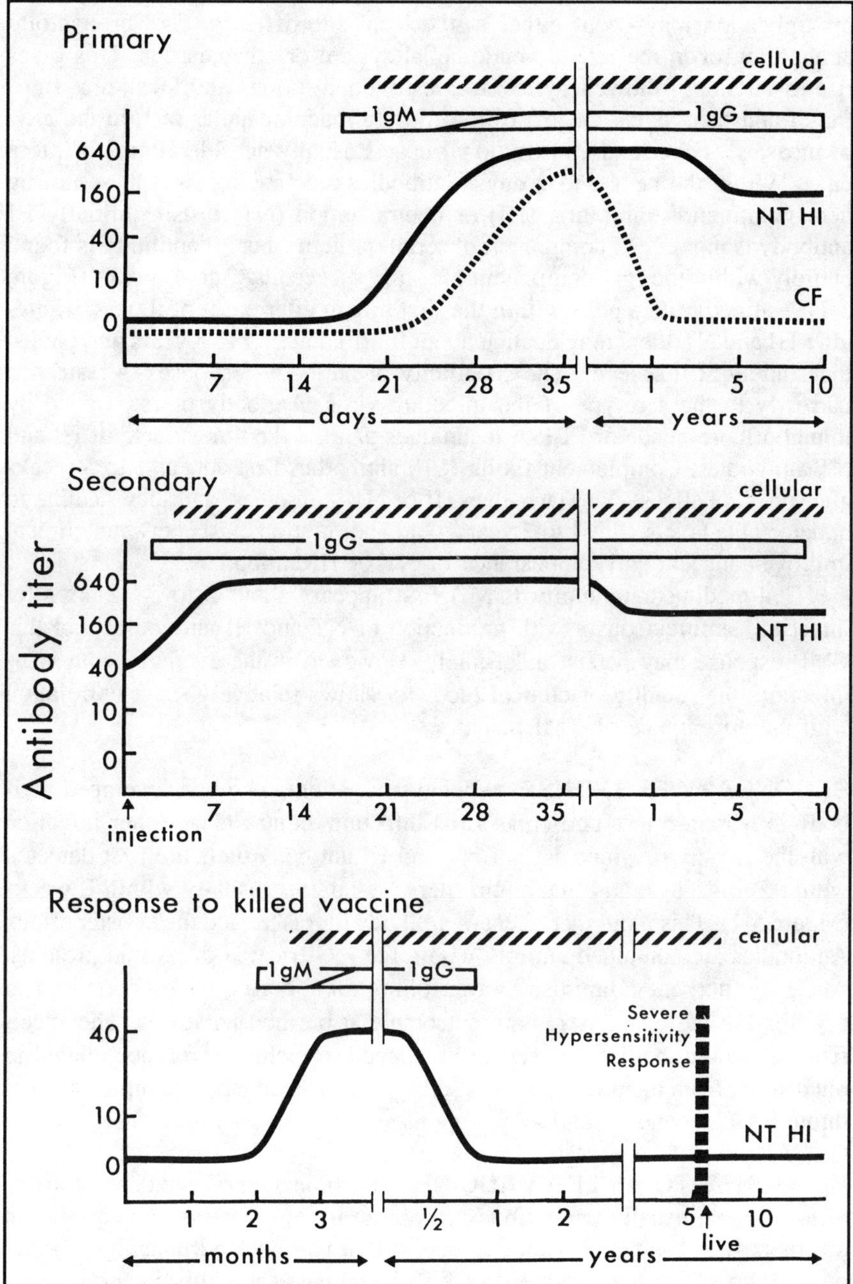

Figure 5-1: Patterns of antiviral antibody responses to: (i) primary (initial) and (ii) secondary (repeat) infection with live virus, (iii) after administration of killed viral vaccine.

multiplication may occur either at the local site of entry, e.g., bronchiolar epithelium, or in the reticulo-endothelial system or other tissues. This gives rise to viremia, followed by fever, constitutional upsets and localizing signs (nasal and pharyngeal catarrh followed by a maculopapular rash in the case of measles). Fever and constitutional upsets usually subside after 2 or more days. Within the next 1 to 2 days, antibodies are first detected in serum by hemagglutination inhibition (HI) or neutralization (NT) tests.[2,3] Initially HI antibody is in the IgM component of serum proteins, but HI antibody is found entirely within the IgG component after the succeeding 2 to 4 weeks (Figure 5-1). Antibody titers peak within the first month after onset of illness. Thereafter HI and NT titers may decline about fourfold after 1 to 5 years and persist indefinitely at that level. The specificity of antibody responses is restricted narrowly to the serotype of the infecting virus. Antibody titers assayed by immunofluorescence or ELISA techniques parallel the time course of HI and NT antibodies. Complement fixing (CF) antibodies first appear 1 to 3 weeks after onset of illness, i.e., later than HI or NT antibodies, and they decline to undetectable levels with 1 to 2 years. Good correlation exists between clinical improvement and early appearance of NT or HI antibodies.[2,3]

Cell-mediated immunity (CMI) first appears about 2 to 3 weeks after infection, simultaneously with production of NT and HI antibodies and this CMI response may persist indefinitely. However, in the average acute virus infection, the rapidity of clinical recovery shows relatively scant correlation with the appearance of CMI responses.

SECONDARY RESPONSE. Whenever a patient, who has developed antibody in response to a particular virus infection, contracts a further infection with the same virus, increases of NT and HI antibody titers are first detected within 2 to 4 days, and maximum titers are attained usually within 2 weeks (Figure 5-1). This rapid increment of antibody titer is termed the booster effect. Antibodies are contained entirely within the IgG fraction of plasma proteins. Antibody titers may diminish by fourfold or more during the succeeding 1 to 5 years, but they usually remain detectable at pre-booster levels. The specificity of the antibody responses is broadened to include serotypes related to but distinct from the infecting virus serotype. Cell-mediated immunity persists through the secondary antibody response.

RESPONSE TO KILLED VACCINE. After injection of one dose of killed virus vaccine, usually the antibody response, if any, remains undetectable in a subject who has never been exposed to that particular virus antigen. After one or two additional injections of killed vaccine at monthly intervals, antibodies are detected by NT or HI tests (Figure 5-1). Antibody titers peak between 3 and 6 months after the initial injection, and decline to undetectable levels within 1 to 2 years. Although antibodies appear in the IgM component of plasma proteins initially, rapidly thereafter they are found only in the IgG component.

Cell-mediated immunity is usually detected within 3 months after the first injection of vaccine and this state may persist indefinitely. For most viruses, e.g., influenza, lack of any adverse clinical response following subsequent exposure to natural infection with the same or related serotype suggests that CMI activity is not expressed clinically. In the case of measles virus however, upon exposure to live virus up to 5 years after initial administration of killed vaccine, cell-mediated immunological responses may be manifested clinically as severe hypersensitivity states such as petechiae and extensive bronchopneumonia.[4] In this example, it appears that the absence of NT antibody permitted unrestricted replication of measles virus which triggered a massive immunological response of T cells which were already primed to recognize measles virus antigen.

REFERENCES

[1]Benacerraf B, Unanue ER: Textbook of Immunology. Williams and Wilkins, Baltimore, 1979.

[2]McLean DM, Best JM, Smith PA, Larke RPB, McNaughton GA: Viral infections of Toronto children during 1965: II. Measles encephalitis and other complications. Can Med Ass J 94:905, 1966.

[3]McLean DM, Larke RPB, Cobb C, Griffis ED, Hackett SMR: Mumps and enteroviral meningitis in Toronto, 1966. Can Med Ass J 96:1355, 1967.

[4]McLean DM, Kettyls GDM, Hingston J, Moore PS, Paris RP, Rigg JM: Atypical measles following immunization with killed measles vaccine. Can Med Ass J 103:743, 1970.

CHAPTER 6

PREVENTION AND TREATMENT

Rational approach both to prevention of virus infections in individuals and communities, and to the treatment of persons with virus-induced illnesses, depends upon (a) prompt and accurate clinical recognition of the causative virus, assisted by same-day laboratory diagnosis[20]; (b) rapid institution of appropriate preventive measures, including isolation of new clinical cases after effective epidemic surveillance and case finding; (c) routine vaccination of the general population against common communicable diseases; plus crash programs of vaccination in the face of threatened or actual epidemics; and (d) the use of antiviral substances or human immune globulins containing antiviral antibodies in selected instances.

EPIDEMIOLOGICAL CONCEPTS

Virus infections may involve single cases *(sporadic)*, or small or large clusters of cases over a narrow time frame *(epidemic)*, or they may affect substantial numbers of cases in many regions and countries of the world for an extensive duration *(pandemic)*. Viruses may continue to persist in communities, causing sporadic cases throughout each year, perhaps with some seasonal fluctuations in the number of cases; i.e., they may be *endemic* within communities. However, viruses which cause epidemics within communities may either be already present within the community from year to year *(indigenous)*, or they may have been imported from another region or country *(exotic)*. A *rate* is a ratio which expresses the number of persons with disease as the numerator and the number of the total population at risk as denominator. Usually rates are expressed either as percentages or as cases per 100,000 population. A rate measures the frequency or risk of occurrence of a virus infection during some specified interval of time *(incidence)* or at some point in time *(prevalence)*.[10]

Some examples will elucidate the meaning of the above concepts. a. *Sporadic*. An infant developed a vesicular eruption over the face during May 1981 due to *Herpesvirus hominis* type 1 which was visualized by electron microscopy and isolated from vesicle fluid.[20] b. *Epidemic*. Clusters of cases of aseptic meningitis due to coxsackievirus B5 or echovirus 9 may affect many communities within the Temperate Zones during the warmer months of several years, but the viruses are rarely detected during winter.[18] c. *Pandemic*. Influenza virus (mainly influenza A (HINI) and to a small extent influenza B), has been detected in many Northern Hemisphere countries during the 1983–84 winter,[7] but substantially fewer cases were encountered than in two former epidemics of 1957–58 due to influenza A (H2N2) and 1968–69 due to influenza A (H3N2). d. *Endemic*. Gastroenteritis due to rotavirus affected infants in Vancouver during all twelve months of the year during a six-year survey.[20] However, during the winter months December through March, the number of hospitalized patients per month was more than twice the monthly rate during summer, and the percentage of virus-positive patients increased from a summertime low of about 15% to exceed 35% per month during winter. These results indicate that rotavirus is endemic in Vancouver but wintertime epidemics occur regularly. Many Temperature Zone communities experience comparable seasonal fluctuations in occurrence of rotavirus gastroenteritis. e. *Indigenous*. Rotavirus is indigenous in Vancouver as shown by the above example. f. *Exotic*. Dengue is the commonest imported arbovirus infection of travellers returning to North America, a non-endemic area, from the Caribbean and Central America where dengue is endemic. A Chicago resident became ill with dengue type 4 virus infection on 1 April 1981, four days after he returned by air from St. Barthelemy in the Caribbean.[5] g. *Prevalence*. On a particular day, 15% or more pupils may be absent from school during an influenza epidemic. The prevalence rate is thus 15 per 100, which measures the impact of influenza virus on the school population at that point in time. h. *Incidence*. During an influenza epidemic, the percentage of deaths per week due to pneumonia and influenza consistently exceeds 6.5%, which is the upper threshold of weekly incidence for the US population.[9] This increased incidence correlates excellently with a high weekly rate of influenza virus isolations within the community.[6]

CLINICAL RECOGNITION

Disease arises from tissue damage as a consequence of growth of viruses in various organs or systems. Clusters of symptoms and signs characteristic of a particular disease are termed *syndromes*. Virus-induced syndromes are classified broadly into those affecting: (i) the respiratory tract, (ii) the serous membranes, (iii) the alimentary tract and accessory viscera, (iv) the skin and mucous membranes (exanthemata), (v) the central nervous system, and (vi) generalized infections (Table 6-1). Involvement of particular areas of a system, e.g., the respiratory tract, by different categories of virus may induce syndromes referable to that portion of the systems, as in common colds

TABLE 6-1
VIRUS-INDUCED SYNDROMES IN PATIENTS

Syndrome	Viruses associated regularly Family	Serotype	less commonly associated virus groupings
Respiratory tract			
coryza	Picornaviridae	Rhinovirus	Enteroviruses Cororaviruses
Pharyngoconjunctival	Adenoviridae	Adenovirus 3, 4 7	
influenza	Orthomyxoviridae	Influenza A, B	
croup	Paramyxoviridae	Parainfluenza 1, 3	Influenza, measles, varicella
bronchiolitis	Paramyxoviridae	Respiratory syncytial	Parainfluenza
bronchopneumonia	Paramyxoviridae	Respiratory syncytial	Parainfluenza, influenza measles, adenovirus, Chlamydia psittaci, Coxiella burnetii
Serous membranes			
Pleurodynia, pericarditis, serous peritonitis	Picornaviridae	Coxsackie B1-B5	
Alimentary Tract			
gastroenteritis	Reoviridae	Rotavirus	Adenovirus, calicivirus, coronavirus, parvovirus
hepatitis A	Picornaviridae	Enterovirus-72	
hepatitis B	Hepadnaviridae	Hepadnavirus-1	
pancreatitis	Paramyxoviridae	Mumps	
Exanthemata: maculopapular			
measles	Paramyxoviridae	Measles	
rubella	Togaviridae (NAR)	Rubella	
enteroviral	Picornaviridae	Echovirus-9	Echovirus-16, 30

TABLE 6-1 (continued)

<u>vesicular</u>			
herpes simplex	Herpesviridae	Herpesvirus hominis-1 (oral)	
		Herpesvirus hominis-2 (genital)	
varicella-zoster	Herpesviridae	Herpesvirus varicellae	
<u>mumps</u>			
mumps (parotitis)	Paramyxoviridae	Mumps	
<u>conjunctivitis</u>			
conjunctivitis	Picornaviridae	Enterovirus-70	Herpesvirus hominis-1
	Adenoviridae	Adenovirus-7	Chlamydia trachomatis

<u>Central nervous system</u>:

aseptic meningitis	Picornaviridae	Coxsackievirus Echovirus	Adenoviruses, togavirus, bunyaviruses
	Paramyxoviridae	Mumps	
paralytic poliomyeltis	Piconaviridae	Poliovirus-1, 2, 3	Enteroviruses
encephalitis	Togaviridae (ARBO)	WEE, SLE	Measles, herpesvirus, rhabdovirus
	Bunyaviridae (ARBO)	LAC	

Generalized infections: ubiquitous

mononucleosis	Herpesviridae	Epstein-Barr virus	cytomegalovirus
cytomegalovirus	Herpesviridae	Cytomegalovirus	
<u>Tropical</u>			
dengue	Togaviridae (ARBO)	Dengue-1, 2, 3, 4	
other tropical and hemorrhagic fevers	Togaviridae (ARBO)	Dengue	Chikungunya, rhabdovirus
	Bunyaviridae (ARBO)	ORO, Congo	Phlebovirus
	Arenaviridae (NAR)	Lassa	Machupo

<u>Rickettsial diseases</u>	Rickettsiae	Rickettsia rickettsii	Coxiella burnetii

<u>Abbrevations</u>: ARBO, arthropod-borne; NAR non-arthropod-borne: LAC, La Crosse; ORO, Oropouche; SLE, St. Louis encephaltis; WEE, western equine encephalomyelitis

(coryza) due to rhinovirus infections of the nasal mucosa and bronchiolitis due to respiratory syncytial virus infections of the bronchiolar mucosa. Detailed clinical descriptions of virus-induced syndromes are provided in chapters 15 through 19; a synopsis will be provided here. Techniques of laboratory diagnosis and described in two separate monographs.[19,20]

RESPIRATORY TRACT INFECTIONS are usually described according to whether the mucous membrane is inflamed above and including the larynx (upper tract), or below the larynx (lower tract). Upper respiratory infections include the common cold and pharyngoconjunctival fever.

COMMON COLDS (coryza) are manifested by intense rhinorrhea (runny nose), nasal stuffiness, some cough and slight malaise, with little or no fever, arising from acute catarrhal inflammation of the nasal and pharyngeal mucosa. Etiological agents include more than 100 serotypes of rhinovirus.

PHARYNGOCONJUNCTIVAL FEVER comprises acute hyperemia of the conjunctivae accompanied by a gritty sensation in the eyes, together with an acutely reddened and sore pharynx, cough and nasal discharge. Etiological agents are regularly adenovirus types 3, 4 or 7.

Lower respiratory tract infections include influenza, croup, bronchiolitis and bronchopneumonia.

INFLUENZA is characterized by high fever, severe malaise accompanied by headache, plus aches and pains in the back and limbs, together with reddened, glazed pharyngeal and nasal mucous membranes and a cough. Symptoms arise from acute inflammation of the nasal and pharyngeal mucosa, and also of the bronchi and bronchioles. Etiological agents comprise serotypes principally within the species influenza virus type A and influenza type B.

CROUP (acute laryngotracheobronchitis) exhibits croupy cough, inspiratory stridor, hoarse voice or cry, and respiratory difficulty on inspiration, accompanied by indrawing of the chest wall, together with diminished air entry into the lungs. Croup usually affects children aged less than three years. Etiological agents are regularly parainfluenza viruses, especially types 1 and 3.

BRONCHIOLITIS develops following a cough and a runny nose for 1 to 2 days. There is an abrupt increase in mucous secretions accompanied by wheezing, increased coughing, and difficulty with respirations resulting in rib-cage retraction, plus a barrel-shaped chest indicating obstruction to outflow of air. Overinflated lungs are observed radiologically. Bronchiolitis usually affects children aged less than 2 years. Respiratory syncytial (RS) virus is the commonest causative agent.

VIRAL BRONCHOPNEUMONIA is diagnosed principally by auscultation of rales over portions of the lung fields, together with a severe cough and difficulty with respiration, accompanied by fever. This contrasts with bronchiolitis and croup, where patients are usually afebrile. All age groups are affected. Radiological examination reveals patchy consolidation throughout the lung fields. Etiological agents are commonly RS virus, but viruses such as influenza, parainfluenza, measles and chicken pox may also induce bronchopneumonia.

SEROUS MEMBRANE INFECTIONS include pleurodynia, pericarditis and serous peritonitis. All arise from infection with group B coxsackieviruses.

PLEURODYNIA is manifested by sudden onset of unilateral sharp pains in the chest on deep inspiration, usually accompanied by a pleural fraction rub over the painful site and mild fever.

PERICARDITIS is characterized by severe precordial pain accompanied by a pericardial friction rub and typical electrocardiographic findings of flattening and inversion of T waves in leads V_3 through V_5.

SEROUS PERITONITIS is characterized by severe generalized abdominal pain and tenderness with fever but normal leukocyte counts, sometimes in association with pericarditis or pleurodynia or acute tenderness of skeletal musculature.

ALIMENTARY TRACT INFECTIONS comprise of gastroenteritis, hepatitis and pancreatitis.

GASTROENTERITIS presents with sudden onset of profuse watery diarrhea, often passing 10 or more loose watery green stools during the initial 24 hours. Patients rapidly become dehydrated with dry flaccid skin, dry glazed buccal mucosa and sunken eyeballs. Diarrhea persists 4 to 7 days in untreated patients, but usually ceases within one day after commencement of intravenous infusion of electrolyte solutions when oral intake of fluids is denied.

Causative viruses are Rotavirus, Adenovirus, Calicivirus and Astrovirus, picornavirus-like agents and Coronavirus, in decreasing order of frequency.

HEPATITIS usually presents with a few days of intense anorexia, together with nausea, vomiting and moderate fever, followed by jaundice, dark urine and pale feces, and characteristic elevation of serum levels of alanine aminotransferase (formerly glutamic pyruvic transaminase) and aspartate aminotransferase (formerly glutamic oxalacetic transaminase). Jaundice and other symptoms may persist for a few days to several weeks. Clinically these are two categories of viral hepatitis. *Hepatitis A* has an incubation period 15 to 40 days and it is transmitted by the fecal-oral route. The causative agent is enterovirus-72. *Hepatitis B* has a mean incubation period about 60 days and it is spread by blood contamination of injection equipment or close mucosal contact. The causative agent is hepadnavirus-1.

PANCREATITIS usually arises as a complication of mumps virus infection. Patients develop severe central abdominal pain accompanied by gross elevation of the serum amylase level.

EXANTHEMATA comprise febrile illnesses, largely of childhood, accompanied by the simultaneous appearance of either maculopapular or vesicular skin rashes. Maculopapular exanthemata, where hypermic red spots (macules), often exhibiting central raised dots (papules) cover various portions of the skin surface, include measles (red measles, rubeola), rubella (German measles) and enteroviral rashes (particularly echovirus-9). Vesicular exanthemata, which exhibit raised round lesions 2–3 mm diameter containing epithelial cells which have undergone liquefactive necrosis, include herpes simplex and varicella-herpes zoster. By convention, mumps which is a febrile illness accompanied by swelling of the parotid or submandibular glands, but without rash, is usually considered along the exanthemata. Conjunctivitis is arbitrarily considered here also.

MEASLES exhibits a blotchy maculopapular rash involving principally the face and trunk, accompanied by moderate fever and runny nose plus conjunctival injection 1 to 2 days before the rash. The incubation period is about 14 days. The sole causative agent is measles virus.

RUBELLA presents with a pinpoint blush resembling peachbloom over the face and trunk, accompanied by slight fever and characteristic enlargement of the postauricular or postcervical lymph nodes. The incubation period is about 18 days. The etiological agent is rubella virus.

ENTEROVIRAL RASHES exhibit blotches over the face and upper trunk, and characteristically red spots appear on the palms of the hands. However there is no nasal or conjunctival catarrh and the cervical lymph nodes are normal. In contrast to measles and rubella which occur mainly during cooler months, enteroviral rashes appear typically during warmer months. The commonest causative agent is echovirus-9, but echovirus types 4, 6, 16 and 30 have caused epidemics of rashes, and enterovirus 70 has caused outbreaks of conjunctivitis.

HERPES. Herpetic eruptions comprise pinpoint vesicles 1 mm or less diameter which occur singly or in clusters. They may affect two principal regions of the body: a. *oral,* involving the face, lips and buccal mucosa due to infection with *Herpesvirus hominis* type 1. b. *genital,* involving the penis (male) or vulva and perineum (female) due to infection with *Herpesvirus hominis* type 2.

VARICELLA exhibits vesicles 1 to 2 mm over the face, scalp and trunk which erupt with successive crops during 3 or 4 days, following an incubation period of about 18 days.

HERPES ZOSTER vesicles involve the cutaneous distribution of one or more sensory nerves. Although herpes zoster may be the initial clinical expression of infection by *Herpesvirus varicellae,* more commonly it occurs many years after primary varicella infection, following severe emotional trauma, or in immunosuppression. Both varicella and herpes zoster are induced by infection with the same agent, *Herpesvirus varicellae* (varicella-zoster virus).

MUMPS usually presents with fever and painful swelling of one or both parotid or submandibular salivary glands after an 18 day incubation period. Complications include pancreatitis, aseptic meningitis, orchitis or oophoritis. Mumps virus is the sole etiological agent.

CONJUNCTIVITIS exhibits reddened conjunctivae with injected blood vessels, serous discharge and gritty sensations in the eyes. Causative viruses include enterovirus-70, coxsackievirus A24 and adenovirus-7.

CENTRAL NERVOUS SYSTEM INFECTIONS comprise aseptic meningitis, poliomyelitis, encephalitis.

ASEPTIC MENINGITIS denotes the syndrome of headache, fever, vomiting, neck stiffness and leukocytosis of the cerebrospinal fluid (CSF), in which more than 50% cells are lymphocytes, and the CSF sugar and protein contents are normal. Causative agents are regularly enteroviruses and mumps virus.

POLIOMYELITIS denotes aseptic meningitis together with flaccid paralysis of some component of the skeletal musculature, accompanied by pain and spasm in the affected muscle groups. Etiological agents are the three serotypes of poliovirus.

ENCEPHALITIS comprises the syndrome of severe headache and high fever, accompanied by drowsiness and disorientation which may progress to stupor or coma, along with twitching and spastic paresis of portions of the skeletal musculature. Causative agents include mosquito-borne and tick-borne arboviruses and certain non-arthropod-borne agents such as rabies, herpes and measles.

GENERALIZED INFECTIONS include certain arthropod-borne virus infections such as dengue (biphasic fever, severe pains in the bones and musculature, frequently accompanied by a maculopapular or hemorrhagic rash) and non-arthropod-borne infections such as Lassa fever.

RICKETTSIAL INFECTIONS present with high fever sometimes accompanied by rashes or bronchopneumonia. Although the causative agents which comprise the genera *Rickettsia* and *Coxiella* are assigned taxonomically to the bacteria, they are normally investigated by virologists because they multiply only inside living cells.

PREVENTIVE MEASURES

Prevention of spread of virus infections in hospitals and other health care facilities is best achieved through adequate case isolation procedures, combined with comprehensive surveillance and prompt, effective case reporting mechanisms.[12]

CASE ISOLATION PROCEDURES

Current practice in North American hospitals provides for 6 types of isolation according to the infecting microorganism and the site in the body infected by it:[15] (i) standard (wound, skin, urine); (ii) enteric; (iii) respiratory; (iv) blood precautions; (v) strict; (vi) protective or reverse (Table 6-2).

STANDARD isolation procedures are applicable to all patients who are hospitalized with communicable infections. They include: nursing the patient in a closed room with in-room handwashing and toilet facilities (two or more patients with the same infecting microorganism may be nursed in the same room for convenience); wearing of gowns by all personnel entering the room and the gowns are deposited in a special laundry bag upon leaving the room; washing of hands by all personnel upon exit from the room; restriction of access to the patient to the minimum number of health care and housekeeping personnel who are essential for exemplary patient care, but including the patients immediate next-of-kin; tableware must be decontaminated in boiling water separately from that of other patients; excreta must be disposed of directly into the sewage system and the containers must be decontaminated before re-use; soiled clothing and bedlinen must be placed in double bags which are leak-proof and these are laundered separately; garbage and soiled dressings must be placed in impervious double bags and disposed of by incineration. The above standard type of isolation is sufficient to contain, i.e., prevent nosocomial (intra-hospital) spread of microbial infections of wounds,

TABLE 6-2
CASE ISOLATION PROCEDURES[15]

Isolation Category	Features	Syndromes	Method of Spread	Causative Viruses
Standard	*Basic to all categories* room with closed door, in-room handwashing and toilet, all personnel wash hands and wear gowns, decontamination of tableware, decontamination of toilet utensils, soiled linen in double bags, garbage incinerated	skin wounds urinary tract	contact	herpesvirus
Enteric	*Additional features* decontamination or disposable tableware, decontamination of toilet receptacles, or decontamination of examination tables etc.	gastroenteritis	fecal soiling	rotavirus
Respiratory	air pressure in room negative with respect to corridor pressure	exanthemata	droplets	measles, varicella mumps
Blood*	autoclaving or boiling of all cutting and blood-collecting equipment	hepatitis B	blood	hepadnavirus −1
Strict*	all of the above, gloves and masks for attendants	Lassa	blood urine	Lassa
Protective (reverse)	air pressure in room positive with respect to corridor pressure, sterile bedding and bedclothes; sterile gloves, gowns, masks for attendants	Stevens-Johnson immunosuppression	contact airborne	prevent virus entry (varicella, herpes)

*This combination is now termed "universal precautions."

the skin and urinary tract. However it is essential that totally enclosed urinary drainage systems be employed in patients with indwelling catheters, and the emptying of urinary containers and insertion of new catheters be performed aseptically.[15] Herpes virus infections of the mouth and skin, which are spread by direct contact with weeping vesicles, are contained effectively by standard isolation procedures.

ENTERIC isolation procedures prevent the spread of viral (and bacterial or amoebic) gastroenteritis. Use of separate gowns and washing of hands between each patient is mandatory, discharge of excreta into the sewage system followed by decontamination of receivers is essential, and disposable eating utensils are required. Immediately after use by patients, care must be taken to launder or discard bedlinen on trolleys for transport of patients, and to chemically decontaminate objects such as x-ray examination tables before they are used by other patients.

RESPIRATORY isolation procedures prevent the spread of airborne virus-laden droplets which are coughed, sneezed or breathed into the environment by patients with measles, respiratory syncytial virus, rubella, chickenpox, mumps and other infections involving the respiratory tract. Special requirements are the operation of the air-conditioning system to achieve an air pressure within the patient's room below that in the corridor, so that airborne microorganisms cannot readily escape into the corridor upon opening the door.

BLOOD precautions prevent the spread of viruses such as hepatitis B which are transmitted by blood contamination of objects. All injection equipment and cutting devices must be sterilized by boiling or autoclaving after each use. Particular care must be taken to ensure that blood or blood products from these patients are not injected or transfused into other patients inadvertently. Blood and secretions for laboratory tests should be tagged to alert laboratory personnel to the possibility of hepatitis B or other blood-borne agent.

STRICT isolation procedures are invoked when a patient has a highly communicable disease transmitted both by air and contact and possibly by the enteric route also. Lassa fever is an example. All of the above procedures are undertaken with the utmost diligence.

PROTECTIVE OR REVERSE isolation procedures reduce the risk of colonization and infection in patients with impaired defenses. Patients are often immunosuppressed either by leukemia or other neoplastic processes, or through large doses of corticosteroids and other immunosuppressive therapy, or they may have extensive areas of denuded skin through thermal burns or from the Stevens-Johnson syndrome. Special requirements are the operation of the air-conditioning system to achieve an air pressure within the patients' room above that in the corridor which restricts entry of the airborne micro-organisms outside the patient's room. Sterile gowns and gloves are worn by all attendants who also wear face masks. The patient is nursed in sterile bedclothes on sterile bedlinen.

SURVEILLANCE AND CASE REPORTING

Since many virus infections are spread from infected patients to their susceptible contacts, either by direct mechanical juxtaposition or by contaminated fomites or by virus-laden airborne droplets, it is essential to locate and document these virus excreters. Several viruses may be spread from healthy carriers, whilst others may be spread from environmental sources such as food or water. In order to prevent the spread of infection, it is essential to report immediately all fresh cases and carriers to a central agency which in turn will notify infection control officers promptly.

Within a hospital, the infection control nurse becomes the key person for surveillance and prevention of nosocomial infections. She receives daily reports of freshly occurring or recurrent infections, i.e., *index cases,* in all clinical facilities. She personally interviews index cases and their immediate families regarding the occurrence of other cases. Furthermore she initiates day-by-day surveillance for fresh cases among adjacent patients and health care personnel during the ensuing incubation period. Each day she notifies health care and administrative personnel the locations and names of patients who require nursing in isolation, and when isolation may be discontinued. The infection control nurse is usually delegated to notify the appropriate municipal, country state or provincial government health officer concerning all communicable diseases.

Within a nation, virus infections may occur simultaneously in several communities or provinces. Prompt transmittal of reports from individual physicians or hospitals through local, county, state or provincial agencies to a national epidemiological bureau, such as the Centers for Disease Control, Atlanta, Georgia for the entire United States, is essential for implementation of effective preventive measures. Equally important is the prompt availability of national disease reports to individual physicians and health officers. For many years, the Centers for Disease Control, US Public Health Service, has disseminated this information most effectively through their weekly publication Morbidity and Mortality Weekly Reports.

Influenza epidemics nationwide or in major geopolitical regions are characterized by an increased rate of death reports per week due to pneumonia and influenza (P + I) above the expected wintertime threshold rate of about 6.5% of all deaths.[9] The excess P and I rate correlates well with other epidemiological markers such as abrupt increases in daily attendances with acute respiratory disease at Emergency Departments of major hospitals in large metropolitan areas,[24] and daily absentee rates exceeding 15% in schools.[21] These epidemiological markers correlate closely with the actual numbers and rate of isolation of influenza virus from patients during epidemics[6,13] (Figure 18-5).

Surveillance of highly communicable airborne infections affecting mainly children such as measles, rubella, mumps and chickenpox is attained largely through detection of fresh cases by school nurses plus medical certificates from absentee students. The local Health Department is notified promptly about these cases. Anecdotal information suggests that only about one-third to one-half of the total cases occurring in a community are detected and reported by this mechanism.

VACCINES: GENERAL PRINCIPLES

Vaccines are biological preparations which prevent development of illness following exposure to virulent naturally occurring (wild) viruses of the same serotype. Vaccines consist either of: (a) live virus without the ability to induce severe or fatal illness (attenuated); or (b) killed (inactivated) virus where the antigenic material comprises either; (i) the whole virus particle, especially its outer coat ("whole virus"), or (ii) small components of the outer coat of the virus ("split product" or "subunit") (Table 6-3). Influenza split product vaccine contains hemagglutinin derived from the outer coat of the influenza virion by

TABLE 6-3
ATTRIBUTES OF VIRUS VACCINES

Property	Live (attenuated) vaccine	Killed (inactivated) vaccine
Antibody persistence	Many years (lifelong)	1–3 years
Doses required	Single[a]	Multiple, with boosters
Route of administration	Parenteral or oral	Parenteral
How stored	Lyophilized 4°C (most vaccines) Liquid 4°C (polio)	Liquid 4°C
Virus excretion after natural challenge	Minimal	Unchanged
Vaccinee as virus excreter	Polio	None
Adverse reactions	Measles (mild rash) Rubella (arthralgia)	Site of infection only[b]

[a]Usually two doses of trivalent oral poliovirus vaccine are administered, with an interval of 2 months between doses, because not all three strains may replicate after the initial dose.
[b]Less severe reactions are observed following influenza split product vaccine than with whole virus vaccine.

treatment with sodium deoxycholate and this vaccine is devoid of nucleic acid. Hepatitis B subunit vaccine contains solely the 22 nm hepatitis B surface antigen particles which become detached readily from the whole virion (Dane particle) during preparation of the vaccine.

LIVE VACCINES multiply within the host and induce antiviral antibodies which persist at least 8 to 10 years and probably lifelong. Antibody titers may decline from their peaks during the initial years after vaccination to levels 4 to 8 fold lower during the succeeding five years, but thereafter they remain stationary for many years unless they are boosted by natural infection or revaccination. Presence of detectable antibody is normally associated with immunity against illness following reinfection with wild virus of the same serotype. When combined vaccines containing several serotypes are administered subcutaneously as one dose, such as measles, mumps and rubella, antibodies to each serotype develop in the same proportion of subjects (97% for each serotype) as that observed after administration of each serotype separately. However when combined vaccines are administered orally, e.g., trivalent oral poliovirus vaccine, one or two serotypes only may multiply and induce antibody production after one dose, but upon administration of further doses of trivalent vaccine 6 to 8 weeks later, antibody to the remaining serotype regularly appears.

Measles, mumps, rubella and yellow fever vaccines are administered subcutaneously, since their viruses induce generalized infections following multiplication in reticuloendothelial cells. Poliovirus vaccine is administered orally, because gut epithelium comprises the initial site for replication of poliovirus.

Viability of virus vaccines is preserved considerably beyond the usual 6-month expiration date when lyophilized vaccine is stored at 4° C. Although storage of lyophilized vaccines continuously at 4° C is highly desirable, no loss of potency is experienced after holding lyophilized vaccines unrefrigerated for 2 days or less. Poliovirus, in contrast to measles and other vaccine viruses, shows substantial loss of infective titer upon lyophilization. Therefore live oral poliovirus vaccine must be stored liquid at 4° C continuously, and this requires transportation between institutions in containers with ice at 4° C, in order to avoid loss of potency.

Vaccine virus may be excreted into the environment following replication within the recipient. For example, a poliovirus vaccine recipient may excrete one or more serotypes of attenuated virus in the feces which may contaminate the household or daycare environment with a sufficiently high dose of virus to induce infection among contacts. However the amount of virus excreted in the pharyngeal or nasal secretions of recipients of measles and rubella vaccine is insufficient to infect close contacts.

Following replication of attenuated measles vaccine virus, a mild rash accompanied by slight fever may affect about 10% of vaccinees, and overall 1 to 3% of rubella vaccinees may develop transient monarticular arthritis, but adverse reactions do not usually affect recipients of the other vaccines. Severe complications such as paralysis following infection of live poliovirus vaccine may involve about 1:30 million recipients,[4] and similarly low rates of severe central nervous system complications have been recorded for measles and yellow fever vaccine. Extremely rare cases of aseptic meningitis have been recorded since live mumps vaccine was first used in 1963.

Efficacy of all currently licensed live vaccines ranges from 95 to 100%, both in terms of antibody conversion rates and in prevention of illness after exposure to wild virus.

KILLED VACCINES stimulate antibody production solely in response to the quantity of antigenic mass deposited during an injection. Usually antibodies appear in serum only after two or more injections of vaccine at intervals of 2 to 4 weeks. Antibodies persist no longer than 1 to 2 years in most instances. Parenteral injection, usually by subcutaneous injection, but occasionally by jet injector, is always required for administration of killed vaccines. Usually vaccines are stored liquid at 4° C, and several vaccines are inactivated by freezing. Full antigenic potency is retained at least 6 months. Virus excretion does not occur after vaccination with killed vaccines. Adverse reactions are confined to the injection site which becomes reddened, hot, swollen and painful during the first day. The use of split product influenza vaccine has minimized local reactions. Improved degrees of purity of vaccine have reduced the incidence rate of adverse reactions.

VACCINES CURRENTLY AVAILABLE

Virus vaccines which are licensed by most jurisdictions and are commonly in use both in private practice and in public health clinics are listed in Table 6-4.

MEASLES VACCINE (live) is manufactured from the Schwarz further attenuated strain of the Edmonston strain of measles virus by propagation in chick embryo tissue cultures. It was licensed in 1967. Administration of a single dose of 1000 TCD_{50} virus subcutaneously evokes an antibody response in the serum within 1 month in at least 95% of vaccines. Antibodies have persisted at least 16 years post vaccination in the absence of natural challenge by wild measles virus, and these subjects are clinically immune, i.e., they do not develop symptoms, upon exposure to wild measles virus. Encephalopathy following measles vaccination has been recorded in fewer than 1 per million recipients, which is substantially lower than 1:1000 rate of measles encephalitis as a regular complication of naturally acquired measles. Between 1967 and 1972, atypical measles which presented with fever, petechiae and bronchopneumonia affected 4 to 5% of children who contracted infection with wild measles virus after having received killed measles vaccine at least one year previously. Following cessation of manufacture of killed measles virus in 1967, this complication is encountered no longer. In the United States, expanded measles vaccination programs including the requirement of documentary evidence of administration of live measles vaccine or physician-diagnosed measles for entry into the school system, together with excellent surveillance and case finding procedures, has virtually eliminated indigenous measles.[8] The lowest ever attack rate of 0.6 cases per 100,000 was encountered in 1983, which was a 99.7% reduction from the average annual rate of 315.2 cases per 100,000 in the pre-vaccine era 1950–1962.

Regularly, live vaccines for measles, mumps and rubella are combined for administration as a single dose to all infants aged 12 to 15 months.

MUMPS vaccine (live) is prepared from the Jeryl Lynn strain of mumps by propagation in a chick embryo cell culture. It was licensed in 1967. Administration of a single dose of 5000 TCD_{50} virus subcutaneously has evoked antibody responses in more than 90% recipients within one month, and antibody has persisted at least 9.5 years. This parallels the 93–98% effectiveness of protection against clinical mumps following natural exposure to wild mumps virus.

RUBELLA VACCINE (live) is manufactured from the RA27/3 isolate by propagation in continuous human diploid cell cultures (WI-38). The present vaccine strain was first licensed in 1979, which superseded vaccines containing other strains propagated in non-human cell systems which were manufactured between 1969 and 1978. Administration of a single dose containing 1000 TCD_{50} virus has evoked antibody responses in more than 95% recipients, with persistence of detectable antibodies for at least 18 years.[22a] Reinfection or excretion of appreciable amounts of rubella virus from the throat is extremely rare in RA27/3 vaccinees following natural exposure to wild rubella virus. Transient arthralgia may affect the small joints of 1 to 3% vaccinees overall, with a higher incidence among women over 20 years of age. To date there is no epidemiological or clinical evidence that rubella-induced congenital anomalies appear in babies born to mothers who had inadvertently received rubella vaccine during the first trimester. However it is recommended that females abstain from pregnancy for 2 months after injection with rubella vaccine.

POLIOMYELITIS VACCINE (live), currently used in USA, Canada and many other jurisdictions, is manufactured from three Sabin attenuated strains of poliovirus by propagation in primary monkey kidney tissue cultures. Plaque-purified stocks of each of three serotypes are mixed to provide single oral doses of vaccine containing 10^6 TCD_{50} poliovirus-1 (LSc 2ab), 10^5 TCD_{50} poliovirus-2 (P712, Ch 2ab), $10^{5.5}$ TCD_{50} poliovirus-3 (Leon 12 ab). In order to exceed 95% seroconversion rates against all three serotypes, two doses of oral vaccine are administered 6 to 8 weeks apart. Vaccine-induced antibodies have persisted at least 10 years. In jurisdictions such as Holland and Sweden, similar high rates of seroconversion have been achieved through subcutaneous

TABLE 6-4
CURRENT VIRUS VACCINES

Vaccine	Type	Preparation	Storage 4°C	Dose	Route
Measles	L	Chick embryo TC	Lyophilized	1000 TCD_{50}	Subcutaneous
Mumps	L	Chick embryo TC	Lyophilized	5000 TCD_{50}	Subcutaneous
Rubella	L	Human Diploid TC	Lyophilized	1000 TCD_{50}	Subcutaneous
Polio-myelitis	L	Monkey Kidney TC	Liquid	Trivalent[c]	Oral
Yellow Fever	L	Chick embryo TC	Lyophilized	1000LD_{50}	Subcutaneous
Influenza	K	Embryonated egg	Liquid	Trivalent[e]	Subcutaneous
Rabies[g]	K	Human diploid TC	Liquid	1.0ml	Intramuscular
HepatitisB	K	Ultracentrifuged human plasma	Liquid	20ug in 1.0ml	Intramuscular

a.   Measles, mumps and rubella (live attenuated) vaccines are usually administered as one dose of a trivalent vaccine.
b.   These live vaccines should not be given to infants aged less than 12 months, due to their neutralization by maternally-acquired antibody in the infant's blood before the first birthday.
c.   Trivalent oral poliovirus vaccine (Sabin) contains $10^{6.0}$ TCD_{50} type 1, $10^{5.0}$ TCD_{50} type 2, $10^{5.5}$ TCD_{50} type 3 per dose.
d.   Rubella vaccine is not teratogenic, but care should be taken to avoid inadvertant administration to pregnant women (MMWR 31:477 and 514, 1982).

TABLE 6-4
CURRENT VIRUS VACCINES

Frequency	Antibody persistence YEARS	Adverse reactions	Severe	Efficacy	MMWR Ref
Once [a, b]	>16	Mild fever, rash 5%	Encepahlitis $1{:}10^6$	$>95\%$	31:217,1982
Once [a, b]	>10	none	none	$>90\%$	31:617, 1982
Once [a,b]	>9	Arthralgia 1-3%	None[d]	$>97\%$	30:37, 1981
Twice	>10	None	Paralysis $1{:}10^6$	$>95\%$	31:22, 1982
Once	$\geqslant 10$	None	Encephalitis $1{:}10^6$	100%	27:268, 1978
Annual	$\geqslant 1$	Local irritation	None[f]	70%	31:348, 1982
3-5	$\geqslant 1$	Local irritation	None	100%	31:279, 1982
3	$\geqslant 1$	Local irritation	None	$>90\%$	31:317,1982

e. Trivalent killed influenza vaccine contains 15 micrograms each of A(H3N2), A(H1N1) and B antigens per dose.

f. During 1976 only, Guillain-Barre syndrome occurred 9 to 14 tmes more frequently among recipients of swine influenza vaccine than in recipients of influenza A plus B vaccine, or no vaccine.

g. For severe, deeply penetrating wounds, rabies hyperimmune golbulin (human) is administered in addition to rabies vaccine.

Abbreviations: L live, K killed, TCD_{50} 50% tissue culture infective doses, LD_{50} 50% mouse lethal doses.

injection of an initial course of 3 doses of trivalent killed poliovirus vaccine (Salk), but booster injections are required at intervals of about 3 years in order to maintain these high antibody prevalence rates. However immunization of entire populations by either procedure has resulted in the virtual elimination of paralytic poliomyelitis among vaccinees, as shown for example in Canada during 1978 when paralytic disease affected only unvaccinated persons following importation of wild poliovirus among family contacts who had recently arrived from overseas.[14] Recipients of oral vaccine may excrete the vaccine strains in feces for 1 to 2 weeks, but this poses no health hazard to close contacts. However upon reinfection of oral vaccines with a wild poliovirus strain, intestinal carriage is fleeting and the amount of virus excreted in feces is trifling. This contrasts with excretion of substantial quantities of virus for 1 to 2 weeks after recipients of killed vaccine have received a natural challenge with wild poliovirus. The safety record of Sabin oral poliovirus vaccine is extremely high, with fewer than 1:4 million cases of paralytic disease directly attributable to the vaccine strains.

YELLOW FEVER vaccine (live) is manufactured from the attenuated 17D strain by propagation in chick-embryo tissue cultures. Each dose of lyophilized vaccine contains 1000 mouse LD_{50} 17D yellow fever virus, which is administered subcutaneously. Immunity to natural challenge commences 10 days after one dose of vaccine and persists at least 10 years. The vaccine is virtually 100% effective. Vaccine safety records indicate the less than 1:1 million recipients may develop mild or moderate encephalitis directly attributable to the 17D vaccine.

INFLUENZA VACCINE (killed) is manufactured, by propagation in allantoic cells of embryonated eggs, of the most recent serotypes of influenza A and influenza B viruses which have caused epidemics around the world. Current influenza vaccines are trivalent, due to the concurrent epidemic activity of both H3N2 and H1N1 serotypes of influenza A, as well as influenza B. Vaccines contain 15 micrograms of hemagglutinin of each serotype per dose. Formulations used during the 1983–84 winter contained A/Philippines/2/82(H3N2), A/Brazil/11/78(HINI) and B/Singapore/222/79. After two initial doses of vaccine about one month apart, annual revaccination with one dose of the updated vaccine is required during each autumn, due to antigenic drift (Chapter 8) and decline of antibody titers one year after killed vaccine. Some vaccines show significant degrees of adverse reactions, i.e., pain and swelling at the site of injection, following administration of vaccine containing whole virus particles. These adverse reactions are minimized through administration of the purified hemagglutinin component ("split product") of the outer coat of the whole virus following treatment with sodium deoxycholate. The effectiveness of trivalent influenza vaccine in reducing the clinical attach rate of influenza is usually about 70%.

Following administration of swine influenza vaccine A/NJ/76(HSWINI) either singly or combined with influenza A (H3N2) and influenza B vaccines in 1976, the attack rate of Guillain-Barre syndrome was observed for the first time to be 9 to 14 times higher among recipients of swine vaccine than the expected normal baseline rate among recipients of influenza A and B vaccine only or in unvaccinated subjects.[2] Following discontinuance of swine influenza vaccine, there has been no association between administration of influenza A plus B vaccine formulations in succeeding years.[17]

RABIES vaccine (killed) is manufactured from a fixed strain of rabies virus by propagation in human diploid cell cultures followed by inactivation with B-propiolactone (Europe) or tri-N-butyl phosphate (USA). It is usually administered in 1.0 ml doses intramuscularly, but intradermal injection of 0.1 ml is considered an adequate alternate for pre-exposure vaccination only. In pre-exposure situations after 3 intramuscular doses administered at 0, 7 and 21 or 28 days, 100% of recipients have developed adequate anti-rabies antibody levels, but it is recommended that veterinarians and other high-risk groups receive boosters every 2 years to maintain adequate antibody levels. After exposure to bites by rabid animals, 5 intramuscular injections should be given at 0, 3, 7, 14 and 28 days, together with rabies immune globulin (human) as soon as possible post-exposure. No severe adverse reactions have been encountered, and neuroparalytic accidents have not been recorded to date.

HEPATITIS B vaccine (killed) is a suspension of inactivated alum-adsorbed 22nm surface antigen (HB$_s$Ag) particles which have been purified from plasma of hepatitis B surface antigen-positive persons by ultracentrifugation and biochemical procedures. Virus inactivation is achieved in three steps using 8M urea, pepsin at pH2 and formalin 1:4000. After 3 intramuscular 1.0 ml doses each containing 20 µg HB$_s$Ag at 0, 1 and 6 months, more than 90% of healthy adults developed anti-hepatitis B antibody, and this has been associated with protection rates of 80 to 95% against occurrence of illness following exposure to live hepatitis B virus.

IMMUNE GLOBULINS

Protection against the occurrence of illness, or a reduction in the severity of symptoms, following exposure to a few virus infections, may be achieved passively by intramuscular administration human immune serum globulin (IG) which contains high titers of specific antiviral antibodies. It is essential to administer IG within 3 days after exposure, and preferably sooner.

Maximum antibody titers are attained in the recipient's serum about 2 days after injection and their half-life is about 20 to 25 days.

Immune serum globulin is a sterile concentrated solution containing 16.5% immune globulins (principally IgG) which is obtained by cold ethanol fraction of pooled human plasma of venous or placental origin. The method of preparation ensures that IG is free from hepatitis viruses. There is no evidence that modern preparations of IG have ever transmitted any virus infection. Most preparations of IG contain specific amounts of antibody against measles and varying amounts of antibodies against hepatitis A and hepatitis B. Some preparations contain high antibody titers to varicella-zoster virus, other lots contain high anti-rabies antibody titers.

MEASLES PROPHYLAXIS is recommended for household or nosocomial contacts with immunodeficiency states or chronic cardiac and pulmonary conditions who may develop severe complications following occurrence of measles in an index case. The dose of IG is 0.25 mg/kg, given as soon as possible after exposure, and followed by administration of live measles vaccine 3 to 4 months subsequently.

CHICKENPOX PROPHYLAXIS is recommended for immunocompromised contacts at home or in hospital, using specially prepared varicella-zoster immune globulin.

RABIES PROPHYLAXIS using a combination of rabies immune globulin plus a course of 5 injections of human diploid cell rabies vaccine is recommended for post-exposure treatment of patients with severe bites by rabid animals.

HEPATITIS A PROPHYLAXIS is recommended for travellers to highly endemic areas of the world, using one intramuscular injection of 0.05ml/kg IG immediately before departure from North America. Injections should be repeated every 4 to 6 months whilst the subject remains in the endemic area.

When 0.02ml/kg IG is administered within 1 to 2 weeks after exposure to hepatitis A infection, the effectiveness of protection against development of jaundice is 80 to 90%.

HEPATITIS B PROPHYLAXIS is required after needlestick exposure or inadvertent infusion of HB_sAg-positive blood. Intramuscular injection of 0.05 to 0.07ml/kg of hepatitis B immune globulin with passive hemagglutination titers exceeding 100,000 has suppressed development of symptomatic infection. In order to prevent development of hepatitis in newborn babies whose mothers have active hepatitis B infection at the time of delivery, it is recommended that babies receive 0.13ml/kg hepatitis B immune globulin.

ANTIVIRAL SUBSTANCES

HERPESVIRUS HOMINIS INFECTIONS

After the first successful demonstration in 1961 that a synthetic antiviral substance, 5-iodo-2'-deoxyuridine (idoxuridine) induced remission of acute herpetic keratoconjunctivitis following hourly instillation of 0.5% preparation on the conjunctiva,[16] efforts have been pursued vigorously to find additional antivirals with enhanced therapeutic efficacy combined with reduced toxicity and greater ease of administration.[1] During the succeeding quarter-century, most research effort and therapeutic trials have been directed successfully towards antiviral chemotherapy of herpesvirus infections, especially infections of the eye, skin, external genitalia, mucous membranes and brain due to both serotypes of *Herpesvirus hominis* (herpes simplex). Limited therapeutic trials of the same range of antiviral substances have been directed towards other species of *Herpesvirus* including varicella-zoster, Epstein-Barr virus (causative agent of mononucleosis) and cytomegalovirus, with generally discouraging results. Thus in 1985, only two synthetic antivirals, idoxuridine and acycloguanosine (acyclovir) are prescribed regularly for treatment of surface infections of *Herpesvirus hominis* type 1 and type 2. Chemical formulae of these two antivirals are shown in Figure 6-1.

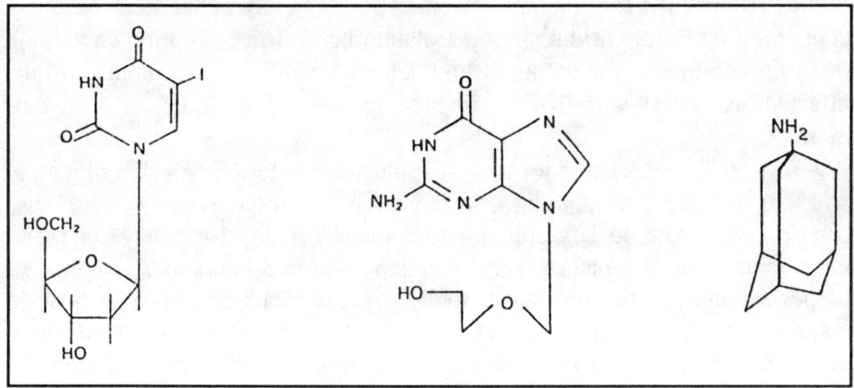

Figure 6-1: Antiviral substances currently licensed for the retail market.

Anti-herpes antivirals inhibit one or more stages in the synthesis of viral DNA.[1] Idoxuridine inhibits thymidine kinase, thymidine monophosphate kinase and DNA polymerase, and is incorporated into DNA. This halts synthesis of completely viable new herpesvirus virions and thus exerts its therapeutic effects in patients. However it also inhibits metabolic activities of the host cell in addition to enzymes induced by the virus, thus exerting a toxic effect on the patient's cells. The difference between therapeutic and toxic concentrations is sufficient to permit the use of idoxuridine in treatment of surface infections of the skin, genitalia and conjunctiva after topical application.

Acyclovir is converted to the monophosphate by the thymidine kinase induced by herpesvirus and further to the triphosphate which inhibits the virus DNA polymerase. Acyclovir is also incorporated into the viral DNA and acts as a chain terminator. However acyclovir has a substantially lower inhibitory activity against DNA polymerase in cells, thus providing a considerably higher ratio of therapeutic (antiviral): toxic (anti-host-cell) concentration. Furthermore acyclovir shows about 10 times greater antiviral activity against *H. hominis* type 1 than idoxuridine and both substances show moderately greater antiviral activity against *H. hominis* type 1 than type 2.

Idoxuridine is retailed through pharmacies in two forms: (a) for topical application to early herpetic eruptions of the skin and lips as 0.1% suspension in polyvinyl alcohol together with dimethyl sulfoxide which facilitates the penetration of the sparingly soluble idoxuridine into epithelial cells (Herplex D Liquifilm®); (b) for ophthalmic application topically either as an ointment containing 0.5% idoxuridine in a petrolatum base or as a solution containing 0.1% idoxuridine in water (Stoxil®). Each medication must be applied to the affected area every 1 to 2 hours (excluding sleeping periods) for 4 days or more.

Acyclovir is marketed for topical application to lesions on skin or genital areas as ointment containing 5% acyclovir in polyethylene glycol base (Zovirax®). It should be applied 4 to 6 times per day for 5 days or more. Commencement of topical acyclovir therapy within 8 hours after eruption of herpes vesicles on the lips substantially reduced virus titers below those in controls who received placebo, but no clinical benefit was noted.[25] Application of topical acyclovir to genital herpetic lesions in both sexes reduced the duration of virus excretion and mean healing times significantly below those observed in placebo recipients with first time genital herpes, but reduction of virus shedding and increased healing time in recurrent genital herpes was observed in men only.[11] Oral administration of acyclovir to patients both with initial and recurrent genital herpes reduced the duration of virus excretion and increased healing time.[22] Intravenous administration of acyclovir to immuno-compromised patients with herpetic eruptions of skin or mucous membranes has significantly reduced virus excretion, shortened the resolution of vesicles and accelerated the relief of the pain.[23] Similar acceleration of healing and relief of pain was observed in varicella-zoster patients who received acyclovir intravenously.[23] Throughout, toxic reactions were negligible.

INFLUENZA VIRUS INFECTIONS

Effectiveness of the antiviral substance 1-adamantanamine hydrochloride (amantadine) in reduction of the clinical attack rate by influenza A (H2N2) virus was first demonstrated clearly in 1964 when subjects received 200 mg per day orally per day for 10 days during an influenza epidemic.[26] Amantadine and its derivative rimantadine have been shown repeatedly to have prophylactic and therapeutic effectiveness during epidemic spread of influenza A viruses, both H3N2 and H2N2 serotypes.[23] More recently, both amantadine and rimantadine induced remission of influenza symptoms within 2 days, instead of 3 days or more in placebo-controls, and virus excretion was reduced substantially in treated subjects after 2 days.[23] The amantadine group of substances inhibit entry of influenza virus into cells. Amantadine antivirals require daily administration to all subjects for 10 days or longer during the currency of an influenza A outbreak in order to achieve 50% or greater prophylactic and therapeutic effectiveness.

REFERENCES

[1]Bauer DJ: The chemotherapy of herpesvirus infections. In Recent Advances in Clinical Virology 2. Ed. AP Waterson, Churchill Livingstone, Edinburgh 1980, p. 111.

[2]Center for Disease Control. Guillain-Barre syndrome - United States. MMWR 25:416, 1976.

[3]Center for Disease Control. Immune globulins for protection against viral hepatitis. MMWR 26:425, 1977.

[4]Center for Disease Control. Poliomyelitis Surveillance Summary 1974–1976. October 1977.

[5]Centers for Disease Control. Dengue type 4 infections in U.S. travellers to the Caribbean. MMWR 30:249, 1981.

[6]Centers for Disease Control. Influenza surveillance summary - United States, 1982–1983 season. MMWR 32:373, 1983.

[7]Centers for Disease Control. Update: Influenza activity - United States. MMWR 33:166, 1984.

[8]Centers for Disease Control. Measles - United States, 1983. MMWR 33:105, 1984.

[9]Choi K, Thacker SB: An evaluation of influenza mortality surveillance, 1962–1979. II Percentage of pneumonia and influenza deaths as an indicator of influenza activity. Am J Epidemiol 113:227, 1981; updated MMWR 38:97, 1989.

[10]Clark DW, MacMahon B, Eds.: Preventive and Community Medicine, Little Brown & Co. Boston 1981, p. 38.

[11]Corey L, Nahmias AJ, Guinan ME, Benedetti JK, Critchlow CW, Holmes KK: A trial of topical acyclovir in genital herpes simplex virus infections. New Eng J Med 306:1313, 1982.

[12]Dixon RE (Ed.): Nosocomial Infections. Yorke Medical Books, New York, 1981. 326 pp.

[13]Frank AL, Taber LH, Glezen WP, Geyer EA, McIlwain S, Paredes A: Influenza B virus infections in the community and the family: the epidemics of 1976–1977 and 1979–1980 in Houston, Texas. Amer J Epidem. 118:313, 1983.

[14]Health and Welfare Canada. Poliomyelitis in contacts of Netherlands travellers - Ontario, Alberta and British Columbia. Canada Diseases Weekly Report 4:157, 1978.

[15]Health Sciences Centre Hospital, University of British Columbia. Infection Control Manual, May 1981.

[16]Kaufman HE: Clinical cure of herpes simplex keratitis by 5-iodo-2'-deoxyuridine. Proc Soc Exp Biol Med 109:251, 1962.

[17]La Montagne JR, Noble GR, Quinnan GV, Curlin GT, Blackwelder WC, Smith JI, Ennis FA, Bozeman FM: Summary of clinical-trials of inactivated influenza vaccine - 1978. Rev Inf Dis 5:723, 1983.

[18]McLean DM: Virology in Health Care. Williams and Wilkins, Baltimore, 1980, p. 70.

[19]McLean DM: Immunological Investigation of Human Virus Disease. Vol. 5, Practical Methods in Clinical Immunology, Series Editor RC Nairn, Churchill Livingstone, Edinburgh 1982, 99 pp.

[20]McLean DM, Wong KK: Same-Day Diagnosis of Human Virus Infections. CRC Press, Boca Raton FL, 1984, 127 pp.

[21]Maynard JE, Dull HB, Hanson ML, Feltz ET, Berger R, Hammes L: Evaluation of monovalent and polyvalent influenza vaccines during an epidemic of type A2 and B influenza. Amer J. Epidemiol 87:148, 1968.

[22]Nilsen AE, Aasen T, Halsos AM, Kinge BR, Tjotta EAL, Wikstrom K, Fiddian AP: Efficacy of oral acyclovir in the treatment of initial and recurrent genital herpes. Lancet 2:571, 1982.

[22a]O'Shea S, Best JM, Banatvala JE, Marshall WC, Dudgeon JA: Persistence of rubella antibody 8 - 18 years after vaccination. Brit Med J 288:1043, 1984.

[23]Oxford JS: The prevention and control of influenza and herpes infections using specific antiviral molecules. In Recent Advances in Clinical Virology 3, Ed. AP Waterson, Churchill Livingstone, Edinburgh 1983, p. 139.

[24]Rubin RJ, Gregg MB: Influenza surveillance in the United States 1972–1974. Amer J Epidemiol 102:225, 1975.

[25]Spruance SL, Schnipper LE, Overall JC, Kern ER, Wester B, Modlin J, Wenerstrom G, Burton C, Arndt KA, Chin GL, Crumpacker CS: Treatment of herpes simplex labialis with topical acyclovir in polyethylene glycol. J Inf Dis 146:85, 1982.

[26]Stanley ED, Muldoon RE, Akers LW, Jackson GG: Evaluation of antiviral drugs: the effect of amantadine on influenza in volunteers. Am NY Acad Sc 130:44, 1965.

PART II

CHAPTER 7

PICORNAVIRIDAE, REOVIRIDAE, CORONAVIRIDAE, CALICIVIRIDAE, PARVOVIRIDAE

GASTROINTESTINAL VIRUSES

Viruses whose principal site of multiplication is the gastrointestinal tract following entry into the human host include serotypes within 5 virus families: Picornaviridae, Reoviridae, Coronaviridae, Caliciviridae, Parvoviridae.

PICORNAVIRIDAE

HISTORICAL

Picornavirus was first recognized as a scientific term to describe 27 nm naked cubically symmetrical RNA-containing virus particles during the VIII International Congress of Microbiology at Montreal, Canada in 1962.[7] The term Picornaviridae was adopted in 1975 to designate a virus family with 3 genera which caused human infections: *Enterovirus, Rhinovirus, Calicivirus*. In 1981, the International Committee on Taxonomy of Viruses at Strasbourg, France designated the genera *Enterovirus* and *Rhinovirus* as members of the family Picornaviridae, and the genus *Calicivirus* was placed in a distinct family Caliciviridae.[14]

The name picornavirus is an acronym derived from pico=very small and RNA=ribonucleic acid; it also may be considered as a mnemonic: P=poliovirus, I=insensitivity to ether (or sodium deoxycholate) C=coxsackievirus, O=orphan (echovirus) R=ribo, NA=nucleic acid (or "Noah's Ark"). The term echovirus is an acronym derived from: E=enteric, C=cytopathic, H=human, O=orphan (unable to be propagated in laboratory animals; some serotypes were not clearly associated with human illness, i.e., a virus without a vertebrate host). The term coxsackievirus was derived from Coxsackie, N.Y., which was the home town of the patients from whom coxsackievirus was first isolated in 1947. The term poliovirus was derived from polio = grey (matter of the central nervous system), myelitis = inflammation of the marrow (brain substance). The term rhinovirus was derived from rhino = nose.

Poliovirus was the first member of the Picornaviridae to be isolated from a patient. This was achieved in 1909 by intracerebral injection of rhesus monkeys with central nervous system (CNS) tissue from a fatal case of paralytic poliomyelitis.[12] Although fecal excretion of poliovirus was initially recorded in 1912, it was not generally recognized until 1937 that poliovirus patients excreted virus in the throat and feces.[21] Whilst it was first recorded in 1931[1] that more than one serotype of poliovirus could cause paralytic disease, and the existence of a third serotype was first recognized in 1937,[8] it was clearly documented only in 1951, that three, and only three serotypes of poliovirus regularly caused paralytic poliomyelitis,[3] through a collaborative effort, sponsored by the National Foundation for Infantile Paralysis ("March of Dimes"). Until that time, laboratory investigators of poliovirus epidemiology were severely restricted by the high cost, inconvenience and lack of regular supplies of rhesus monkeys which provided the only suitable laboratory test system. However by 1949, Enders, Robbins and Weller demonstrated that all three serotypes of poliovirus multiplied in tissue cultures of human and monkey cells, causing cytopathic effects[17] which were inhibited specifically by antibody to the same serotype. This provided a cheap, rapid and convenient laboratory technique for epidemiological investigations and a means for propagation of vaccine. Development of safe and effective inactivated poliovirus vaccine by Salk and associates[20] was first reported in 1954 and the effectiveness of live poliovirus vaccine was first documented by Sabin[18] in 1959. Following implementation of universal vaccination programs throughout industrialized nations of the north and south Temperate Zones in the 1960's paralytic poliomyelitis has been virtually eliminated except among small groups of conscientious objectors.[2] However in tropical countries where poliovirus vaccine is not available routinely, paralytic poliomyelitis continues to pose a significant health hazard.

Coxsackieviruses were first isolated during investigations of a poliomyelitis outbreak at Coxsackie, N.Y. (near Albany) in 1947.[5] Initially termed Coxsackie viruses, these isolates from feces of patients were pathogenic for suckling mice aged less than 48 hours. By means of neutralization tests in mice, numerous isolates were assigned either to group A (23 serotypes) which regularly induced myositis (necrosis of skeletal muscle) or to group B (6 serotypes) which mainly caused encephalitis, sometimes accompanied by myositis.

Echoviruses were initially termed orphan viruses because they were not associated with human illness.[4] They were first isolated from feces of groups of normal children in 1951, during surveys for enterovirus prevalence using the recently introduced tissue culture techniques. Shortly thereafter, several serotypes including echovirus 6[6] and echovirus 9[13] were clearly demonstrated as causative agents in epidemics of aseptic meningitis. Enterovirus 69 etc.[15] is used to designate new serotypes identified beyond echovirus 34. One serotype, originally termed ECHO-10, induced a different category of cytopathic effect with enlarged nuclei due to inclusion formation, and this was subsequently designated reovirus-1.[19] Reovirus is an acronym for R = respiratory, E = enteric, O = orphan.

Successful propagation in tissue cultures of viruses causing common colds was first reported in 1960,[19] after repeated attempts over many years. These viruses, now termed rhinoviruses, induced cytopathic effects in monolayer cultures of primary human embryonic kidney or monkey kidney under mild acidic conditions after incubation at 33° C. Currently more than 100 serotypes have been described.

ENTEROVIRUS

BIOLOGICAL ATTRIBUTES
Properties Common to all Enteroviruses
1. Picornavirus particles are roughly spherical naked nucleo-capsids 22–30 nm diameter with an almost featureless surface and no core, and each contains one molecule of infectious positive-sense single-stranded RNA (An electron micrograph of purified poliovirus-3 is shown in Figure 7-1).
2. Viruses retain infectivity after treatment with diethyl ether overnight at 4° C or with sodium deoxycholate 1:1000 for 1 hour at 22° C.
3. Infectivity is retained after treatment with molar concentrations of $CaCl_2$ or $MgCl_2$ for 1 hour at 50° C (stabilization by divalent cations).
4. Full infectivity is retained after storage for several years frozen at −20° C (or −70° C), but substantial loss of infectivity occurs upon lyophilization unless special precautions are observed. Infectivity is retained after holding liquid for 1–2 weeks at 4° C and for several days at 22° C.
5. Enterovirus infectivity is retained at pH 3, in contrast to Rhinovirus infectivity which is inactivated at pH<5. However enteroviruses are inactivated at pH 2.
6. Some enterovirus serotypes agglutinate human group O erythrocytes in buffered media at pH 5.8 or 7.4 after incubation at 4° C or 37° C. Hemagglutination is inhibited specifically by antiserum to the same serotype after removal of non-specific inhibitors by pretreatment with kaolin.

Properties of Individual Species
Laboratory characteristics
Poliovirus. This species contains three serotypes, poliovirus types 1, 2, 3. All multiply in primary monolayer tissue cultures prepared by trypsinization of kidneys from rhesus or cynomolgus monkeys with production of cytopathic

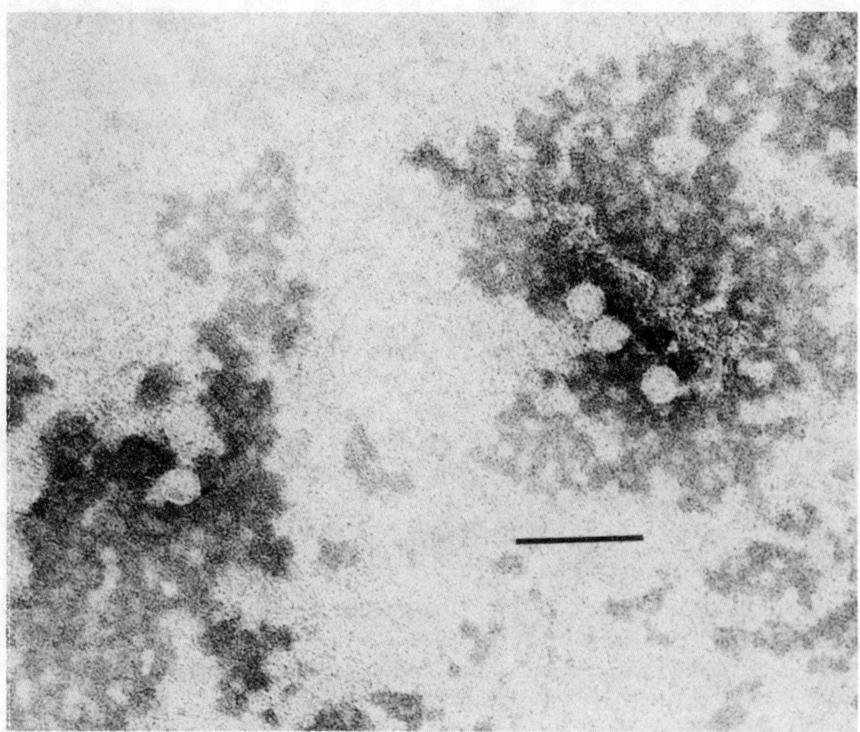

Figure 7-1: Poliovirus 3 Leon 12ab vaccine strain (X 196,350). Purified by centrifugation through a sucrose density gradient after propagation in primary monkey kidney cells. Reproduced with permission from McLean DM and Wong KK, 1984. Same-day Diagnosis of Human Virus Infections. CRC Press, Boca Raton, FL, p. 80.

effects (Figure 7-2). Infected cells become shrunken and rounded, with deeply stained pyknotic nuclei, and cells eventually become detached from the surface of the glass or plastic container. Virus infectivity is neutralized specifically by antiserum to the same serotype, which is demonstrated by lack of induction of cytopathic effect after inoculation of tissue cultures.

Polioviruses induce flaccid paralysis after intracerebral injection of rhesus monkeys. Some strains of poliovirus-2 induce encephalitis after intracerebral injection of suckling mice aged less than 48 hours. Virulent strains of each serotype induce encephalitis after intraspinal injection of suckling mice or rhesus monkeys, but attenuated strains do not induce symptoms in monkeys. Virulent strains viruce infection of tissue cultures in low (0.11%) concentrations of sodium bicarbonate (d+), after incubation at 40° C (rct 40+), attenuated

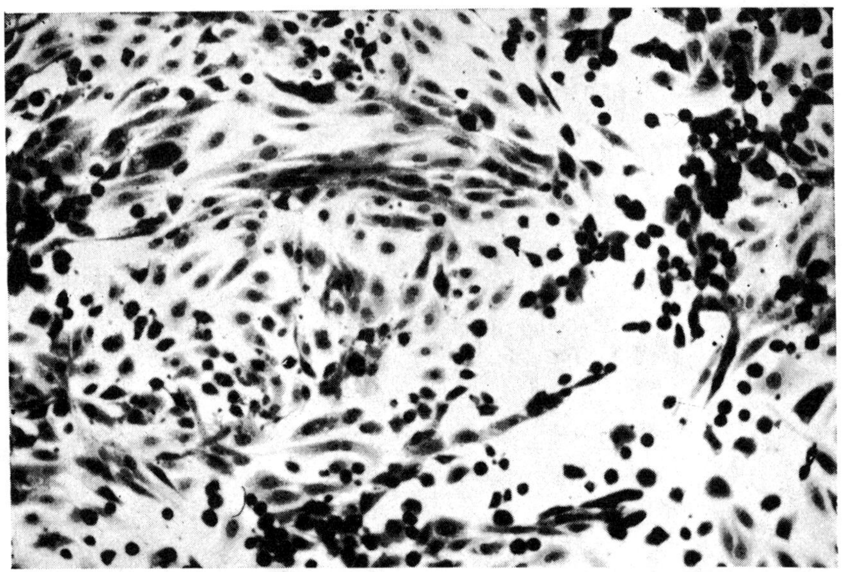

Figure 7-2: Cytopathic effect induced by poliovirus after growth in primary monkey kidney tissue culture H and E (x 113). Pyknotic cells are observed particularly on the right; intact cells are observed in the middle. Reproduced with permission from Rhodes AJ and Van Rooyen CE, 1968. Textbook of Virology 5th edition. Williams and Wilkins, Baltimore, p. 88.

strains do not multiply under these conditions. However infectivity of attenuated strains of poliovirus-1 is stabilized by heating in 20 mM.A1C1$_3$ for 1 hour at 50° C, infectivity of virulent strains is inactivated.

Poliovirus antibodies in patients' sera are routinely detected by neutralization tests. Using highly purified poliovirus antigens, the enzyme immunoassay (ELISA) technique offers a same-day alternative procedure for titration of poliovirus antibodies. Polioviruses do not agglutinate erythrocytes. The complement fixation test is not sufficiently serotype-specific for routine antibody titrations.

PATHOGENESIS

Poliovirus normally enters the body by ingestion of virus-contaminated food or water. Upon swallowing, the virus passes through the stomach and duodenum to enter the jejunal mucosa in which it multiplies without obvious destruction of cells. Most of the newly formed virus enters the jejunal lumen and in due course it is conveyed through the gastrointestinal tract to reach the exterior in the feces. Some virus reaches Peyer's patches (collections of lymphoid tissue in the submucosa). A limited amount of virus multiplication may occur in pharyngeal epithelium covering lymphoid tissue comprising the tonsils and adenoids, from which it may be excreted in the throat. Virus released after replication in jejunal or pharyngeal epithelium may enter the blood, inducing transient viremia, by which it is conveyed to the central nervous system which constitutes the target organ (Figure 7-3). Virus multi-

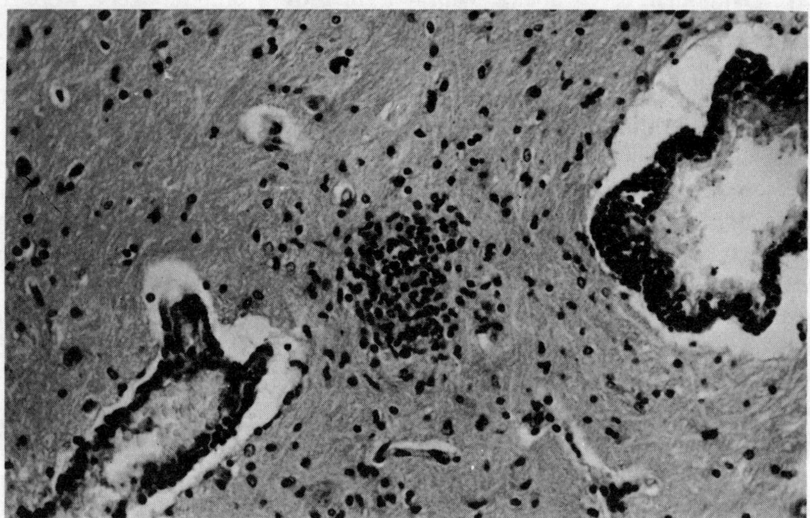

Figure 7-3: Focal lesion in brain caused by coxsackievirus B5 showing perivascular cuffing and a knot of proliferating glial cells from a case of neonatal meningoencephalitis and myocarditis. Reproduced with permission from McLean DM, 1980. Virology in Health Care. Williams and Wilkins, Baltimore, p. 69.

plication occurs both in the meninges, including hyperemia of cerebral blood vessels and outpouring of lymphocytes with CSF (aseptic meningitis), and also in motor neurones of the anterior horns of the spinal cord and the base of the brain, inducing neuronal destruction which gives rise to the pathological findings of neuronophagia and cuffing of cerebral blood vessels (Figure 4-2). This evokes clinical manifestation of flaccid paralysis of muscles supplied by the particular neurones. Virus excretion in feces may persist as long as one month. Neutralizing antibodies first appear in serum less than one week after onset of symptoms and they persist lifelong.

SYMPTOMATOLOGY

Poliomyelitis is characterized by flaccid paralysis of one or more skeletal muscle groups, usually accompanied by intense pain and spasm, regularly commencing 1–2 days after onset of aseptic meningitis (see next section). Lymphocytosis is observed in CSF during the initial week after onset. Minor febrile illness may sometimes precede the onset of paralysis. Characteristically patients are alert and apprehensive. Flaccid paralysis arises from selective destruction of groups of motor neurones in the anterior horn of the grey matter of the spinal cord or the base of the brain. The incubation period is 4 to 10 days. Although fever abates within a few days and recovery from the meningeal phase occurs within one week, mild to severe degrees of flaccid paralysis may persist indefinitely in limb muscles. Involvement of the basal ganglia of the brain may affect the respiratory and cardiovascular centers which may terminate fatally especially during pregnancy.

Coxsackievirus, Echovirus, Enterovirus
LABORATORY CHARACTERISTICS

Members of the genus *Enterovirus* apart from poliovirus are distinguished serologically from each other by neutralization tests. The 1982 Report of the International Committee on the Taxonomy of Viruses[14] designates human coxsackieviruses with serotypes A1–22 and 24 (coxsackievirus A23 is serologically identical with echovirus 9), human coxsackievirus B1–6, human echovirus 1–9, 11–27, 29–34, human enterovirus 68–71, human enterovirus 72 (hepatitis A virus) and additional enteroviruses which are pathogenic for mice, monkeys, cattle or pigs, exclusively.

Echoviruses and enteroviruses induce cytopathic effects in tissue cultures of primary monkey kidney and continuous human diploid cells (Figure 7-2). However hepatitis A virus from clinical material is not readily propagated in tissue cultures; one strain has multiplied in primary explant cultures of marmoset livers and in a normal fetal rhesus monkey kidney cell line (FRhK6).[16] Echoviruses except echovirus 9 are not pathogenic for newborn mice.

Coxsackieviruses B1–6 multiply and induce cytopathic effects in primary monkey kidney and continuous human diploid cell cultures. They also induce fatal encephalomyelitis after intracerebral injection of newborn mice aged less than 48 hours (suckling mice), together with varying degrees of necrosis of skeletal muscle (myositis). Coxsackieviruses A7, A9 and A16 are cytopathic for primary monkey kidney tissue cultures, other group A coxsackieviruses do not normally multiply in tissue culture systems used routinely. All group A coxsackieviruses multiply in newborn mice after intracerebral or intraperitoneal injection, inducing widespread myositis.

PATHOGENESIS

Enteroviruses, for example echovirus 9, enter the body through ingestion of virus-contaminated food or fluids. They multiply initially in the jejunal mucosa, from which they are excreted into the intestinal lumen and eventually they are excreted in feces for as long as 1–2 weeks after onset of illness (Figure 7-4). After initial replication in the intestinal mucosa and submucosal Peyer's

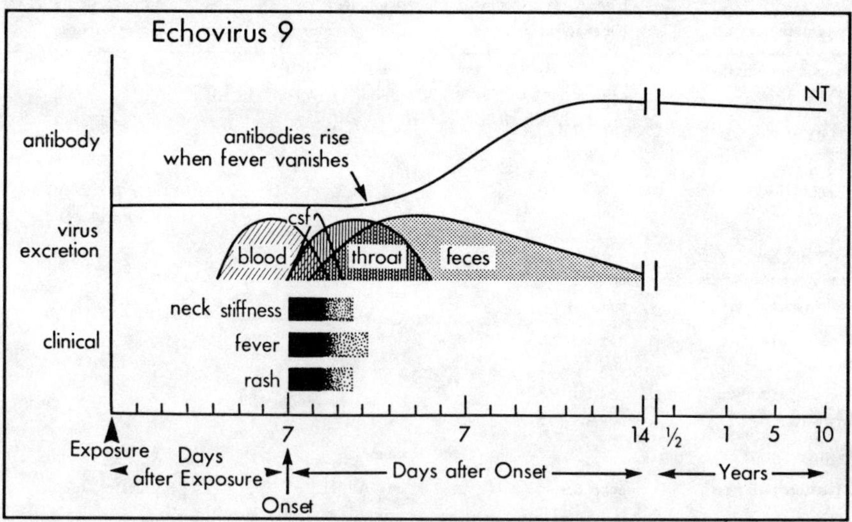

Figure 7-4: Time course of infection by echovirus 9. Reproduced with permission from McLean DM, 1980. Virology in Health Care. Williams and Wilkins, Baltimore, p. 69.

patches, virus may enter the blood stream briefly, by which it is conveyed to target organs such as the meninges where further viral multiplication occurs, inducing an acute inflammatory response with fever and clinical evidence of meningitis. Fever and meningeal signs usually abate after 2–4 days and thereafter convalescence is rapid and complete in most instances. Neutralizing antibodies characteristically are detected first in sera of patients within 1–2 days after remission of fever, coinciding with clinical recovery. Antibodies usually persist lifelong.

SYMPTOMATOLOGY

Syndromes associated with enterovirus infections are listed in Table 7-1. Although a particular syndrome such as aseptic meningitis may be induced by a wide range of enterovirus serotypes, in practice only relatively few serotypes have been associated regularly with recorded outbreaks of the disease during the past 3 decades. Furthermore a particular enterovirus serotype such as coxsackievirus B5 may induce a wide spectrum of clinical manifestations, whilst others such as coxsackievirus A16 may be restricted to one syndrome only, a vesicular exanthem.

TABLE 7-1
CLINICAL ASSOCIATIONS OF ENTEROVIRUS INFECTIONS

Syndrome	Commonly associated Enteroviruses	Less commonly associated Enteroviruses	Viruses apart from Enteroviruses
Aseptic meningitis	cox A9, B1–B5 echo 4,6,9,30	pol 1,2,3; cox B6 echo 7,11,14,16,17,18,33	mumps
Paralytic poliomyelitis	pol 1,2,3	cox A7, B5 echo 9, 11	
Encephalitis		pol 1,2,3	measles, herpes arboviruses
Neonatal meningoencephalitis and myocarditis	cox B1–B5 echo 11		
Pleurodynia	cox B1–B5		
Pericarditis	cox B1–B5		
Serous peritonitis	cox B1–B5		
Myositis	cox B1–B5		
Gastroenteritis		echo 18	rotavirus
Maculopapular rash	echo 6,9,16	cox A9,B1,B5	measles, rubella
Vesicular rash	cox A16	echo 9	herpes
Herpangina	cox A2, A4, A5, A6, A8, A10		
Conjunctivitis	ent 70		adenovirus
Hepatitis	ent 72 (hepatitis A)		
Croup		echo 11	parainfluenza
Coryza		cox A21	rhinoviruses

cox: coxsackievirus; echo: echovirus; ent: enterovirus; pol: poliovirus.

Aseptic Meningitis. Patients suddenly develop severe headache accompanied by vomiting and fever with temperatures above 38.5° C, together with stiffness of the neck and back, Kernig's sign (pain and spasm in the hamstring muscles on straightening the knee beyond a right angle) and Brudzinski's sign (when the head and neck are raised, the legs move upwards). The incubation period is 4–8 days. Regularly the CSF exhibits lymphocytosis with cell counts frequently exceeding 500 per mm^3 (CSF normally shows less than 10 lymphocytes per mm^3). Occasionally during the first few hours of illness, a higher proportion of polymorphonuclear leukocytes than lymphocytes may be observed in CSF. The glucose and protein levels in CSF remain unchanged. If patients are untreated, headache and neck stiffness may persist 3–5 days, but following lumbar puncture these symptoms may abate within 1 day.

Although complete clinical recovery occurs regularly within 5–7 days with no sequelae, rare examples of moderate or severe neurological sequelae have been reported. Transient muscle weakness has been noted during several outbreaks of aseptic meningitis due to non-polio enteroviruses. Usual causative enteroviruses are coxsackievirus A9 and B1–B5, together with echovirus types 4, 6, 9, 30. Aseptic meningitis may also arise from mumps virus infections (Chapter 8).

Encephalitis. Rarely, polioviruses may induce substantial damage among neurones at the base of the brain, causing sudden onset of hyperpyrexia (temperature above 40° C) with severe headache, clouding of consciousness, convulsions, irregular respiration and rapid irregular heart rate. This disease may terminate fatally. Encephalitis is also associated rarely with infection by other enterovirus serotypes, or with measles or herpesvirus, but arthropod-borne viruses are the usual causative agents (Chapter 10).

Neonatal Meningoencephalitis and Myocarditis. Infants born to mothers who contract group B coxsackievirus infections during the week immediately preceding delivery may develop elevated temperature, irritability, twitching, bulging of the anterior fontanelle and inability to take oral feedings within the first week of life. Neck stiffness and lymphocytosis of CSF indicate concomitant meningitis. A few days later, rapid respirations, rapid heart rate and hepatomegaly appear, which denote damage to the myocardium (myocarditis) and this terminates fatally. Extensive areas of necrosis of heart muscle is observed post-mortem. Each group B coxsackievirus serotype has induced this syndrome.

Pleurodynia. Patients develop sharp pains in the chest unilaterally which are aggravated by deep breathing or coughing. A pleural friction rub is frequently heard over the painful area, but pleural effusions are uncommon. The temperature is elevated to 38–39° C. Often patients experience severe pain in skeletal muscles of the trunk and limbs (myositis). Clinical recovery usually occurs within one week. Group B coxsackieviruses are causative agents.

Pericarditis. Sudden onset of severe pain in the precordium, accompanied by a pericardial friction rub, together with flattening and inversion of the T waves in leads V3 through V5 of the electrocardiogram is characteristic of coxsackievirus pericarditis. Usually there is no pericardial effusion, but occasional patients develop profuse serous effusions which may require removal by pericardial aspiration in order to prevent embarrassment to the circulation through cardiac tamponade. Although the pericarditis usually resolves completely within 2 weeks, constrictive pericarditis is an occasional complication. Group B coxsackieviruses are causative agents.

Serous Peritonitis. Patients develop severe generalized abdominal pain and tenderness accompanied by fever but the leukocyte counts remain normal.

Pleurodynia or pericarditis may sometimes occur simultaneously. Tenderness may become localized to the right lower abdominal quadrant, suggesting acute appendicitis, but if laparotomy is performed, the only abnormality detected is excessive serous fluid with or without enlarged mesenteric lymph nodes. Resolution of symptoms usually occurs within 3–5 days. Group B coxsackieviruses are the etiological agents.

Myositis denotes exquisitely tender skeletal muscles of the trunk and limbs, so that patients experience acute discomfort during routine nursing procedures or from the weight of the bed sheets. Occasionally this is the sole clinical manifestation of a group B coxsackievirus infection; in other patients the pleura or other serous membranes may be affected concomitantly. Summer grippe was the term formerly employed to describe summertime epidemics of coxsackievirus myositis, since muscle tenderness resembles that experienced during wintertime epidemics of influenza (grippe).

Gastroenteritis is a rare clinical manifestation of infection with enteroviruses. Outbreaks of watery yellow-green diarrhea affecting infants in newborn nurseries, together with their nursing attendants, have been attributed to echovirus 18 infection. However, most epidemics and individual cases of non-bacterial gastroenteritis are induced regularly by rotaviruses or other virions which are observed readily by electron microscopy of feces, but they are not isolated in tissue culture systems used routinely.

Maculopapular Rash. Blotchy or punctate maculopapular rashes may occur over the trunk and particularly the extremities including the palms of the hands, but without nasal catarrh or conjunctivitis. These epidemics usually occur during summertime. Echovirus 9 is the commonest causative enterovirus, but echovirus types 6 and 16, and some coxsackieviruses, have occasionally induced similar rashes. These enterovirus rashes are readily distinguished from two wintertime viral exanthemata, measles and rubella. Measles regularly induces nasal catarrh and conjunctivitis and the rash does not frequently extend to the palms; rubella induces a fine peach-bloom rash over the trunk but not the palms, and the post-auricular lymph nodes are always enlarged.

Vesicular Rash. Summertime outbreaks of febrile illnesses accompanied by vesicular eruptions over the hands and feet and also the oropharyngeal mucous membrane have been attributed to coxsackievirus A16 in several centers, and occasionally echovirus 9 infections induce vesicular rashes. Vesicles are readily distinguished clinically from herpes.

Herpangina denotes large (2–4 mm) painful vesicles in the posterior one-third of the oropharynx, accompanied by fever and constitutional upset. Several group A coxsackieviruses are the causative agents.

Conjunctivitis. Epidemics of acute hemorrhagic conjunctivitis have affected communities within tropical regions of Africa and Asia, extending northwards into Europe and Japan since 1969.[9,10,11] Common manifestations are sub-conjunctival hemorrhages and fever after an incubation period of 24 hours, sometimes accompanied by transient neurological disorders such as lumbosacral radiculitis. Enterovirus 70 has been identified regularly as the causative agent. Outbreaks are not related to the use of swimming pools, as in adenovirus conjunctivitis. Coxsackievirus A24 has also been implicated recently.

Hepatitis. After a few days of intense anorexia, elevation of the temperature to 38–39° C occurs, accompanied by nausea, vomiting and sudden onset of jaundice (yellow staining of skin and conjunctivae). This is sometimes accompanied by hepatomegaly or abdominal pain. The incubation period ranges from 15 to 40 days, average 30 days. The urine contains bilirubin and urobilinogen, which becomes darkened, and the feces become pale due to lack of bile pigments. Characteristically the serum levels of alanine aminotransferase (ALT) (formerly serum glutamic pyruvic transaminase, normal 6–35 units/ml) and aspartate aminotransferase (AST) (formerly serum glutamic oxalacetic transaminase, normal 15–40 units/ml) become elevated 4–7 days before onset of jaundice and remain elevated one week or more after disappearance of jaundice. In children, clinical recovery with disappearance of jaundice usually occurs within one week; adults may require longer durations to achieve full recovery. Occasional patients may develop acute yellow atrophy (massive liver necrosis) with death a few days after sudden onset of severe constitutional disturbances progressing through stupor and coma accompanied by increasing degrees of jaundice. Enterovirus 72, commonly termed hepatitis A virus, is the causative agent of acute hepatitis. Virions have been visualized by electron microscopy of feces collected before or at the onset of jaundice, but this virus cannot be cultured routinely.

Respiratory Tract Infections are rare clinical manifestations of enterovirus infections. Occasional cases of croup (acute laryngotracheobronchitis, see Chapters 8, 14) have been attributed to infection with echovirus 11 (U virus), whilst a few outbreaks of nasal catarrh resembling common colds (coryza) have been induced by coxsackievirus A21 (Coe virus).

REFERENCES - ENTEROVIRUSES

[1]Burnet FM, Macnamara J: Immunological differences between strains of poliomyelitis virus. Brit J Exp Path 12:57, 1931.

[2]Center for Disease Control: Poliomyelitis Surveillance. Summary 1974–1976, issued October 1977.

[3]Committee on Typing of the National Foundation for Infantile Paralysis: Immunologic classification of poliomyelitis viruses. I. A cooperative program for the typing of one hundred strains. Am J Hyg 54:191, 1951.

[4]Committee on the ECHO viruses: Enteric cytopathogenic human orphan (ECHO) viruses. Science 122:1187, 1955.

[5]Dalldorf G: The Coxsackie group of viruses. Science 110:594, 1949.

[6]Davis DC, Melnick JL: Association of ECHO virus type 6 with aseptic meningitis. Proc Soc Exp Biol Med 92:839, 1956.

[7]International Enterovirus Study Group: Picornavirus group. Virology 19:114, 1963.

[8]Kessel JF, Moore FJ, Pait CF: Differences among strains of poliomyelitis virus in *Macaca mulatta*. Am J Hyg 43:82, 1946.

[9]Kono R: Apollo 11 disease or acute hemorrhagic conjunctivitis: a pandemic of a new enterovirus infection of the eyes. Am J Epidemiol 101:383, 1975.

[10]Kono R, Miyamura K, Tajiri E, Shiga S, Sasagawa A, Irani PF, Katrak SM, Wadia NH: Neurologic complications associated with acute hemorrhagic conjunctivitis virus infection and its serologic confirmation. J Infect Dis 129:590, 1974.

[11]Kono R, Miyamura K, Yamazaki S, Sasagawa A, Kurahashi H, Tajiri E, Takeda N, Robin Y, Renaudet J, Ishii K, Nakazono N, Sawada H, Uchida Y, Minami K: Seroepidemiologic studies of acute hemorrhagic conjunctivitis virus (enterovirus type 70) in West Africa. II. Studies with human sera collected in West African countries other than Ghana. Am J Epidemiol 114:274, 1981.

[12]Landsteiner K, Popper E: Ubertragung der poliomyelitis acuta auf affen. Z. Immunitatsforsch. Orig. 2:377, 1909.

[13]McLean DM, Melnick JL: Association of mouse pathogenic strain of ECHO virus type 9 with aseptic meningitis. Proc Soc Exp Biol Med 94:656, 1957.

[14]Matthews REF: Classification and nomenclature of viruses. Intervirology 17:1, 1982.

[15]Melnick JL, Tagaya I, von Magnus H: Enteroviruses 69, 70 and 71. Intervirology 4:369, 1974.

[16]Provost PJ, Hilleman MR: Propagation of human hepatitis A virus in cell culture in vitro. Proc Soc Exp Biol Med 160:213, 1979.

[17]Robbins FC, Enders JF, Weller TH, Florentino GL: Studies on the cultivation of poliomyelitis viruses in tissue culture. V. The direct isolation and serologic identification of virus strains in tissue culture from patients with nonparalytic and paralytic poliomyelitis. Am J Hyg 54:286, 1951.

[18]Sabin AB: Present position of immunization against poliomyelitis with live virus vaccines. Brit Med J 1:663, 1959.

[19]Sabin AB: Reoviruses. A new group of respiratory and enteric viruses formerly classified as ECHO type 10 is described. Science 130:1387, 1959.

[20]Salk JE, Krech U, Youngner JS, Bennett BL, Lewis LJ, Bazeley PL: Formaldehyde treatment and safety testing of experimental poliomyelitis vaccines. Am J Pub Health 44:563, 1954.

[21]Trask JD, Vignec AJ, Paul JR: Poliomyelitis virus in human stools. JAMA 111:6, 1938.

[22]Tyrrell DAJ, Parsons R: Some virus isolations from common colds: III. Cytopathic effects in tissue cultures. Lancet 1:239, 1960.

RHINOVIRUS

BIOLOGICAL ATTRIBUTES

Rhinoviruses have particles 22–30 nm diameter which are naked and show icosahedral symmetry, and they contain RNA. Other physiochemical properties resemble those of enteroviruses (p. 100), except that rhinovirus infectivity is destroyed at pH 5 or lower, but enterovirus infectivity is retained below pH 5.

Rhinoviruses are isolated from human nasal or throat secretions by inoculation of tissue cultures of human diploid cells (MRC-5 or WI-38) or primary rhesus monkey kidney cells after incubation at 33° C in the presence of low concentrations (0.03%) of sodium bicarbonate. Cytopathic effects appear 2–7 days later, and these are inhibited by type-specific antiserum. Rhinoviruses have been adapted to growth in continuous cultures of human polyploid cells (HeLa).

A numbering scheme[1] for fresh rhinovirus isolates was developed in 1967 on the basis of cross-neutralization tests in tissue culture[2] and currently 113 serotypes are recognized internationally.[5] Each serotype has induced coryza (the common cold).

PATHOGENESIS

Rhinoviruses exert their pathological effects at the site of entry into the human host. Intense catarrhal inflammation of the nasal turbinate epithelium evokes a profuse watery nasal discharge which persists 1–2 days, but thereafter the discharge becomes mucopurulent due to secondary bacterial overgrowth.

SYMPTOMATOLOGY

After an incubation period of usually 2 days, human volunteers infected with rhinoviruses develop sneezing, watery nasal discharge requiring 15 or more tissue paper handkerchiefs per day, nasal obstruction, sore dry or scratchy throat, cough, headache, malaise and chilliness, but usually the temperature is elevated only slightly.[4,6] Symptoms may persist for 3–5 days. However bacterial superinfection rapidly causes the secretions to become mucopurulent. The above syndrome is termed coryza or the common cold. It is important to distinguish clinically between it and more extensive infections involving the tracheobronchial tree due to influenza and parainfluenza viruses. Contaminated hands, in addition to aerosols induced by sneezing, may transmit rhinoviruses.[3]

REFERENCES - RHINOVIRUSES

[1]A collaborative report: Rhinoviruses - extension of the numbering system. Virology 43:524, 1971.

[2]Conant RM, Hamparian VV: Rhinoviruses: basis for a numbering system. II. Serologic characterization of prototype strains. J Immunol 100:114, 1968.

[3]Gwaltney JM, Hendley JO: Rhinovirus transmission. One if by air, two if by hand. Am J Epidemiol 107:357, 1978.

[4]Hendley JO, Edmondson WP, Gwaltney JM: Relation between naturally acquired immunity and infectivity of two rhinoviruses in volunteers. J Infect Dis 125:243, 1972.

[5]Matthews REF: Classification and Nomenclature of Viruses. Intervirology 17:1, 1982.

[6]Tyrrell DAJ, Bynoe ML: Some further virus isolations from common colds. Brit Med J 1:393, 1961.

REOVIRIDAE

Reoviridae[10] contain three genera of viruses which induce human illness: Reovirus, Rotavirus, Orbivirus.

HISTORICAL

Reoviruses were first isolated from feces of normal high school children in Cincinnati, Ohio during summer 1953,[11] using tissue culture techniques for surveys of the prevalence of poliovirus. Formerly the initial isolate of reovirus 1 was designated echovirus 10,[13] but this designation was changed in 1959. Subsequently reoviruses were isolated from anal or throat swabs of children at a child care center in Washington D.C. during longitudinal surveys for the prevalence of viruses in mild febrile illnesses between 1955 and 1957.[12] Although they are encountered occasionally in patients with a wide variety of illnesses involving the gastrointestinal, respiratory or central nervous systems, their role in the causation of these illnesses is frequently obscure.

Orbiviruses have been implicated as the causative agents in the sheep disease bluetongue and the horse disease, African horse sickness, for many years. They are transmitted in nature by *Culicoides* sp. This group also contains tick-borne viruses: (a) Colorado tick fever[6] which was first described in 1944 in the Rocky Mountain region of the United States; and (b) viruses of the Kemerovo group[3] in eastern Europe, north Africa and western United States.

Rotaviruses were first visualized in 1973 during electron microscopic examination of duodenal mucosa obtained by biopsy[1] and from feces[2] of infants with gastroenteritis in Melbourne, Australia. Subsequently rotavirus particles have been observed regularly in feces of 20% or more of cases of acute gastroenteritis in many Temperate Zone communities throughout the world.[4,8,9] However, in the absence of any convenient technique for their propagation in the laboratory, their detection depends entirely on their visualization by electron microscopy[8] or demonstration of their antigens by enzyme immunoassay.[16]

BIOLOGICAL ATTRIBUTES
Properties Common to all Reoviruses

Reoviridae have cubically symmetrical (icosahedral) naked particles 60–80nm diameter with two protein coats; the inner coat is termed the core.[10] Particles contain 10–12 pieces of linear double stranded RNA with molecular weight $12–20 \times 10^6$. Virion protein contains 6–10 polypeptides, including transcriptase and other enzymes. Transcriptase activity is associated with the core. Cores have 12 spikes with fivefold symmetry arranged icosahedrally. Viruses multiply in the cytoplasm of infected cells.

PROPERTIES OF INDIVIDUAL GENERA

Reovirus. All 3 serotypes of reovirus propagate readily in primary monolayer cultures of rhesus or cynomolgus monkey kidney cells in which they induce the characteristic cytopathic effects of cell granularity and shrinkage, but the cells usually remain attached to the surface. Cytopathic effects are inhibited by mixture of reovirus with its serotype - specific antiserum. Reoviruses agglutinate human group 0 erythrocytes in unbuffered saline after holding at bench temperature 23° C for 1 hour. Hemagglutination is inhibited by type-specific antiserum after removal of non-specific inhibitors by absorption with kaolin. All reoviruses share a common complement fixing antigen.

Reoviruses induce encephalitis after intracerebral injection of newborn mice. Reovirus 3 infections are common within mouse colonies, inducing diarrhea (the oily hair effect). Although reoviruses have been isolated from patients with a variety of gastrointestinal and respiratory symptoms, their role as disease - inducing agents is not clear.

Orbivirus. Of the 12 currently recognized serological subgroups,[10] one subgroup contains the important human pathogen, Colorado tick fever virus, but some members within the Kemerovo (tick-borne) and the Changuinola (sandfly-borne) subgroups may also induce human illnesses. Colorado tick fever virus induces fatal encephalitis after intracerebral injection of newborn mice. It is transmitted biologically by *Dermacentor andersoni* ticks after infection in the field or the laboratory. It induces symptomless long-sustained viremia in small mammals of the Rocky Mountain region of U.S.A., especially golden mantled ground squirrels *(Citellus lateralis)*.

Antibodies to Colorado tick fever virus are detected by neutralization tests in mice or by complement fixation tests using as antigen a sucrose-acetone extract of infected suckling mouse brain.

Rotavirus. Rotavirus particles have total diameters 65–75 nm.[5,10] They contain negatively stained hubs 36–38 nm diameter, bounded by membranes from which an inner layer of capsomeres radiates outwards like short spokes and these are surrounded by an additional layer of capsomeres, giving the appearance of wheels[5] from which the name rotavirus is derived (rota=wheel). In feces obtained from children 2 or more days after onset of acute gastroenteritis,[8] both the typical double-shelled arrangement of capsomeres and those with outer shells only ("empty" particles) are observed regularly (Figure 7-5) but

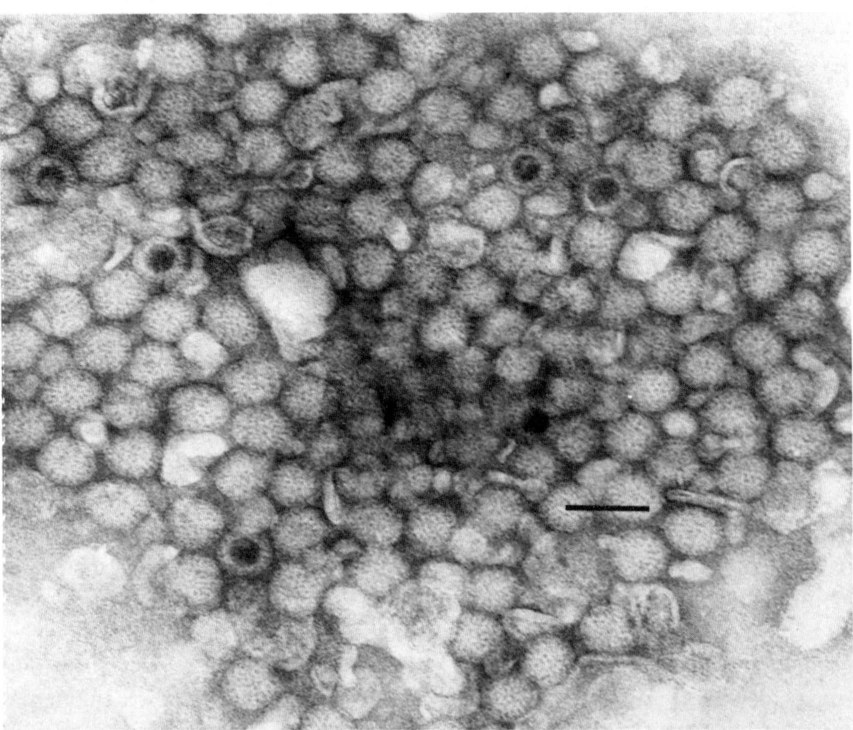

Figure 7-5: Rotavirus virions in feces of an infant aged 20 months with acute gastroenteritis (X120,120). Reproduced with permission from McLean DM and Wong KK, 1984. Same-day Diagnosis of Human Virus Infections. CRC Press, Boca Raton, FL, p. 94.

in a few patients, electron microscopy of feces may reveal 45 nm diameter particles consisting of cores surrounded by the inner layer of capsomeres only.

Rotaviruses differ morphologically from reoviruses, antigen grown in embryonic kidney cells has been employed in complement fixation tests to detect antibodies to human rotavirus in patients sera.[7] Using antisera prepared in guinea pigs and goats by injection of human rotavirus purified ultracentrifugally, an ELISA test has been developed and used extensively to detect rotaviruses in feces of patients.[16] By this technique 25% of Washington D.C. patients with infantile gastroenteritis excreted Rotavirus type 1 and 75% excreted type 2. Antibodies in patients sera are assayed best by an ELISA test. An additional 3 rotavirus serotypes have been defined subsequently.[4a]

PATHOGENESIS (ROTAVIRUS)

Rotaviruses enter patients through oral ingestion of foodstuffs and fluids contaminated with virus. Viral replication occurs in the mucosa of the small intestine, including catarrhal inflammation with outpouring of fluid rich in sodium ions. This stimulates peristalsis and the explusion of many watery yellow-green stools containing high concentrations of rotavirus particles. The duration of excretion ranges from about 2 days to 2 weeks (Figure 7-6). Generalized viremic infections are rare, and rotavirus is not usually excreted in the throat.

SYMPTOMATOLOGY (ROTAVIRUS)

Sudden onset of frequent watery yellow-green stools (as many as 10 or more per day) accompanied by moderate to severe degrees of dehydration is characteristic of infection with rotaviruses and other non-cultivatable electron-microscopically visible virions. The incubation period is about 2 days. Watery diarrhea usually abates within 1–2 days after total withdrawal of oral feedings and administration of adequate fluids and electrolytes intravenously, after which oral feedings are commenced gradually. Rotavirus excretion usually ceases 5–7 days after onset of diarrhea, but it may persist as long as 12 days.[8]

PATHOGENESIS (REOVIRUS)

Reoviruses probably enter the body through consumption of contaminated foodstuffs or fluids, or by children placing contaminated objects in the mouth. They are excreted for several days in feces, and thus they may be disseminated in nurseries and daycares by fecal contamination of fomites. Their multiplication within the human body appears to be confined to the gastrointestinal mucosa.

SYMPTOMATOLOGY (REOVIRUS)

Reoviruses have been isolated repeatedly from rectal or throat swabs of institutionalized children with mild febrile disorders or no discernible illness, but occasionally these children may have mild diarrhea or runny nose.

PATHOGENESIS (COLORADO TICK FEVER)

Colorado tick fever virus is introduced into the body through saliva of infected ticks which induce formation of a pool of blood subcutaneously where the mouthparts pierce the skin. Virus enters the blood stream, multiplies in endothelial cells and viremia appears 2–3 days later, persisting for 3–4 days. Thus induces fever, which may be biphasic, but it subsides with the appearance of antibody.

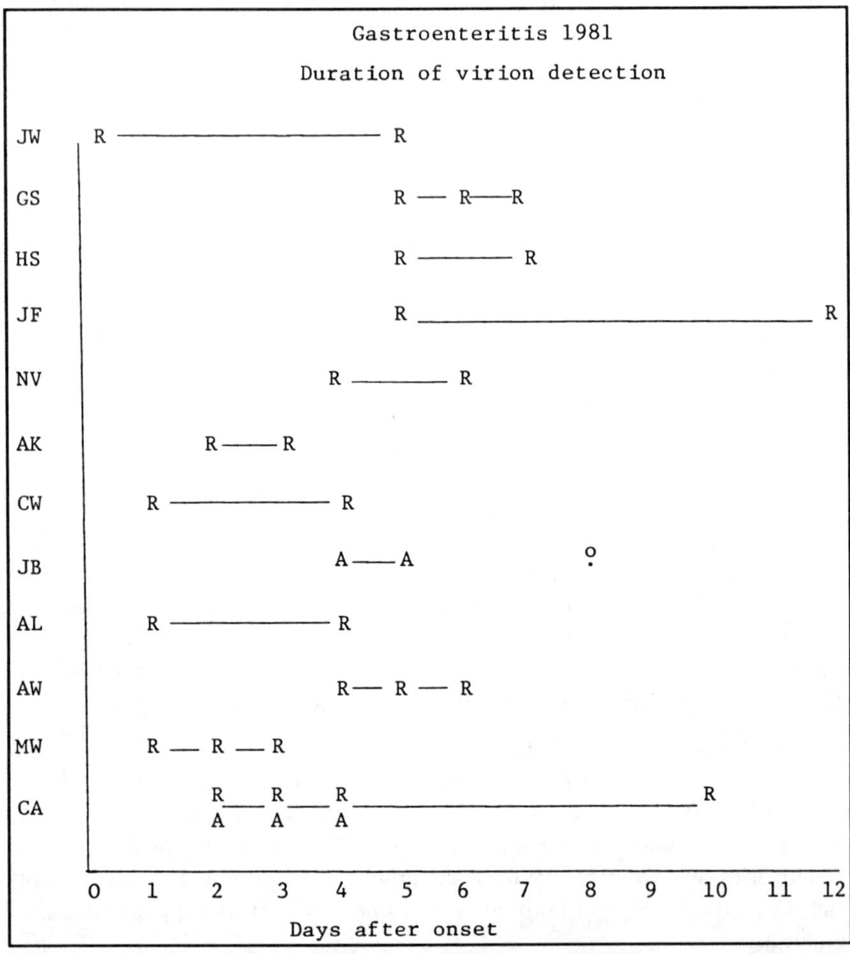

Figure 7-6: Duration of rotavirus excretion in feces of 12 infants with gastroenteritis. Reproduced with permission from McLean DM and Wong KK, 1984. Same-day Diagnosis of Human Virus Infections. CRC Press, Boca Raton, FL, p. 119.

SYMPTOMATOLOGY (COLORADO TICK FEVER)

Fever with temperatures as high as 39–40° C appears after an incubation period of about 7 days. Characteristically the fever shows a biphasic course during the ensuing 3–4 days, accompanied by severe muscle pains in the back and limbs, but usually there is no rash. Typically Colorado tick fever occurs during spring in the Rocky Mountain Region of USA where *Dermacentor andersoni* ticks are prevalent. Complete recovery is the rule.

REFERENCES - REOVIRIDAE

[1]Bishop RF, Davidson GP, Holmes IH, Ruck BJ: Virus particles in epithelial cells of duodenal mucosa from children with acute non-bacterial gastroenteritis. Lancet 2:1281, 1973.

[2]Bishop RF, Davidson GP, Holmes IH, Ruck BJ: Detection of a new virus by electron microscopy of faecal extracts from children with acute gastroenteritis. Lancet 1:149, 1974.

[3]Borden EC, Shope RE, Murphy FA: Physicochemical and morphological relationships of some arthropod-borne viruses to bluetongue virus—a new taxonomic group. Physicochemical and serological studies. J Gen Virol 13:261, 1971.

[4]Brandt CD, Kim HW, Yolken RH, Kapikian AZ, Arrobio JO, Rodriguez WJ, Wyatt RG, Chanock RM, Parrott RH: Comparative epidemiology of two rotavirus serotypes and other viral agents associated with pediatric gastroenteritis. Am J Epidemiol 110:243, 1979.

[4a]Dupont HL: Rotaviral gastroenteritis—some recent developments. J Infect Dis 149:663, 1984.

[5]Flewett TH, Bryden AS, Davies H, Woode GN, Bridger JC, Derrick JM: Relation between viruses from acute gastroenteritis of children and newborn calves. Lancet 2:61, 1974.

[6]Florio L, Stewart MD, Mugrage ER: The experimental transmission of Colorado tick fever. J Exp Med 80:165, 1944.

[7]Kapikian AZ, Cline WL, Mebus CA, Wyatt RG, Kalica AR, James HD, VanKirk D, Chanock RM, Kim HW: New complement fixation test for the human reovirus-like agent of infantile gastroenteritis. Lancet 1:1056, 1975.

[8]McLean DM, Wong KK: Same-day diagnosis of human virus infections. CRC Press, Boca Raton, FL, 1984.

[9]Madeley CR, Cosgrove BP, Bell EJ, Fallon RJ: Stool viruses in babies in Glasgow. I. Hospital admissions with diarrhea. J Hyg 78:261, 1977.

[10]Matthews REF: Classification and nomenclature of viruses. Intervirology 17:1, 1982.

[11]Ramos-Alvarez M: Cytopathogenic enteric viruses associated with undifferentiated diarrheal syndrome in early childhood. Ann NY Acad Sci 67:326, 1957.

[12]Rosen L, Hovis JF, Mastrota FM, Bell JA, Huebner RJ: An outbreak of infection with a type 1 reovirus among children in an institution. Am J Hyg 71:266, 1969.

[13]Sabin AB: Reoviruses. A new group of respiratory and enteric viruses formerly classified as ECHO 10 is described. Science 130:1387, 1959.

[14]Torres-Medina A, Wyatt RG, Mebus CA, Underdahl NR, Kapikian AZ: Diarrhea caused in gnotobiotic piglets by the reovirus-like agent of human infantile gastroenteritis. J Infect Dis 133:22, 1976.

[15]Wyatt RG, Kapikian AZ, Thornhill TS, Sereno MM, Kim HW, Chanock RM: In vitro cultivation in human fetal intestinal organ culture of a reovirus-like agent associated with non-bacterial gastroenteritis in infants and children. J Infec Dis 130:523, 1974.

[16]Yolken RH, Wyatt RG, Zissis G, Brandt CD, Rodriguez WJ, Kim HW, Parrott RH, Urrutia JJ, Mata L, Greenberg HB, Kapikian AZ, Chanock RM: Epidemiology of human rotaviruses types 1 and 2 as studied by enzyme-linked immunosorbent assay. New Eng J Med 299:1156, 1978.

CORONAVIRIDAE

HISTORICAL

Coronavirus isolations from nasal washings of subjects with common colds were first reported using organ cultures of human tracheal epithelium (B 814) in 1965 in England,[13] tissue cultures of human embryonic kidney cells (229E) in 1966 in Chicago,[4] and cultures of human tracheal epithelium (OC 43) in 1967 in Washington, DC.[6] These strains were morphologically identical to infectious bronchitis virus of chickens.[1] Subsequently the 229E strain was adapted to growth in continuous human diploid cells WI-38 with production of cytopathic effects,[4] and the OC 43 strain was adapted to a growth in suckling mouse brains.[7] The latter procedure provided a convenient source of antigens for complement fixation and hemagglutination inhibition which were used successfully in serological surveys of coronaviruses in children in Atlanta, Georgia[5] and Chicago.[8] Coronaviruses virions were first visualized in feces of young adults affected by an epidemic of gastroenteritis in Bristol, England during 1975.[3]

BIOLOGICAL ATTRIBUTES

Coronavirus particles are pleomorphic with diameters ranging from 75 to 160 nm.[11] Club-like projections 12–24 nm high protrude from the viral envelope (Figure 7-7). They contain one molecule of single stranded RNA with molecular weight $5.5 - 6.1 \times 10^6$. They show helical symmetry of the ribonucleoprotein strands with diameter 11–13 nm. The family Coronaviridae contains 11 viruses within one genus which infect humans or other vertebrates.[12]

Some coronavirus strains isolated from the throat are propagated with difficulty in tissue cultures of continuous human diploid cells (MRC-5 or WI-38) with production of cytopathic effects; other respiratory strains multiply in organ cultures of tracheal epithelium. Most enteric strains do not propagate in convenient laboratory tissue culture systems, and their detection depends on their visualization by electron microscopy of negatively stained preparations.[10]

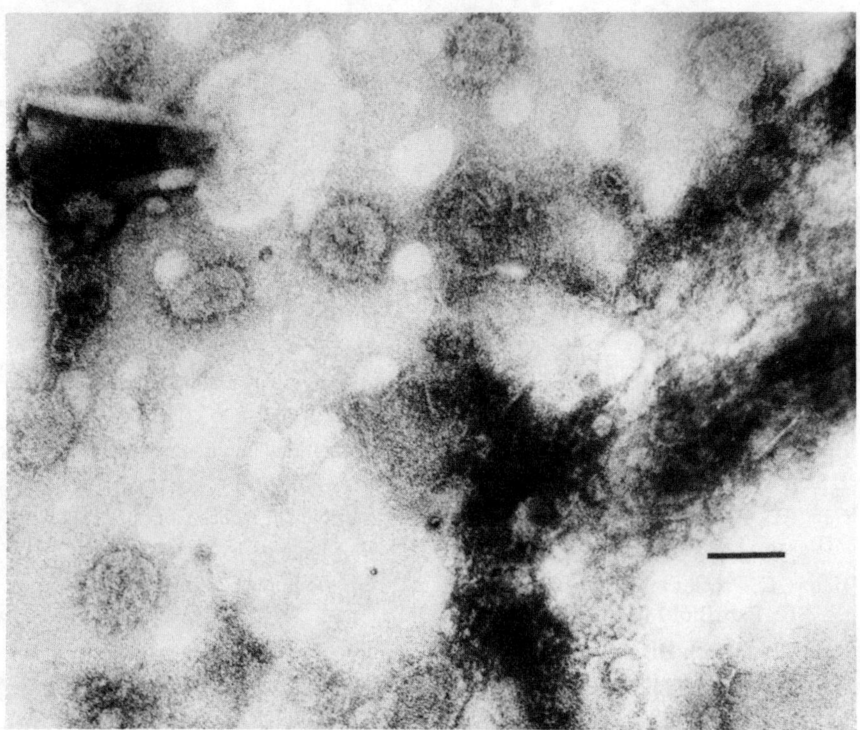

Figure 7-7: Coronavirus virions in feces from a 7-month-old boy with gastroenteritis, fever and rhinorrhea (X120,120). Reproduced with permission from McLean DM and Wong KK, 1984. Same-day Diagnosis of Human Virus Infections. CRC Press, Boca Raton, FL, p. 39.

PATHOGENESIS

After inhalation of virus-laden droplets or ingestion of virus-contaminated foodstuffs, coronaviruses appear to multiply in the mucosa of the respiratory and gastrointestinal tracts, from which they are discharged into the environment through the nasopharyngeal secretions and feces respectively. Recent observations in Vancouver pediatric patients[9] suggest that coronaviruses multiply preferentially in the gut of patients with histopathological anomalies such as Hirschspring's disease and ulcerative colitis, or in patients with immunosuppression after corticosteroid administration.

SYMPTOMATOLOGY

Respiratory infections with coronaviruses acquired naturally or after intranasal instillation of 229E virus[2] may exhibit runny nose and sneezing, together with mild fever, which is indistinguishable from the common cold due to rhinovirus infection.

Enteric infections with coronaviruses may show frequent watery yellow-green stools similar to diarrhea induced by rotavirus infection. However some patients may exhibit hemorrhagic colitis with frequent blood-stained stools, and symptoms may persist longer than one week.

REFERENCES - CORONAVIRIDAE

[1]Almeida JD, Tyrrell DAJ: The morphology of three previously uncharacterized human respiratory viruses that grow in organ culture. J Gen Virol 1:175, 1967.

[2]Bradburne AF, Bynoe ML, Tyrrell DAJ: Effects of a "new" human respiratory virus on volunteers. Brit Med J 2:767, 1967.

[3]Caul ED, Paver WK, Clarke SKR: Coronavirus particles in faeces from patients with gastroenteritis. Lancet 1:1192, 1975.

[4]Hamre D, Procknow JJ: A new virus isolated from the human respiratory tract. Proc Soc Exp Biol Med 121:190, 1966.

[5]Kaye HS, Marsh HB, Dowdle WR: Seroepidemiologic survey of coronavirus (strain OC 43) related infections in a children's population. Am J Epidemiol 94:43, 1971.

[6]McIntosh K, Dees JH, Becker WB, Kapikian AZ, Chanock RM: Recovery in tracheal organ cultures of novel viruses from patients with respiratory disease. Proc Nat Acad Sc USA 57: 933, 1967.

[7]McIntosh K, Becker WB, Chanock RM: Growth in suckling - mouse brain of "IBV-like" viruses from patients with upper respiratory tract disease. Proc Nat Acad Sc 58:2268, 1967.

[8]McIntosh K, Chao RK, Krause HE, Wasil R, Mocega HE, Mufson MA: Coronavirus infection in acute lower respiratory tract disease of infants. J Infect Dis 130:502, 1974.

[9]McLean DM: Viral gastroenteritis in Vancouver children 1983—British Columbia. Canada Dis Wkly Rep 10:17, 1984.

[10]McLean DM, Wong KK: Same-day diagnosis of Human Virus Infections. CRC Press, Boca Raton, FL, 1984.

[11]Matthews REF: Classification and nomenclature of viruses. Intervirology 17:1, 1982.

[12]Siddell SG, Anderson R, Fujiwara K, Klenk HD, Macnaughton MR, Pensaert M. Stohlman SA, Sturman L, van derZeijst BAM: Coronaviridae. Intervirology 20:181, 1983.

[13]Tyrrell DAJ, Bynoe ML: Cultivation of a novel type of common-cold virus in organ cultures. Brit Med J 1:1467, 1965.

CALICIVIRIDAE (and other small round viruses)

HISTORICAL

Small round viruses about 35 nm total diameter with crenated surfaces typical of the family Caliciviridae[9] have been isolated from the gastrointestinal tract and other organs of a variety of domestic animals such as cats, dogs and swine; one strain is associated with vesicular exanthema of swine. Since 1975 they have been observed in about 1% of human patients with acute gastroenteritis by electron microscopy of feces.[8] Other small round viruses with smooth surfaces and star-shaped internal markings termed Astroviruses,[7] or devoid of obvious features resembling picornaviruses, or with electron dense cores typical of parvoviruses[9] have also been observed in feces of gastroenteritis patients. Norwalk virus[3] was first reported in 1972 as a small round virus inducing an outbreak of gastroenteritis. Although initially considered to be a parvovirus, currently it is classified within the Caliciviridae.[9]

BIOLOGICAL PROPERTIES

Caliciviruses are round non-enveloped particles 35–39 nm total diameter with 32 cup-like depressions over the surface arranged in icosahedral symmetry.[9] They contain positive sense single strand RNA. When present, they are visualized in feces by negative-strain electron microscopy. To date there is no routine tissue culture system for propagation of human caliciviruses in the laboratory, but some strains have propogated in LLC-MK2 cells.

Human caliciviruses are visualized by electron microscopic examination of feces from patients with acute gastroenteritis.[5,6] All appear to multiply in the gut epithelium after ingestion of virus-contaminated foodstuffs or fluids. They are excreted in high concentrations in feces where they may be visualized either singly or in clusters, or as structured particles in addition to rotavirus virions. Morphologically, two distinct categories are recognized: (i) typical calicivirus (Figure 7-8) with the crenated outline, this probably includes Norwalk virus which was the first member of the family to be implicated as the causative agent in an epidemic of gastroenteritis; (ii) astrovirus (Figure 7-9) which has a smooth round outline and internal markings reminiscent of a star.[6]

Other small round viruses which are observed occasionally in feces of patients with gastroenteritis are picornavirus-like particles with total size about 28 nm, featureless outline and no obvious internal markings. These particles and the caliciviruses should be distinguished morphologically from parvoviruses which are 18–26 nm particles with smooth outline but they show electron dense cores 14–17 nm diameter.[9]

Parvoviridae are round non-enveloped particles 18–26 nm total diameter with icosohedral symmetry and they contain single stranded DNA.[9] They show

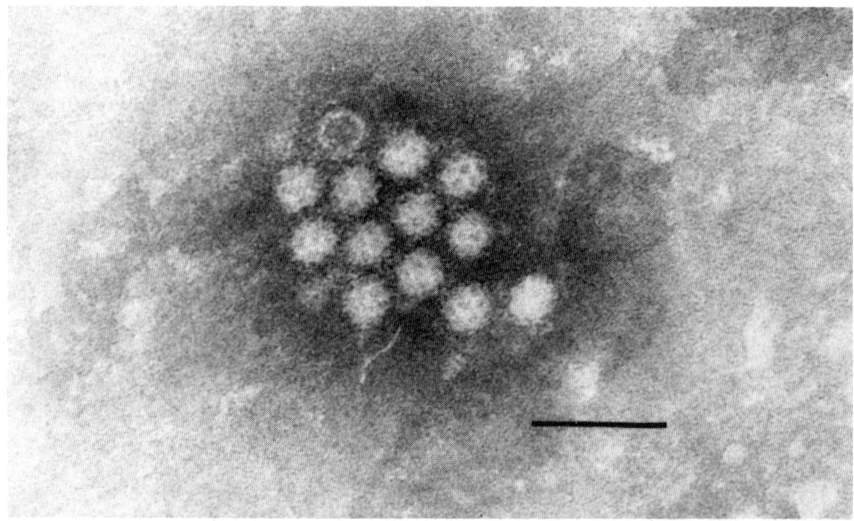

Figure 7-8: Calicivirus virions in feces of a gastroenteritis patient aged 2-1/2 years (X207,900). Reproduced with permission from McLean DM and Wong KK, 1984. Same-day Diagnosis of Human Virus Infections. CRC Press, Boca Raton, FL, p. 35.

smooth outlines and electron-dense cores 14–17 nm diameter. Currently they are classified into 3 genera: (a) *Parvovirus* which contains parvoviruses of cats (feline panleukopenia virus), dogs (canine parvoviruses causing severe enteritis), rats (Kilham's rat virus) and other vertebrates; (b) *Dependovirus* which contains the Adeno-associated virus group; (c) *Densovirus* which contains the insect parvovirus group which infect moths, mosquitoes and other insects. Although human parvoviruses have been visualized in feces of gastroenteritis patients in some communities, recent evidence indicates that they are more commonly associated with outbreaks of erythema infectiosum.[10]

SYMPTOMATOLOGY

Acute gastroenteritis, which clinically is indistinguishable from the syndrome induced by rotaviruses,[2] usually affects children, and less commonly adults, following infection by caliciviruses and other small round viruses.[1,8] Norwalk virus-induced gastroenteritis was acquired during swimming in recreational freshwater in Michigan.[4]

Parvoviruses have been demonstrated in the blood of two young adults with acute fever 9 days after being tattooed.[11] Serological evidence has implicated human parvovirus B19 as the causative agent in outbreaks of fifth disease (erythema infectiosum) in London suburbs and elsewhere in Great

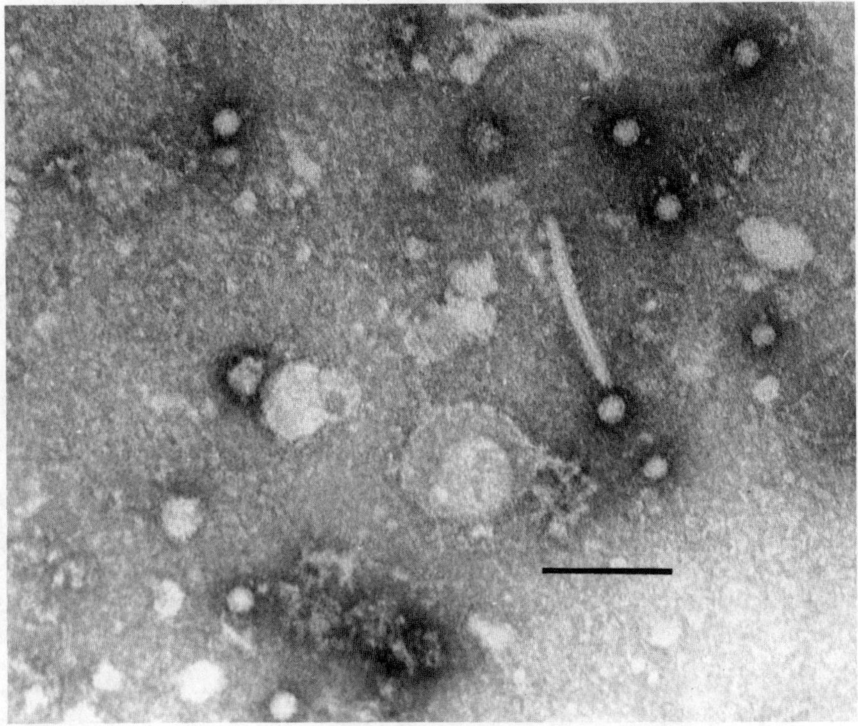

Figure 7-9: Astrovirus virions in feces of a girl aged 3-1/2 years with lipid storage disease and loose stools (X192,050). Reproduced with permission from McLean DM and Wong KK, 1984. Same-day Diagnosis of Human Virus Infections. CRC Press, Boca Raton, FL, p. 34.

Britain between 1980 and 1984.[10] Characteristic features of erythema infectiosum comprise malar flush ("slapped cheek") and a serpiginous, often recurrent, erythema on the trunk and limbs, together with transient fever, malaise and arthralgia which occur after an incubation period of about 10 days.[10]

REFERENCES - CALICIVIRIDAE
(small round viruses)

[1]Cubbitt WD, McSwiggan DA: Calicivirus gastroenteritis in Northwest London. Lancet 2:975, 1981.

[2]Dupont HL: Rotaviral gastroenteritis - some recent developments. J Infect Dis 149:663, 1984.

[3]Kapikian AZ, Wyatt RG, Dolin R, Thornhill TS, Kalica AR, Chanock RM: Visualization by immune electron microscopy of a 27 nm particle associated with acute infectious non-bacterial gastroenteritis. J Virol 10:1075, 1972.

[4]Koopman JS, Eckert EA, Greenberg HB, Strohm BC, Isaacson RE, Monto AS: Norwalk virus enteric illness acquired by swimming exposure. Am J Epidemiol 115:173, 1982.

[5]McLean DM, Wong KK: Same-day diagnosis of human virus infections. CRC Press Inc., Boca Raton, FL, 1984.

[6]Madeley CR: Comparison of the features of astroviruses and caliciviruses seen in samples of feces by electron microscopy. J Infect Dis 139:519, 1979.

[7]Madeley CR, Cosgrove BP: 28 nm particles in faeces in infantile gastroenteritis. Lancet 2:451, 1975.

[8]Madeley CR, Cosgrove BP: Caliciviruses in man. Lancet 1:199, 1976.

[9]Matthews REF: Classification and nomenclature of viruses. Intervirology 17:1, 1982.

[10]Public Health Laboratory Service: Fifth disease and the human parvovirus (B19). Communicable Disease Report 84/07, 1984.

[11]Shneerson JM, Mortimer PS, Vandervelde EM: Febrile Illness due to a parvovirus. Brit Med J 280:1580. 1980.

CHAPTER 8

ORTHOMYXOVIRIDAE, PARAMYXOVIRIDAE

RESPIRATORY VIRUSES

Respiratory tract infections are frequently caused by influenza virus (Orthomyxoviridae family) and parainfluenza and respiratory syncytial viruses (Paramyxoviridae family). Important childhood infections, measles and mumps are caused by two additional viruses within the Paramyxoviridae family. For convenience, these two virus families will be considered together.

HISTORICAL

Influenza virus was first isolated from throat washings of a medical scientist who contracted influenza in London, England during 1933, by intranasal inoculation of ferrets which subsequently developed fever and sneezing.[26] This was termed the WS strain. This procedure offered the first reliable laboratory technique for identification of viruses responsible for influenza epidemics. Following the great pandemic of 1919, influenza epidemics have continued to command world-wide attention due to disruption of normal community activities through sharply increased absentee rates at work and school, together with higher case-fatality rates among young adults and elderly citizens.[20] Both the WS strain and a 1934 isolate from Puerto Rico termed PR8[11] were adapted readily to mice which developed fatal bronchopneumonia after intranasal inoculation. Isolation of the MEL strain during an epidemic of influenza in Melbourne, Australia in 1935[3] demonstrated the prevalence of influenza virus in both hemispheres. These 3 topotypes were shown subsequently to share a common ribonucleoprotein antigen (S-antigen) in complement fixation tests,[19] but antigenic differences have been detected between isolates from different epidemics since 1936.[22] This shared S-antigen was designated type A which distinguished the above strains from ribonucleoprotein antigen of the Lee isolate termed type B which was first encountered during the 1940 epidemic of influenza in New York.[12] Currently most influenza epidemics are caused principally by influenza A or influenza B virus but occasional cases may be caused by influenza C which was first isolated from a single individual in New York during 1949.[13] Although the virus of swine influenza, first isolated in 1931[25] has caused repeated outbreaks among swine during subsequent years, it has been isolated only rarely from human cases of influenza in the mid-west[27] and New Jersey.[24]

Technical developments since 1940 greatly facilitated virological investigation of influenza epidemics and development of effective vaccines. During 1940, Burnet[4] reported the efficacy of amniotic inoculation of chick embryos for isolation of influenza viruses from patients. The 1941 report that influenza virus agglutinated chick erythrocytes, but that hemagglutination was inhibited by prior mixture of virus and corresponding antibody[15] provided a most convenient and rapid tool for virus identification and serological surveys. Inoculation of chick embryos remained the principal technique for isolation of influenza virus until superseded some 20 years later by tissue cultures.

Enhanced rates for isolation of influenza B virus using primary monkey kidney tissue cultures were first described in 1954[23] when cytopathic effects were observed. This was followed in 1955 by the first isolation of parainfluenza -2 virus from children with croup[7] and in 1956 by the initial isolations of respiratory syncytial virus from a child with pneumonia and another child with croup.[8] Development of the hemadsorption test[28] in 1957 facilitated the isolation of influenza virus during an epidemic in the same year and provided a new technique for the isolation of two additional serotypes of parainfluenza virus, types 1 and 3.[9]

Tissue culture techniques have also provided the key to our present understanding of the epidemiology of two common childhood virus infections, measles and mumps, both of which have been controlled effectively through the development and widespread administration of live virus vaccines.[5,6] Isolation of mumps virus was first achieved by inoculation of monkeys in 1935,[16] and hemagglutination after growth in chick embryos was demonstrated in 1945.[18] Since the late 1950's tissue cultures have been used routinely for mumps virus isolations.[21] Measles virus was first isolated using tissue cultures in 1954.[10]

The term "myxovirus"[1] was first applied in 1955 to the group of viruses comprising influenza (types A, B and C) and mumps which infect humans, together with Newcastle disease and fowl plaque which infect mainly birds. These viruses agglutinated erythrocytes by virus attachment to mucoproteins on the red cell surfaces, and they eluted (detached) from erythrocytes through degradation of the mucoprotein receptors by neuraminidase[14] which is an enzyme on the surface of the virus particles. (The term, myxo=mucus, denotes the close associations between these viruses and mucoproteins). Development and standardization of the phosphotungstic acid negative staining technique in 1959[2] permitted detailed studies of viral ultrastructure so that by 1962 the existence of two main categories within the myxovirus group became obvious.[29] The influenza subgroup contained the viruses of human influenza which showed total particle diameters of 80–120nm and a nucleocapsid diameter of 9nm. The Newcastle disease subgroup contained the human viral pathogens parainfluenza, measles and respiratory syncytial virus, plus the avian pathogen Newcastle disease virus which may cause conjunctivitis in humans infected accidentally. Total particle diameters of viruses in the latter subgroup were 150–300nm and a nucleocapsid diameter was 18nm. By 1971, the term "paramyxovirus"[30] was advocated to describe the Newcastle disease subgroup, but in 1976 this designation was superseded by the family name Paramyxoviridae.[17]

REFERENCES

[1]Andrewes CH, Bang FB, Burnet FM: A short description of the myxovirus group (influenza and related viruses). Virology 1:176, 1955.

[2]Brenner S, Horne RW: A negative staining method for high resolution electron microscopy of viruses. Biochim Biophys Acta 34:103, 1959.

[3]Burnet FM: Virus isolated from Australian epidemic. Med J Aust 2:651, 1935.

[4]Burnet FM: Influenza virus infections of the chick embryo by the amniotic route. I. General character of the infections. Aust J Exp Biol Med Sci 18:353, 1940.

[5]Centers for Disease Control: Mumps - United States, 1980–1983. MMWR 32:545, 1983.

[6]Centers for Disease Control: Measles - United States, 1983. MMWR 33:105, 1984.

[7]Chanock RM: Association of a new type of cytopathogenic myxovirus with infantile croup. J Exp Med 104:555, 1956.

[8]Chanock RM, Finberg L: Recovery from infants with respiratory illness of a virus related to chimpanzee coryza agent (CCA). I. Isolation, properties and characterization. Am J Hyg 66:281, 1957.

[9]Chanock RM, Parrott RH, Cook MK, Andrews BE, Bell JA, Reichelderfer T, Kapikian AZ, Mastrota FM, Huebner RJ: Newly recognized myxoviruses from children with respiratory disease. New Eng J Med 258:207, 1958.

[10]Enders JF, Peebles TC: Propagation in tissue cultures of cytopathogenic agents from patient with measles. Proc Soc Exp Biol Med 86:277, 1954.

[11]Francis T Jr: Transmission of influenza by a filterable virus. Science 80:457, 1934.

[12]Francis T Jr: A new type of virus from epidemic influenza. Science 92:405, 1940.

[13]Francis T Jr, Quilligan JJ Jr, Minuse E: Identification of another epidemic respiratory disease. Science 112:495, 1950.

[14]Gottschalk A: Neuraminidase: the specific enzyme of influenza virus and *Vibrio cholerae*. Biochim Biophys Acta 23:645, 1957.

[15]Hirst GK: The agglutination of red cells by allantoic fluid of chick embryos infected with influenza virus. Science 94:22, 1941.

[16]Johnson CD, Goodpasture EW: An investigation of the etiology of mumps. J Exp Med 59:1, 1934.

[17]Kingsbury DW, Bratt MA, Choppin PW, Hanson RP, Hosaka Y, Ter Muelen V, Norrby E, Plowright W, Rott R, Wunner WH: Paramyxoviridae. Intervirol 10:137, 1978.

[18]Levens JH, Enders JF: The hemagglutinative properties of amniotic fluid from embryonated eggs infected with mumps virus. Science 102:117, 1945.

[19]Lief FS, Henle W: Methods and procedures for use of complement-fixation technique in type- and strain-specific diagnosis of influenza. Bull WHO 20:411, 1959.

[20]Loosli CG, Portnoy B, Myers EC: International bibliography of influenza 1930–1959. University of Southern California Press 1978, 348 pp.

[21]McLean DM, Walker SJ, Wyllie JC, McQueen EJ, McNaughton GA: Infections of the central nervous system with mumps and enteroviruses in Toronto, 1960. Can Med Ass J 84:941, 1961.

[22]Magill TP, Francis T Jr: Antigenic differences in strains of human influenza virus. Proc Soc Exp Biol Med 35:463, 1936.

[23]Mogabgab WJ, Green IJ, Dierkhising DC, Phillips IA: Isolation and cytopathogenic effect of influenza B viruses in monkey kidney cultures. Proc Soc Exp Biol Med 89:654, 1955.

[24]Seal JR, Sencer DJ, Meyer HM Jr: A status report on national immunization against influenza. J Infec Dis 133:715, 1976.

[25]Shope RE: Swine influenza III. Filtration experiments and etiology. J Exp Med 54:373, 1931.

[26]Smith W, Andrewes CH, Laidlaw PP: A virus obtained from influenza patients. Lancet 2:66, 1933.

[27]Smith TF, Burgert EO Jr, Dowdle WR, Noble GR, Campbell R, Van Scoy RE: Isolation of swine influenza virus from autopsy lung tissue in man. New Eng J Med 249:708, 1976.

[28]Vogel J, Shelokov A: Adsorption-hemagglutination test for influenza virus in monkey kidney tissue culture. Science 126:358, 1957.

[29]Waterson AP: Two kinds of myxovirus. Nature (London) 193:1163, 1962.

[30]Wildy P: Classification and nomenclature of viruses. Monographs in Virology vol. 5, p. 47, Karger, Basel 1971.

INFLUENZA VIRUSES

BIOLOGICAL ATTRIBUTES

Influenza viruses are classified within the virus family Orthomyxoviridae[11] which contains 2 genera, influenza A and B and a possible third genus influenza C. Each genus is distinguished by the antigenic category of the helically symmetrical nucleocapsid (S-antigen) which contains 8 molecules of linear negative-sense single stranded RNA with total molecular weight 5×10^6. Enveloped virions are pleomorphic with total diameters 80–120nm, but the length is up to several micrometers ("filamentous form"). Nucleocapsid strands with diameter 9nm and cross striations every 4nm which comprise the virus core are arranged helically within the lipoprotein envelope which contains 2 categories of surface projections: (a) hemagglutinins (HA) which are protein rods 14nm length x 4nm diameter; (b) neuraminidase (NA) which are club-shaped proteinaceous structures with heads 4 x 8.5nm attached to stalks 10 x 4nm. The lipoprotein envelope is termed the V-antigen (Figure 8-1).

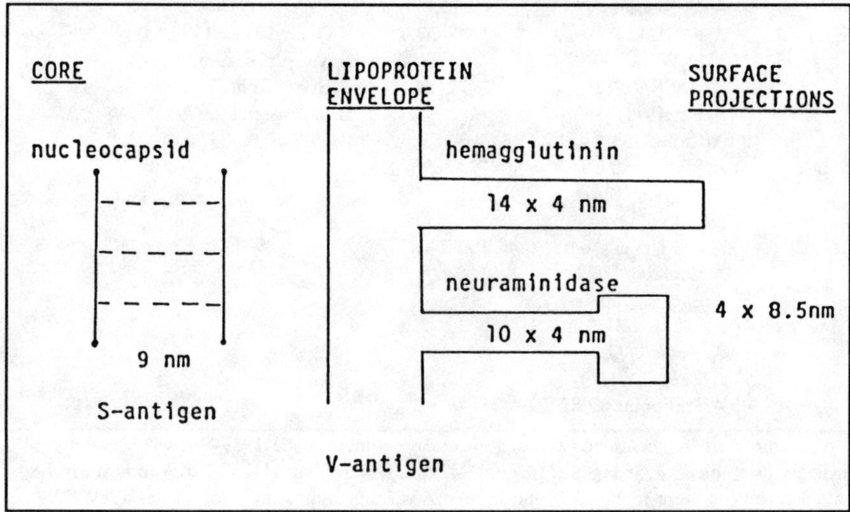

Figure 8-1: Diagram of antigenically active components of influenza virion.

Influenza viruses are named using the scheme approved by the World Health Organization for implementation in January 1972.[12] For example, the influenza strain with biological properties typical of those isolated during the 1972 epidemic throughout England was selected as the topotype (reference strain) and named A/England/42/72/(H3N2). The name includes the country or locality of the epidemic (England), the antigenic type of the ribonucleoprotein (A), the accession number of the isolate in the laboratory (no. 42), the year of isolation (1972), together with the antigenic category of the hemagglutinin (H3) and the neuraminidase (N2) (Table 8-1). For influenza viruses of non-human origin, the vertebrate species is designated thus: swine influenza hemagglutinin ($H_{SW}1$), avian influenza neuraminidase ($N_{AV}2$). Hemagglutinin and neuraminidase categories are always included with influenza A virus names, but they are omitted from influenza B and C names.

Influenza viruses are isolated readily from throat secretions of infected

TABLE 8-1

ANTIGENIC SHIFT AND DRIFT OF HUMAN INFLUENZA VIRUSES 1933–1984*

	Influenza A		*Influenza B*	
H,N category	*Reference Strain*	*Year of prevalence*	*Reference Strain*	*Year of prevalence*
H0N1[§]	A/WS/1/33	1933–46	B/Lee/40	1940–53
	A/PR/8/34		B/Melbourne/4/53	
	A/Melbourne/1/35			
H1N1	A/FM/1/47	1947–57	B/Great Lakes 1739/54	1954–84
	A/FLW/1/52		B/Massachusetts/3/66	
	A/USSR/90/77	1977–84	B/Hong Kong/5/72	
	A/Brazil/11/78		B/Singapore/222/79	
	A/Chile/1/83		B/USSR/100/83	
H2N2	A/Singapore/1/57	1957–67		
	A/England/12/64			
	A/Tokyo/3/67			
H3N2	A/Hong Kong/8/68	1968–84		
	A/England/42/72			
	A/Port Chalmers/1/73			
	A/Victoria/3/75			
	A/Texas/1/77			
	A/Bangkok/1/79			
	A/Philippines/2/82			

*Antigenic drift has continued through successive winters until 1989–90, when current isolates resembled: A/Shanghai/11/87 (H3N2), A/Taiwan/1/86 (H1N1), B/Yamagata/16/88. All 3 serotypes were included in the influenza vaccine formulation for winter 1989–90.
[§]After 1980, these were designated as H1N1 strains.

humans by inoculation of primary rhesus monkey kidney tissue cultures. After incubation of some cultures at 33° C and others at 35–37° C for 3 or more days, hemadsorption is demonstrated by removal of tissue culture supernatant and addition of 0.1% saline suspensions of erythrocytes from humans (group 0), guinea pigs, geese or chickens (Figure 8-2).[10] All type B isolates and some type A strains agglutinate mammalian and avian erythrocytes at the same titer, i.e., they are in the D-phase (derived) whilst other type A isolates agglutinate mammalian erythrocytes at higher titers than avian cells, i.e., they are in the O-phase (original) of Burnet and Bull,[3] from which they usually change into the D-phase after several passages at high multiplicity of infection. This O- D transformation of influenza A isolates was first reported in 1943 using amniotic inoculation of chick embryos which was the standard procedure for isolation of influenza virus from 1940 until superseded by tissue cultures around 1960. After primary isolation using either of the above techniques, influenza viruses grow to high titer following allantoic inoculation of chick

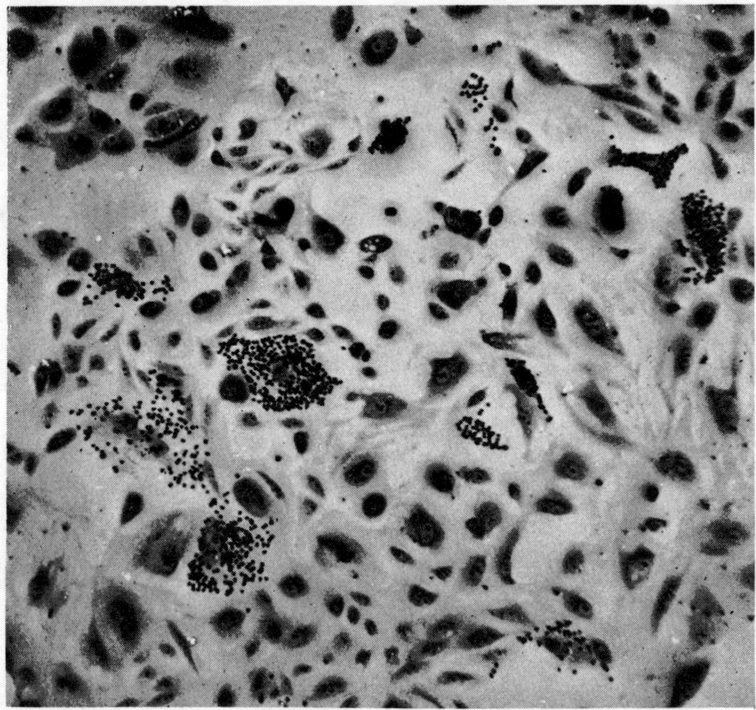

Figure 8-2: Hemadsorption following growth of influenza A virus in primary monolayer culture of monkey kidney cells. Leishman's stain (x120). Reproduced with permission from Rhodes AJ and Van Rooyen CE, 1968. Textbook of Virology, 5th edition, Williams and Wilkins, Baltimore, p. 86.

embryos (Figure 8-3). Allantoic fluid provides an excellent source of influenza virus, relatively free of extraneous material, for conduct of hemagglutination inhibition (HI) and complement fixation (CF) tests and for the manufacture of influenza vaccine.

Influenza viruses propagate in the mucous membranes of the nasal turbinates of ferrets after intranasal inoculation, inducing fever and sneezing, and followed by production of high titer serotype-specific HI antibody. Influenza viruses multiply throughout the tracheobronchial trees of mice, and some strains have been adapted to induce bronchopneumonia. Serotype-specific antibody is produced readily after intravenous injection of rabbits or chickens, usually in the absence of fever or other symptoms.

When the envelopes of influenza virus particles are disrupted by treatment with lipid solvents such as ether or sodium deoxycholate, virus particles lose

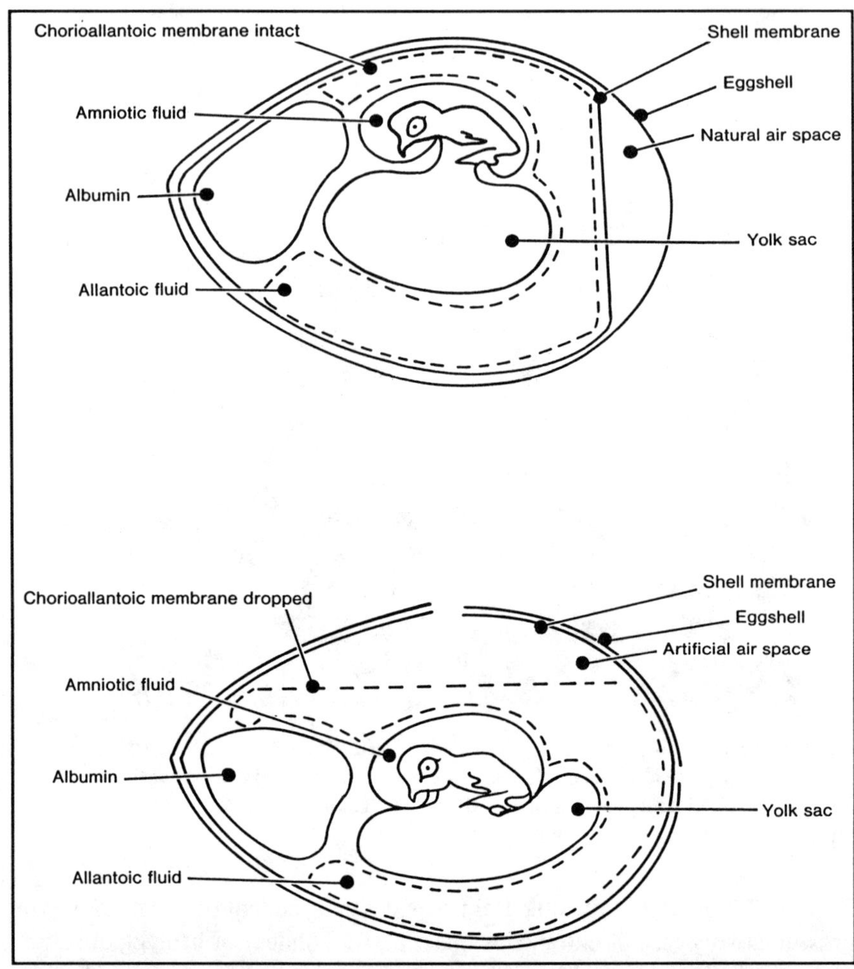

Figure 8-3: Diagram of fertile hen egg (chick embryo) after 11 days incubation. Reproduced with permission from McLean DM, 1980. Virology in Health, Williams and Wilkins, Baltimore, p. 36.

their infectivity and the nucleocapsid is liberated into suspension. The nucleocapsid antigen, termed the soluble (S-antigen), due to its low sedimentation coefficient (30 S) in contrast to the whole virus particle (600 S), is detected readily by complement fixation. All influenza A isolates show the same antigenic determinants of the S-antigen, which differ those of influenza B isolates. Lipoprotein envelopes contain the virus (V-antigen) which is detected by complement fixation. Isolates of a particular year share the same V-antigen.

Hemagglutinin and neuraminidase glycoproteins have been isolated from viral envelopes by additional biochemical and biophysical procedures. Morphologically, both these subunits appear as spikes protruding from the viral envelope (Figure 8-4). Hemagglutinin attaches to a mucoprotein receptor on

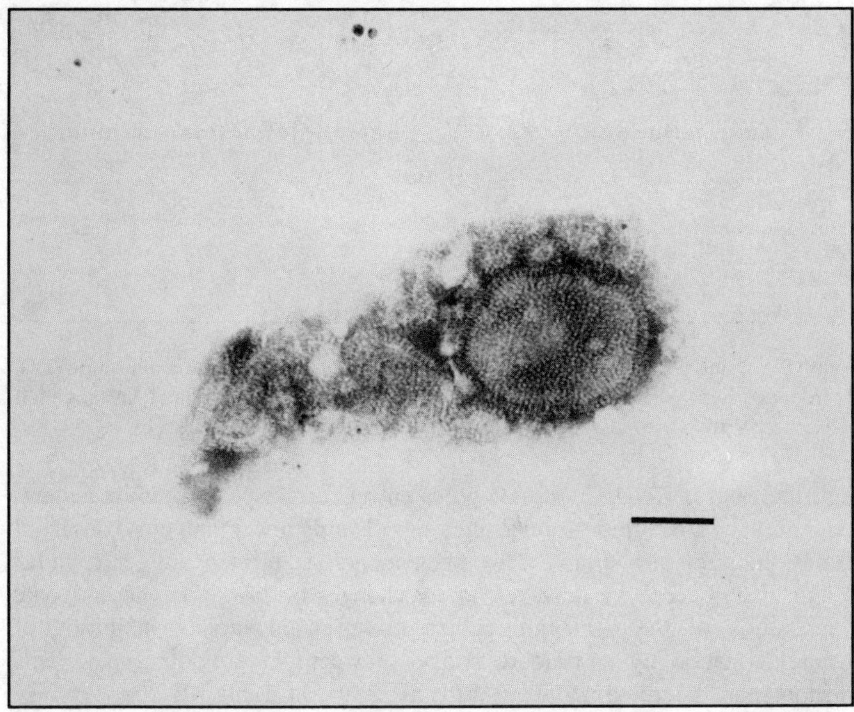

Figure 8-4: Influenza A (H3N2) virion isolated from the sputum of an infant with bronchiolitis (X120,120). Reproduced with permission from McLean DM and Wong KK, 1984. Same-day Diagnosis of Human Virus Infections, CRC Press, Boca Raton, FL, p. 60.

the surface of erythrocytes, causing hemagglutination through the binding of one virus particle to two erythrocytes (dimer formation) (Figure 8-5). Hemagglutination is inhibited by addition of antiserum to the same serotype of influenza virus before addition of erythrocytes.

Substantial changes in the antigenic composition of the hemagglutinin, have occurred at intervals of 10 years or more. Antibody to the current year's virus serotype inhibits hemagglutination by isolates of all previous years at

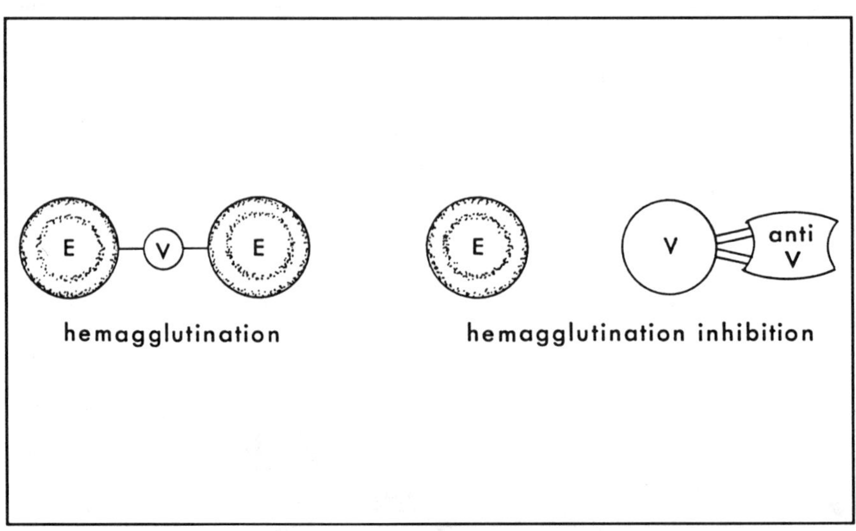

Figure 8-5: Principle of hemagglutinination (HA) and hemagglutination inhibition (HI). Reproduced with permission from McLean DM, 1982. Immunological Investigation of Human Virus Diseases, Churchill Livingstone, Edinburgh, p. 9.

high titer, but antibody to strains prevalent in former years inhibits hemagglutination by the current strain at titers significantly lower than those observed against homologous strains. This phenomenon is termed antigenic shift.[2] Within this 10-year era however, minor changes occur within the antigenic composition of the hemagglutinin resulting in incomplete inhibition of hemagglutination by antisera to strains prevalent in previous years. This phenomenon is termed antigenic drift, as shown in Table 8-1.

Antigenic shift and drift have occurred more frequently with influenza A than influenza B viruses. After the initial isolation of influenza A/WS/1/1933 (HON1) in 1933, HON1 strains remained prevalent until 1946, when a shift occurred to HINI early in 1947. Some antigenic drift was noted during subsequent years, but this category remained dominant until 1956. Antigenic shift to H2N2 was noted during the 1957 pandemic, with emergence of strains resembling A Singapore/1/57 (H2N2). Antigenic drift was observed among H2N2 isolates during successive years until 1967. Strains causing the 1968 pandemic showed antigenic shift to H3N2, but antigenic drift has been observed in epidemic strains during subsequent years to 1990. During the 1977-78 winter,H1N1 strains which had not been encountered since 1957, emerged concurrently with H3N2 strains in many Northern Hemisphere epidemics. Antigenic drift of H1N1 strains was noted during 1978 and 1983, but these strains have continued to co-exist alongside H3N2 strains through 1990 in both Hemispheres.[5]

Antigenic shift and drift have been noted less frequently among influenza B strains. After the initial isolate B/Lee/40 during 1940, isolates during subsequent years showed some degree of antigenic drift until B/Melbourne/4/53. Antigenic shift was first detected with the emergence of strains resembling B/Great Lakes/1739/54 during the 1954-55 winter. Antigenic drift has been observed among epidemic strains during subsequent years through 1990.[6]

PATHOGENESIS

Influenza viruses typically induce surface infections (Chapter 4).[1] After inhalation in droplet nuclei, influenza virus multiplies within epithelial cells of the nasopharyngeal and tracheobronchial mucosa, slowing ciliary action and causing cellular desquamation plus increased exudate. Accumulation of bronchial exudate at the bifurcation of the trachea stimulates coughing, thereby expelling droplets laden with influenza virus. These are disseminated into the air within a 2 meter radius of the patient, thereby providing ample opportunity for spread of infection through inhalation by close contacts.

Influenza virus is excreted in the throat for 2 to 5 days after onset of illness. The incubation period is 2 days. Antibodies are first detected by complement fixation using the S-antigen about 7 days after onset, and subsequently by hemagglutination inhibition and by complement fixation using the V-antigen about 10 to 14 days after onset. Antibodies to the S-antigen persist 3 to 6 months; antibodies titrated by HI and V-CF techniques persist 1 to 2 years. Influenza vaccines (killed) induce antibody responses which are detected by HI and V-CF tests only, not S-CF tests.

Upon reinfection of a subject several years after a previous influenza virus infection, HI antibody titers against the serotype which caused the first infection are significantly higher than those against the current virus strains. This principle is termed the doctrine of "original antigenic sin".[8]

SYMPTOMATOLOGY

Influenza denotes the symptoms and signs arising from infection of the respiratory tract with influenza A, B or C viruses. In children and young adults, after an incubation period of about 2 days, headache and lassitude occur, followed in a few hours by fever (temperatures 38–40° C), and subsequently by aches and pains in the back and legs, feelings of weakness, dry hacking cough and reddened glazed mucous membranes of the mouth and nose. Fever usually persists 2-3 days, but myalgia and weakness may persist an additional

2 days, and the average period off duty is usually about 5 days.[9] Symptoms are frequently more severe in infants and especially in the elderly who regularly experience high mortality rates due to influenza and pneumonia during epidemics.[1] Secondary bacterial infection of the respiratory tract frequently complicates the primary catarrhal inflammation of the bronchiolar mucosa due to influenza virus, inducing loose cough with production of copious mucopurulent sputum and accompanied in some instances by clinical and radiological evidence of bronchopneumonia. Other complications are rare, but Reye syndrome comprising acute onset of encephalopathy and liver dysfunction, eventually leading to fatty degeneration in fatal cases, has been associated with 1:2000 to 1:100,000 cases of influenza.[4]

Influenza characteristically occurs during the cooler months of the year. Typically it occurs in epidemics of 4–6 weeks duration. Usually it affects simultaneously most countries in the same climatic zone, between October and March in the North Temperate Zone and between May and August in the South Temperate Zone. Peaks of influenza prevalence are also observed in the tropics, despite the relative lack of seasonal temperature variations.

The most useful epidemiological parameter of an influenza epidemic is the increase of the percentage weekly rate of mortality attributed to pneumonia and influenza above the expected average rate for the period,[7] which in mid-winter is about 6.5% in the United States (Figure 8-6). Additional epidemiological parameters include abrupt increases of: (a) daily school absentee rates more than 2 standard deviations above the average daily expected rate for the period; (b) emergency room attendances or physician office visits with influenza-like illnesses.

REFERENCES - INFLUENZA

[1]Beveridge WIB: Immunity to viruses: a general discussion with special references to the role of allergy. Lancet 2:299, 1952.

[2]Burnet FM: Principles of Animal Virology, pp. 380–382. Academic Press, New York 1955.

[3]Burnet FM, Bull DR: Changes in influenza virus associated with adaptation to passage in chick embryos. Aust J Exp Biol Med Sc 21:55, 1943.

[4]Centers for Disease Control: National Reye syndrome surveillance - United States 1982 and 1983. MMWR 33:41, 1984.

[5]Centers for Disease Control: Influenza activity - Mississippi, United States, World-wide, MMWR 33:131, 1984.

[6]Centers for Disease Control: Prevention and control of influenza. MMWR 33:253, 1984.

[7]Choi KW, Thacker SB: An evaluation of influenza mortality surveillance 1962–1979.

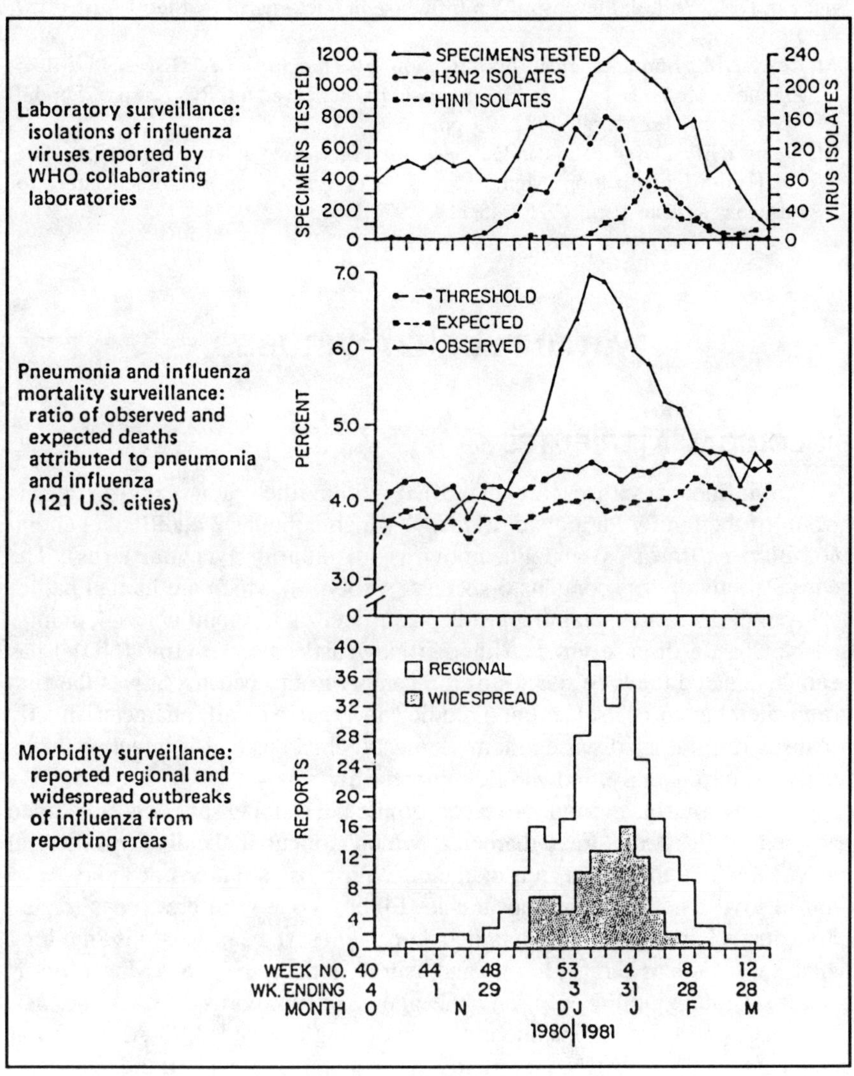

Figure 8-6: Influenza surveillance in the United States, 1980–1981. Reproduced with permission from Centers for Disease Control: Influenza Surveillance Report No. 94, issued June 1984, p. 17. Threshold was increased to 6.5% for 1989–90.

II. Percentage of pneumonia and influenza deaths as an indicator of influenza activity. Am J Epidemiol 113:227, 1981.

[8]Francis T Jr: On the doctrine of original antigenic sin. Proc Am Phil Soc 104:572, 1960.

[9]McLean DM, White J, Stevenson WJ: Influenza in Victoria, 1954. Med J Aust 1:257, 1955.

[10]McLean DM: Immunological Investigation of Human Virus Diseases. Vol. 5, Practical Methods in Clinical Immunology, series editor RC Nairn, Churchill Livingstone, Edinburgh 1982, 99 pp.

[11]Matthews REF: Classification and nomenclature of viruses. Intervirology 17:1, 1982.

[12]World Health Organization: Memorandum. A revised system of nomenclature for influenza viruses. Bull WHO 45:119, 1971.

PARAINFLUENZA VIRUSES

BIOLOGICAL ATTRIBUTES

Parainfluenza viruses are classified within the Paramyxovirus genus (group)of the family Paramyxoviridae,[6,11] which contains 2 additional genera: Morbillivirus (measles) and Pneumovirus (respiratory syncytial virus). The genus Paramyxovirus contains 6 species (serotypes) which are human pathogens: parainfluenza-1, parainfluenza-2, parainfluenza-3, parainfluenza-4, mumps and Newcastle disease virus. Although Newcastle disease virus (NDV) has been designated the type species of the genus (group) because it was the first group member to be isolated and studied in greater detail, characteristically it causes respiratory disease among domestic chickens and it infects humans relatively infrequently, inducing conjunctivitis.

Paramyxoviridae virions are pleomorphic but roughly spherical enveloped particles, 120–300nm total diameter, which contain helically symmetrical nucleocapsid strands 12–17nm diameter, with cross striations at intervals of 4nm to give a herringbone appearance (Figure 8-7). Viral envelopes (coats) of the genus Paramyxovirus contain glycoprotein surface projections 8nm long which serve both as hemagglutinin and neuraminidase, the genus Morbillivirus contains hemagglutinin only, and the genus Pneumovirus contains neither. Each virus particle contains one molecule of single stranded RNA, molecular weight $5-7 \times 10^6$ with RNA regularly as a negative sense strand. Particles contain 5–7 polypeptides, molecular weight $35-200 \times 10^3$ and lipids 20–25% by weight with composition mainly host dependent. The hemagglutinin and the neuraminidase, if present, are each represented by a single glycoprotein species; cell fusion and hemolysis are mediated by another glycoprotein species. Within the Paramyxovirus genus, the nucleocapsid antigen, which is specific for each serotype, is detected by complement fixation tests comparable to the S-CF antigen of influenza virus (see p. 127).

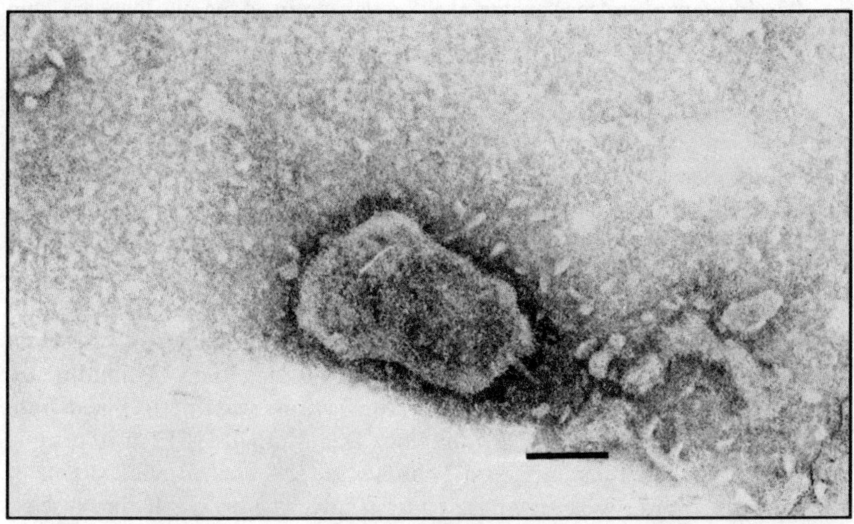

Figure 8-7: Parainfluenza-1 virion in nasopharyngeal secretion of a girl aged 10 months with croup (X120,120). Reproduced with permission from McLean DM and Wong KK, 1984. Same-day Diagnosis of Human Virus Infections, p. 75.

Parainfluenza viruses propagate readily after inoculation of primary monolayer tissue cultures of rhesus or cynomolgus monkey kidney cells and are detected after incubation at 35–37° C for 3–7 days by hemadsorption (Figure 8-2). Tissue culture fluid agglutinates erythrocytes of guinea pigs, chickens and geese. Hemagglutination is inhibited by mixture of serotype-specific antiserum with virus-laden tissue culture fluid before addition of erythrocytes. Viral envelope (V-CF) antigen within tissue culture fluid may be detected by complement fixation. Viral antigen within infected tissue culture cells is detected readily by indirect immunofluorescence using serotype-specific antisera prepared in rabbits or guinea pigs. Parainfluenza virions are visualized readily in nasopharyngeal secretions of infected humans by direct electron microsopy of preparations stained negatively with phosphotungstic acid.[9] However this procedure reveals the presence of a member of the Paramyxoviridae family; further serotypic identification requires the use of one or more of the serological tests described above.

Parainfluenza viruses, with the exception of parainfluenza 2 and the Sendai strain of parainfluenza 1, do not regularly induce cytopathic effects in monkey kidney tissue cultures. The latter two serotypes induce syncytia formation; Sendai virus is used regularly in laboratory experiments to induce cell-fusion between cells of different animal species.

Parainfluenza viruses, except the Sendai strain of parainfluenza 1 and the shipping fever strain of parainfluenza 3, do not induce disease in any laboratory animals; Sendai virus induces pneumonia in rodents after intranasal instillation and shipping fever strains induce respiratory infection in calves.

Parainfluenza 1 virus, initially termed hemadsorption type 2 virus, was first isolated from a throat swab from a boy aged 3 years with acute laryngotracheobronchitis (croup) in Washington, D.C. during 1957.[4] It was antigenically identical with the Sendai strain, first isolated from the lung of a fatal case of newborn pneumonitis in Sendai, Japan during 1952.[7] Parainfluenza 2 virus was first isolated from nasopharyngeal secretions of an infant aged 11 months with croup in Cincinnati, Ohio during 1955.[3] Parainfluenza 3 virus, initially termed hemadsorption type 1 virus, was first isolated from an infant with pneumonia in Washington, D.C. during 1957,[4] in the same outbreak from which parainfluenza 1 virus was recovered. Bovine strains of parainfluenza 3 virus were first isolated from calves with a respiratory disease termed shipping fever in Maryland during 1958[12] and they have been recovered during subsequent outbreaks of shipping fever, Parainfluenza 4 virus was first isolated from the throat swab of a college student with mild upper respiratory tract illness in Washington, D.C. during 1958,[5] but it has been isolated relatively infrequently during subsequent years.

After propagation of parainfluenza viruses in the mucosa of the tracheobronchial tree of children aged more than 3 years, antibodies detectable by hemagglutination inhibition or neutralization appear in the serum 1 to 2 weeks subsequently, and they are detectable by complement fixation 2 to 3 weeks after infection. However in children aged less than 3 years, antibody production is frequently delayed until patients have contracted repeated parainfluenza virus infections over the course of a year or more. It is important to remove both heat-labile and heat-stable inhibitors of hemagglutination, using techniques identical to those for influenza antibody detection, before commencing hemagglutination inhibition tests on patients' sera.

PATHOGENESIS

Parainfluenza viruses enter new susceptible hosts by inhalation of virus-laden droplet nuclei. Virus multiplication occurs throughout the tracheobronchial tree inducing catarrhal inflammation with excessive production of mucus. The aryepiglottic folds of the larynx become grossly swollen, causing obstruction to the inflow of air, which is manifested by inspiratory stridor and indrawing of the soft tissues around the rib cage. Infection does not spread beyond the respiratory tract.

SYMPTOMATOLOGY

Croup, also termed acute laryngotracheobronchitis ("tracheitis"), is the commonest clinical manifestation of infection with the parainfluenza viruses in children, particularly those aged less than 3 years.[1,8] Typical clinical features comprise inspiratory stridor, croupy cough, hoarse voice or cry, and respiratory difficulty on inspiration accompanied by indrawing of the chest wall in the subcostal, intercostal or subclavicular areas. About 80% of patients exhibit a cough and runny nose 1 to 3 days before onset of croup. Patients are usually afebrile. Air entry to the chest is diminished, scattered rhonchi may be heard over the chest fields in the absence of crepitations, and diminished inflation of the lungs is revealed by radiological examination. Bronchopneumonia is uncommon. The throat is frequently sore and red. Occasionally the epiglottis is grossly swollen and reddened, due to infection either by parainfluenza viruses or *Haemophilus influenza* type b. Severe airway obstruction arising either from acute laryngotracheobronchitis or acute epiglottitis may require emergency tracheotomy to restore an adequate airway. Respiratory symptoms usually subside within 1 to 2 days after onset, when patients are nursed in transparent plastic tents in an atmosphere of humidified oxygen.

Respiratory disease syndromes apart from croup are uncommon following infection with parainfluenza viruses (Table 8-2). In contrast to children, symptomatic infections with parainfluenza viruses in adults are uncommon,[2] but the usual clinical manifestation is an influenza-like illness.[10]

REFERENCES - PARAINFLUENZA

[1]Banatvala JE, Anderson TB, Reiss BR: Parainfluenza infections in the community. Brit Med J 1:537,1964.

[2]Buynak EB, Hilleman MR: Live attenuated mumps virus vaccine: I. Vaccine development. Proc Soc Exp Biol Med 123:768, 1966.

[3]Chanock RM: Association of a new type of cytopathogenic myxovirus with infantile croup. J Exp Med 104:555, 1956.

[4]Chanock RM, Parrott RH, Cook MK, Andrews BE, Bell JA, Reichelderfer T, Kapikian AZ, Mastrota FM, Huebner RJ: Newly recognized myxoviruses from children with respiratory disease. New Eng J Med 258:207, 1958.

[5]Johnson KM, Chanock RM, Cook MK, Huebner RJ: Studies of a new human hemadsorption virus. I. Isolation, properties and characterization. Am J Hyg 71:81, 1960.

[6]Kingsbury DW, Bratt MA, Choppin PW, Hanson RP, Hosaka Y, Ter Muelen V, Norrby E, Plowright W, Rott T, Wunner WH: Paramyxoviridae. Intervirology 10:137, 1978.

[7]Kuroya M, Ishida N. Shiratori T: Newborn virus pneumonitis (type Sendai). II. The isolation of new virus possessing hemagglutinin activity.

Yokohama Med Bull 4:217, 1953.

[8]McLean DM, Bach RD, Larke RPB, McNaughton GA: Myxoviruses associated with acute laryngotracheobronchitis in Toronto, 1962–63. Canad Med Ass J 89: 1257, 1963.

[9]McLean DM, Wong KK: Same-day diagnosis of human virus infections. CRC Press, Boca Raton, FL 1984, 125 pp.

[10]McKinney RW, England BL, Froede S: Studies with hemadsorption virus type 1. I Recovery from two cases of influenza-like disease in military personnel and related investigations. Am J Hyg 70:280, 1959.

[11]Matthews REF: Classification and nomenclature of viruses. Intervirology 17:1, 1982.

[12]Reisinger RC, J Am Vet Med Ass 135:147, 1959.

TABLE 8-2
PARAINFLUENZA VIRUS ISOLATES FROM CHILDREN WITH
ACUTE LOWER RESPIRATORY INFECTIONS

| | | Percentage virus isolation in each clinical category | | | |
Serotype	Location	Croup	Tracheo-bronchitis	Bronchiolitis	Pneumonia
Parainfluenza-1	Newcastle 1969–70[a]	19.1	1.5	2.1	1.1
	Washington 1957–61[b]	20.0	1.0	1.0	0.6
	Seattle 1966-71[c]	12.9	—	2.6	0.2
	Chapel Hill 1966-75[d]	23.8*	5.9	5.5	20.0
Parainfluenza-2	Newcastle	10.6	0.0	0.0	0.0
	Washington	4.4	0.4	0.3	0.1
	Seattle	1.4	—	1.3	0.0
	Chapel Hill	*	*	*	*
Parainfluenza-3	Newcastle	5.3	2.7	6.4	3.2
	Washington	4.4	2.0	4.0	1.6
	Seattle	1.4	—	1.3	1.1
	Chapel Hill	*	*	*	*
Respiratory syncytial	Newcastle	10.6	+	40.8[+]	+
	Washington 1959–61[e]	3.0	2.0	25.0	10.0
	Seattle	1.0	—	9.8	2.3
	Chapel Hill	3.4	4.7	7.5	26.1

a   Gardner et al., Brit Med J 2:7, 1971.
b   Parrott et al., Am J Pub Health 52:907, 1962.
c   Foy et al., Am J Epidemiol 97:80, 1973.
d   Chapman et al., Am J Epidemiol 114:786, 1981.
e   Chanock et al., Am J. Pub Health 52:918, 1962.
*   Serotypes were not stated in the publication.
+   Overall RS isolation rate from respiratory infections other than croup.

MUMPS VIRUS

BIOLOGICAL ATTRIBUTES

Mumps virus is a species containing a single serotype within the genus Paramyxovirus.[4] Mumps virus particles are indistinguishable from parainfluenza virus when negatively stained preparations are examined by electron microscopy (Figure 8-8).

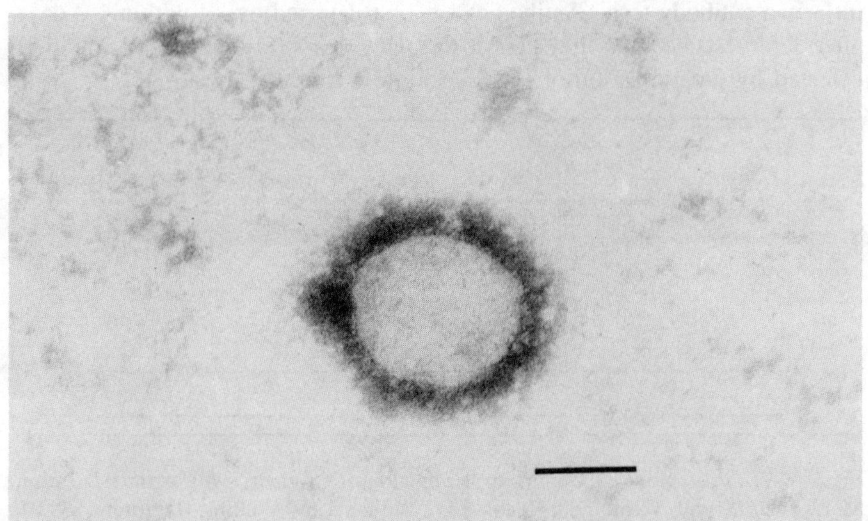

Figure 8-8: Mumps virion in CSF of infant with meningoencephalitis (X150,150). Reproduced with permission from McLean DM and Wong KK, 1984. Same-day Diagnosis of Human Virus Infections, CRC Press, Boca Raton, FL, p. 67.

Mumps virus propagates readily in tissue cultures of primary monkey kidney cells, inducing syncytia formation after 3 to 5 days incubation at 37° C and hemadsorption is detected readily using erythrocytes from geese or chickens. Mumps virus also multiplies in chick embryo fibroblast tissue cultures, with induction of cytopathic effects and hemadsorption. Although earlier strains of mumps virus were isolated from patients by amniotic inoculation of chick embryos,[1] this technique has been superseded virtually completely by 1960 through the use of tissue cultures which have provided both a higher rate of virus isolation from patients combined with ease of performance.[2]

Hemagglutination is inhibited specifically by mumps antibody in sera from patients convalescent from mumps, or in sera of experimental animals such as guinea pigs 3-4 weeks after intranasal inoculation with mumps virus. Supernatant fluid from infected tissue cultures provides the best source of virus for hemagglutination of 0.5% suspensions of goose or chicken erythrocytes in unbuffered 0.15M saline. Removal of non-specific inhibitors of hemagglutination from all sera, either by heating at 56° C for 30 minutes followed by treatment with M/100 KIO$_4$, or by overnight treatment with receptor destroying enzyme (neuraminidase), is required before conduct of mumps HI tests, as in influenza antibody tests. Antibodies are first detected by HI within 1-2 days after defervescence and they persist for many years (Figure 8-9). Antibodies detected by neutralization or ELISA follow a similar pattern.

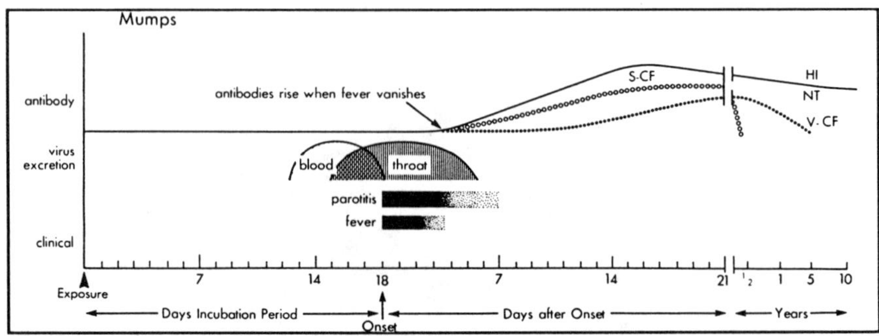

Figure 8-9: Time course of mumps virus infection. Reproduced with permission from McLean DM, 1980. Virology in Health Care, Williams and Wilkins, Baltimore, p. 110.

Mumps antibodies may be detected by complement fixation. Antibody to the nucleocapsid (S-CF) appears less than one week after onset of illness and persists about 6 months. Antibody to the viral envelope (V-CF) appears 2-3 weeks after onset and may persist for one year or more.

PATHOGENESIS

Mumps virus enters a new host by inhalation of virus-laden droplets, and enters the blood stream within the first week, presumably after an initial cycle of multiplication somewhere in the respiratory tract. Virus is conveyed to target organs by the blood, wherein it undergoes extensive multiplication, for example in the parotids resulting in catarrhal inflammation of acinar cells and outpouring of virus-laden saliva, and also in the meninges inducing elaboration of CSF with high concentrations both of lymphocytes and virus. Virus is excreted in urine for at least 5 days after onset of parotitis.

SYMPTOMATOLOGY

Painful swelling of one or both parotid glands, accompanied by temperatures of 38–39° C occur after an incubation period of 18–21 days. Parotid swelling is accompanied by redness and pouting of the orifices of the parotid (Stensen's) ducts and dryness of the mouth. Bilateral parotitis occurs in about 70% of cases; swelling of submandibular glands may also occur in 5–10% of cases. Fever persists 2–3 days, parotitis may persist for 4–7 days. The period of communicability ranges from about 6 days before to 4 days after onset of parotitis.

Complications of mumps commonly include: (a) orchitis affecting overall about 5% of males, but attaining 18% in adult men; (b) oophoritis affecting about 5% postpubertal women; (c) pancreatitis affecting about 7% cases; (d) meningitis (meningoencephalitis) affecting 0.5–2% of cases. Rare complications include presternal edema or thyroiditis, arthritis, polyneuritis plus central hypertension, encephalitis with perivascular demyelination which may terminate fatally. Although rare, mumps deafness due to damage of cochlear cells of the inner ear, is permanent.

Mumps meningitis occurs 2–3 times more frequently among males than females. Meningitis begins 6 days before 14 days after onset of parotitis, and it may occur in one-third of laboratory confirmed cases without parotitis.[3] Clinical features include high fever, neck stiffness, positive Kernig or Brudzinski signs, vomiting, headache, irritability and a high count of lymphocytes in CSF ($500–3000\text{mm}^{-3}$) without significant alteration of glucose, protein or chloride levels. Convulsions may affect 5–10% pediatric patients. Although meningeal signs usually resolve within 2–3 days, especially after lumbar puncture, symptoms may persist as long as 2 weeks in 10% of patients. Antibodies are detected by HI within 1–2 days after resolution of meningeal signs. Laboratory investigation is essential to distinguish between meningitis induced by mumps and enteroviruses.

REFERENCES - MUMPS

[1]Levens JH, Enders JF: The hemagglutinative properties of amniotic fluid from embryonated eggs infected with mumps virus. Science 102:117, 1945.
[2]McLean DM, Walker SJ, Wyllie JC, McQueen EJ, McNaughton GA: Infections of the central nervous system with mumps and enteroviruses in Toronto, 1960. Can Med Ass J 84:941, 1961.
[3]McLean DM, Larke RPB, Cobb C, Griffis ED, Hackett SMR: Mumps and enteroviral meningitis in Toronto, 1966. Can Med Ass J 96:1355, 1967.
[4]Matthews REF: Classification and nomenclature of viruses. Intervirology 17:1, 1982.

NEWCASTLE DISEASE VIRUS

BIOLOGICAL ATTRIBUTES

Newcastle disease virus (NDV) is the type species comprising a single serotype within the genus Paramyxovirus.[3] Enveloped virions are spheres about 100 nm diameter which contain helical nucleocapsid strands 17nm diameter, and both hemagglutinin and neuraminidase projections are included in the envelope. The virus multiples in tissue cultures of primary monkey kidney, primary chick embryo fibroblasts and continuous polyploid human (HEp-2) cells inducing plaque formation; virus also propagates after allanatoic inoculation of chick embryos. Hemagglutinin for erythrocytes of geese or chickens is found in high titer in supernatant fluid from infected tissue cultures and in allantoic fluid.

SYMPTOMATOLOGY

Newcastle disease virus is essentially a pathogen causing severe and often fatal disease involving the respiratory and nervous systems of domestic chickens and turkeys.[2] Many cases of acute conjunctivitis following accidental splashing of virus-laden fluids in the eyes of laboratory workers have been documented since the initial report in 1943.[1] The incubation period is 1–2 days. Conjunctivitis is sometimes hemorrhagic, but without corneal involvement. Conjunctivitis may be accompanied by preauricular lymphadenopathy and generalized mild constitutional upset with fever. Full recovery occurs within 2 weeks or less.

REFERENCES - NEWCASTLE DISEASE VIRUS

[1]Burnet FM: Human infection with the virus of Newcastle disease of fowls. Med J Aust 2:313, 1943.
[2]Hanson RP, Brandly CA: Newcastle disease. Ann NY Acad Sc 70:595, 1958.
[3]Matthews REF: Classification and nomenclature of viruses. Intervirology 17:1, 1982.

MEASLES VIRUS

BIOLOGICAL ATTRIBUTES

Measles virus is one of 4 species within the genus *Morbillivirus* of the family Paramyxoviridae.[9] It is the only species pathogenic for humans. Measles virus is distributed world-wide as a single serotype. All species of Morbillivirus contain hemagglutinin within the viral envelope but they are devoid of neuraminidase. Although measles virus particles are somewhat large in overall dimensions, they closely resemble parainfluenza virions in negatively stained preparations examined by electron microscopy (Figure 8-10).

Measles virus propagates in primary tissue cultures of cercopithecus (African green) and rhesus monkey kidney cells[14] and in human kidney[5] and

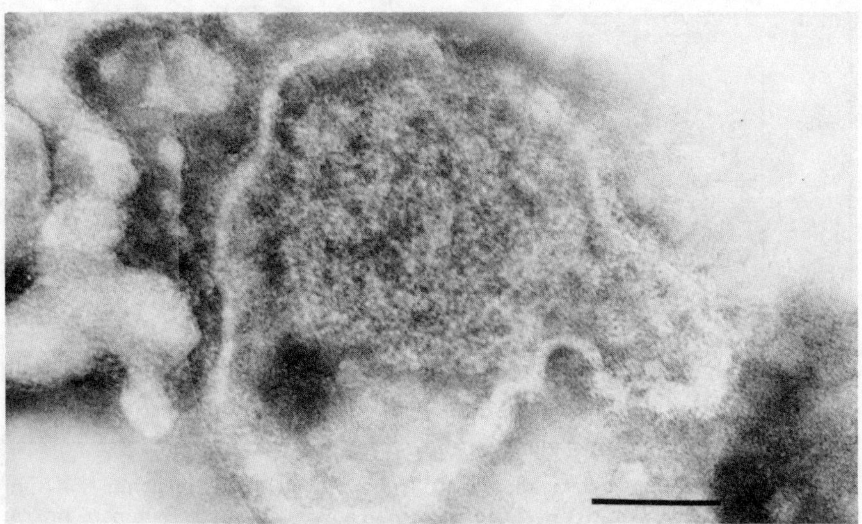

Figure 8-10: Measles virion in nasopharyngeal secretion from a girl aged 1-3/4 years with measles (X192,050). Reproduced with permission from McLean DM and Wong KK, 1984. Same-day Diagnosis of Human Virus Infections, CRC Press, Boca Raton, FL, p. 62.

amnion cells with production of syncytia after about 1 week of incubation at 37° C. Tissue culture supernatant fluids contains hemagglutinin for cercopithecus and rhesus monkey erythrocytes at pH7 and 37° C.[13] In tissues of patients persistently infected with measles virus, such as brains in subacute sclerosing panencephalitis, measles virus has been isolated by co-cultivation of lightly trypsinized brain tissue with susceptible lines of human polyploid cells HeLa or HEp-2.[6] Virus-infected brain cells fuse with HeLa cells, permitting virus transfer and subsequent induction of syncytia following virus multiplication. However virus has not been recovered from suspensions of ground up brain tissue.

Hemagglutinin is inhibited by antibodies in sera of patients convalescent from measles infection. Non-specific lipid inhibitors of hemagglutination must be removed by adsorption with 12.5% kaolin suspension before use in HI tests. Antibodies are first detected by HI within 1–2 days after abatement of fever and they persist many years (Figure 8-11). Antibodies detected by neutralization or ELISA tests show a similar time course of appearance and persistence. However complement fixing antibodies to the whole virus (V-CF) first appear 10–14 days after onset of rash and persist 6–12 months.

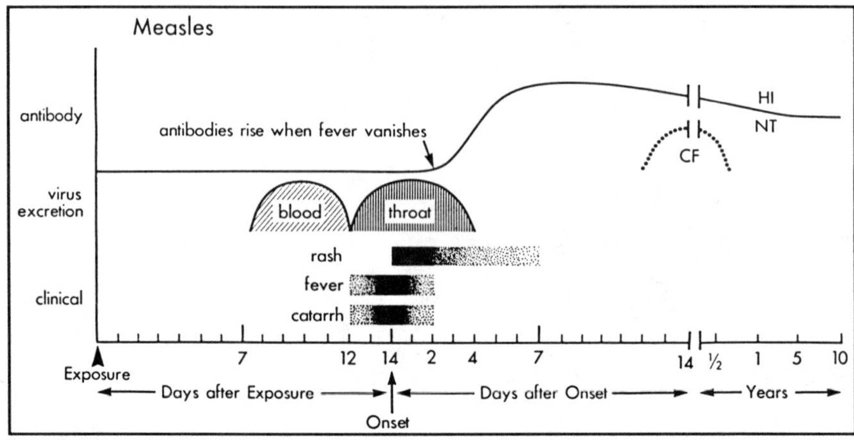

Figure 8-11: Time course of measles virus infection. Reproduced with permission from McLean DM, 1980. Virology in Health Care, Williams and Wilkins, Baltimore, p. 123.

PATHOGENESIS

Measles virus enters the respiratory tract by inhalation of virus-laden droplet nuclei. Shortly thereafter it enters the reticulo-endothelial system in which it undergoes replication, with the appearance of viremia during the second week. This disseminates virus widely throughout the body, inducing fever and nasopharyngeal catarrh, accompanied by Koplik spots, about 12 days after exposure. The rash appears about 14 days after exposure and it persists for 7 days, but it shows brownish discoloration after 4 days. Fever persists for about 2 days after onset of the rash, and upon defervescence HI antibody is detected in the serum. Viremia persists for 3–4 days before, to 1 day after onset of rash. Virus is excreted from the throat during the catarrhal stage 2 days before onset of rash until 2 or more days after onset of rash, and this corresponds to the period of transmissibility.

SYMPTOMATOLOGY

Measles denotes a blotchy maculopapular rash affecting mainly the face, trunk and proximal portions of the extremities, accompanied by a moderate constitutional upset with the temperature elevated to 38–39° C, after an incubation period about 14 days. Red blotches, 2–4 mm diameter, are scattered over the skin resembling cement thrown against a stucco wall. Characteristically some 2 days before appearance of the external maculopapular rash (exanthem), Koplik spots comprising white dots 1 mm diameter resembling fine grains of white sand against a bluish red background appear internally on the buccal mucosa (enanthem). Koplik spots are accompanied by watering eyes with drooping eyelids, giving a dejected appearance (the "measly" look), and there is usually a runny nose plus harsh cough. Fever usually abates after 2–3 days. The maculopapular rash shows bronze staining after 3–4 days and disappears within 7 days, without desquamation.

Atypical measles has affected children who contracted an infection with wild measles virus 1–5 years after receiving one or more doses of killed measles vaccine.[9] Constitutional upset is more severe, the rash is petectial or vesicular, bronchopneumonia is demonstrated radiologically, rales are heard throughout the chest and there is respiratory distress.

The case fatality rate from measles in developed countries such as Great Britain[10] and the United States[2] ranges from 0.7–1.8 per 1000 reported cases. This is due mainly to complications involving the respiratory and nervous systems. However in underdeveloped rural areas of tropical Africa, the mortality rate was 5.7–21%,[12] where malnutrition may be an important contributing factor.

Complications have been reported in 1 of 15 (6.7%) cases of measles in Britain.[10] Commonly the respiratory tract is affected, giving rise to croup, bronchopneumonia and otitis media. Among fatal cases, 55–60% have died with pneumonia [1,2] and 21% have died with encephalitis. Nationwide, encephalitis has affected 0.6–1.4 per 1000 reported cases of measles,[10] but among hospitalized patients, encephalitis has affected 4.7%.[1] Febrile convulsions without encephalitis may affect another 1.4 per 1000 reported cases.[10]

Encephalitis usually begins 2–7 days after onset of measles rash.[7] Elevation of the temperature above 39° C is accompanied by drowsiness deepening into stupor or coma, irritability, neck stiffness, CSF cell counts exceed 10 per mm^3 in 75% of cases, and virtually all patients show diffuse abnormalities of the electroencephalogram. The case fatality rate has ranged from 7 to 29% throughout the United States.[2] Neurological sequelae including paresis, athetosis, loss of speech, dementia and personality changes such as emotional lability and temper tantrums, may be present in 18–23% of patients upon discharge from hospital. No clearly defined therapeutic effects have been demonstrated following administration of corticosteroids, adrenocorticotrophic hormone or human immune serum globulin.

Subacute sclerosing panencephalitis (SSPE) is a slowly progressing encephalopathy which usually terminates fatally within 2 years. It complicates 5.2–9.7 per million reported cases of measles,[2] but is has also been encountered among 0.48–1.13 per million live measles vaccine recipients. The syndrome comprises progressive dementia, myoclonic jerks, pyramidal and extrapyramidal signs, an electroencephalogram with regular periodic complexes, and a paretic type of colloidal gold reaction in CSF.[3] Characteristically, measles antibody titers in both IgM and IgG components are found in CSF, usually at 8- to 32-fold lower titers than in serum.[4]

Immunosuppressed conditions, such as leukemia, may predispose to unusually severe attacks of measles, resulting in giant cell pneumonia.[11] Radiologically there may be extensive bilateral nodular infiltration of the lung fields.

REFERENCES - MEASLES VIRUS

[1]Broughton CR: Morbilli in Sydney: A review of 3601 cases with consideration of morbidity, mortality and measles encephalomyelitis. Med J Aust 2:859, 1964.

[2]Center for Disease Control: Measles Surveillance Report No. 10 1973–1976, issued July 1977.

[3]Connolly JH, Allen IV, Hurwitz LT, Miller JHD: Measles virus antibody and antigen in subacute sclerosing panencephalitis. Lancet 1:542, 1967.

[4]Connolly JH, Haire M, Hadden DSM: Measles immunoglobulins in subacute sclerosing panencephalitis. Brit Med J 1:23, 1971.

[5]Enders JR, Peebles TC: Propagation in tissue cultures of cytopathogenic agents from patients with measles. Proc Soc Exp Biol Med 86:277, 1954.

[6]Horta-Barbosa L, Fucillo DA, Sever JL, Seman W: Subacute sclerosing panencephalitis: isolation of measles virus from a brain biopsy. Nature 221:974, 1969.

[7]McLean DM, Best JM, Smith PA, Larke RPB, McNaughton GA: Viral infections of Toronto children during 1965. II. Measles encephalitis and other complications. Can Med Ass J 94:905, 1966.

[8]McLean DM, Kettyls GDM, Hingston J, Moore PS, Paris RP, Rigg JM: Atypical measles following immunization with killed measles vaccine. Can Med Ass J 103:743, 1970.

[9]Matthews REF: Classification and nomenclature of viruses. Intervirology 17:1, 1982.

[10]Miller DL: Frequency of complications of measles. Brit Med J 2:75, 1964.

[11]Mitus A, Enders JF, Craig JM, Holloway A: Persistence of measles virus and depression of antibody formation in patients with giant-cell pneumonia after measles. New Eng J Med 261:882, 1959.

[12]Morley D: Severe measles in the Tropics. Brit Med J 1:297 and 363, 1969.

[13]Rosen L: Hemagglutination and hemagglutination - inhibition with measles virus. Virology 13:139, 1961.

[14]Underwood GE: Studies on measles virus in tissue culture. I. Growth rates in various cells and development of a plaque assay. J Immunol 83:198, 1959.

RESPIRATORY SYNCYTIAL VIRUS

BIOLOGICAL ATTRIBUTES

Respiratory syncytial (RS) virus is one of 3 species within the genus Pneumovirus of the family Paramyxoviridae.[10] It is the only species pathogenic for humans. Although minor antigenic variants have been isolated during some epidemics, it is generally agreed that RS virus exists as a single serotype. Pneumovirus species differ from Paramyxovirus and Morbillivirus because hemagglutinin and neuraminidase are absent. Although RS virus particles show larger overall dimensions, they resemble the appearance of parainfluenza virions in negatively stained preparations examined by electron microscopy.

Respiratory syncytial virus propagates readily in tissue cultures of continuous human heteroploid cells such as HEp-2, HeLa or KB[2,3,6] and in continuous human diploid cells such as WI-38[1] or foreskin fibroblasts[9] with induction of syncytia after 3–7 days incubation at 35–37° C, but RS virus multiplies less readily in primary monkey kidney cells. Infected cells within cell sheets show points of fluorescence within the cytoplasm when examined by the indirect immunofluorescent technique.[6] Since the infectivity of RS virus in nasopharyngeal secretions from patients deteriorates rapidly, efforts should be made to inoculate tissue cultures within 1/2 to 3 hours after collection of specimens. Cytoplasmic fluorescence due to the presence of RS antigen in cells of the respiratory epithelium[7] are observed readily in smears of nasopharyngeal or throat secretions after treatment with anti-RS serum prepared in guinea pigs followed by application of fluorescein-labelled anti-guinea pig serum, thus providing a same-day diagnostic test. Respiratory syncytial virus infects but does not induce disease in the usual laboratory animals, except chimpanzees which may develop coryza.[11]

Antibodies are detected in patients' sera by neutralization and CF tests some 2–3 weeks after onset of illness, and they persist several years.

PATHOGENESIS

Catarrhal inflammation involves the epithelium throughout the tracheo-bronchial tree, inducing obstruction to outflow of air through the smaller bronchioles by excessive secretion of mucus. This induces the characteristic over-inflation of the chest which is demonstrated radiologically, plus the typical rhonchi (wheeze) and rales which are heard throughout the chest.

SYMPTOMATOLOGY

Respiratory syncytial virus is regularly associated with outbreaks of bronchiolitis and bronchopneumonia which affect many industrialized communities each winter.[3,5]

Bronchiolitis characteristically affects infants aged 2 years or less. After a runny nose and cough for 1–2 days, there is copious output of mucous secretions accompanied by wheezing, increased coughing and difficulty with respirations resulting in rib-cage retraction plus a barrel-shaped chest indicating obstruction to the outflow of air. Fever is minimal. Chest x-rays reveal over-inflated lungs. Bronchoscopic suction may be required to remove excessive mucous secretions. Nursing in humidified tents (Croupettes) promotes resolution of symptoms after 2–3 days. Typically bronchiolitis occurs in short sharp peaks towards the end of winter.

Bronchopneumonia is recognized principally by auscultation of rales over portions of the lung fields, together with severe cough, respiratory distress and fever. Patchy consolidation throughout the lung fields is observed on chest x-ray examination. Clinical remission usually occurs within 4–7 days. Occasional cases terminate fatally.

Acute upper respiratory illness affecting infants during winter and spring presents with cough, increased nasopharyngeal secretions, runny nose, mild fever, irritability and crankiness. Young infants may refuse feedings. Clinical remission usually occurs within 2–5 days. Tracheobronchitis, comprising deep cough and rhonchi audible over the large airways, also affects mainly children under 6 years of age during the cooler months, and RS virus is the commonest agent isolated from these patients[4] (Table 8-2).

A syndrome resembling the common cold has been induced in adult human volunteers following intranasal instillation of RS virus.[7] Clinical features are nasal discharge, nasal obstruction, sneezing, redness of nostrils, malaise and pharyngitis.

REFERENCES - RESPIRATORY SYNCYTIAL VIRUS

[1]Anderson JM, Beem MO: Use of human diploid cell cultures for primary isolation of respiratory syncytial virus. Proc Soc Exp Biol Med 121:205, 1966.

[2]Chanock RM, Finberg L: Recovery from infants with respiratory illness of a virus related to chimpanzee coryza agent (CCA). I. Isolation, properties and characterisation. Am J Hyg 55:281, 1957.

[3]Chanock RM, Kim HW, Vargosko AJ, Deleva A, Johnson KM, Cumming C, Parrott RH: Respiratory syncytial virus. I. Virus recovery and other observations during 1960 outbreak of bronchiolitis, pneumonia and minor respiratory diseases of children. JAMA 176:647, 1961.

[4]Chapman RS, Henderson FW, Clyde WA Jr, Collier AM, Denny FW: The epidemiology of tracheobronchitis in pediatric practice. Am J Epidemiol 114:786, 1981.

[5]Clarke SKR, Gardner PS, Poole PM, Simpson H, Tobin J O'H: Respiratory syncytial virus infection: Admissions to hospital in industrial, urban and rural areas. Brit Med J 2:796, 1978.

[6]Gardner PS, McQuillan J: Application of immunofluorescent antibody technique in rapid diagnosis of respiratory syncytial virus infection. Brit Med J 3:340, 1968.

[7]Gardner PS, McQuillan J: Rapid virus diagnosis. Application of immunofluorescence, 2nd ed. 1980. Butterworth, London, 317 pp.

[8]Kravetz HM, Knight V, Chanock RM, Morris JA, Johnson KM, Rifkind D, Utz JP: Respiratory syncytial virus III. Production of illness and clinical observations in adult volunteers. JAMA 176:657, 1961.

[9]McLean DM: Immunological investigation of human virus diseases. 1982. Churchill Livingstone, Edinburgh, 99 pp.

[10]Matthews REF: Classification and nomenclature of viruses. Intervirology 17:1, 1982.

[11]Morris JA, Blount RE Jr, Savage RE: Recovery of cytopathogenic agent from chimpanzees with coryza. Proc Soc Exp Biol Med 92:544, 1956.

CHAPTER 9

RUBELLA

Rubella virus exists throughout the world as a single serotype, which causes the disease rubella (German measles), and also congenital anomalies in babies born to mothers who develop rubella during the first trimester of pregnancy, termed the congenital rubella syndrome (CRS).

HISTORICAL

Maculopapular rashes mainly affecting children were first described as two distinct clinical entities during the early 19th century.[31] Rubella (German measles) had a longer incubation period, milder constitutional upset, shorter duration of rash and less frequent complications than typical measles (red measles). Rubella was considered to be a trivial but unavoidable infectious disease of childhood, at least in the developed countries, until the occurrence of a cluster of infants with congenital cataracts in the practice of a Sydney, Australia ophthalmologist in 1941.[8] Upon detailed questioning of the mothers of these affected infants, a history was elicited of maternal rubella during the first trimester of pregnancy in each instance. Subsequently, it became clear in Australia and elsewhere[11] that any combination of cataracts, deafness and congenital heart lesions, usually patent ductus arteriosus, could affect infants whose mothers contracted rubella at any time during the initial four months of gestation. By 1958 on clinical grounds,[9] it was established that the risk of congenital rubella syndrome in infants approached 50% in those born to mothers who contracted rubella at 1–4 weeks of gestation, decreased to about 11% when rubella occurred at 13–16 weeks, and became negligible after the 24th week.

Isolation of rubella virus from throat secretions of military recruits who developed rubella during winter 1961,[20] through the use of tissue culture techniques, provided the scientific means for adequate epidemiological investigations and laid the groundwork for production of a successful live rubella vaccine which was licensed for human administration in 1969.[6,21] Meanwhile the occurrence of a major rubella pandemic in 1964 which was followed by numerous CRS cases among infants in 1965,[13] provided adequate stimulus for the development in 1969 of a strategy to eliminate rubella from North America through a program of universal vaccination of infants after their first birthdays.[10] By 1983, reported cases of clinical rubella reached an all-time low rate[6] and only 4 fresh cases of CRS were encountered during 1983.

BIOLOGICAL ATTRIBUTES

Rubella virus is the sole member of the genus Rubivirus within the family Togaviridae.[16] Rubella virus is not arthropod-borne. Humans comprise the sole vertebrate host for rubella virus. In common with other Togaviridae, the rubella virus particle contains a single molecule of positive sense ss RNA with molecular weight about 4×10^6, comprising 5–8% by weight of the virus, and 3–4 polypeptides. Lipoprotein viral envelopes contain virus-specific glycopeptides. Particles have total diameters 40–50nm diameter with spherical nucleocapsids 25–35nm diameter which exhibit presumed icosahedral symmetry. Rubella virus multiplies in the cytoplasm of infected cells.

Rubella virus multiplies readily in monolayer tissue cultures of grivet (*Cercopithecus sp.* or African green) monkey kidney cells without production of cytopathic effects. However, when cultures are challenged after one week of incubation at 37° C with 100 TCD_{50} of echovirus-11, they interfere with the multiplication of the second virus. This cumbersome system still provides the best technique for isolation and serotyping of rubella virus from patients. Rubella virus induces cytopathic effects in continuous polyploid tissue cultures of rabbit kidney (RK 13 cell line) which are convenient for many purposes, especially neutralization tests on patient's sera. Large quantities of rubella virus are obtained by propagation in continuous polyploid-baby hamster kidney (BHK) cells maintained in spinner cultures.

Rubella virus agglutinates erythrocytes of geese and newly hatched chicks under defined conditions of temperature and pH. For demonstration of hemagglutination, rubella virus is propagated in spinner cultures of BHK cells containing Eagle's minimal essential medium and 10% fetal bovine serum from which lipoprotein inhibitors have been removed by prior adsorption with kaolin. Virus released into the supernatant fluid is concentrated 10- to 50-fold by centrifugation at 100,000 x g for 1 hour.

For hemagglutination inhibition (HI) tests, patients' sera are adsorbed with kaolin to remove non-specific inhibitors, then serial two-fold dilutions commencing 1:10 are mixed with 4 hemagglutinating doses of rubella virus in borate saline pH9. After holding at 4° C for 15 minutes, equal volumes of 0.25% suspension of goose erythrocytes in phosphate-buffered virus adjusting diluent are added to give a final pH 6.2. The mixtures are incubated at 4° C and the pattern of hemagglutination is read after 45–60 minutes. Antibody response in the IgM and IgG components of patients' sera may be determined after ultracentrifugation through a discontinuous sucrose gradient 10–60% at 100,000 x g until equilibrium is reached 2 hours later. Usually antibody is detected first by HI (mainly in the IgM component) 2–4 days after onset of rash and fever, but after 3–4 weeks HI antibody is found mainly in the IgG component. Antibodies probably persist lifelong.

Antibodies measured by neutralization or ELISA or radioimmunoassay (RIA) tests show times of appearance and persistence parallel with those of HI tests. Antibodies measured by RIA have persisted for 8–18 years after rubella vaccination.[19]

Antibodies measured by complement fixation (CF) tests appear some 1–3 weeks after onset of rash and persist for 1–2 years. An adaptation of the CF test to a solid phase system, termed the single radial hemolysis test, has been employed widely in serological surveys for prevalence of rubella antibodies.[14]

PATHOGENESIS

Rubella virus normally enters the susceptible human host by inhalation of infected droplet nuclei expelled in nasopharyngeal secretions from close contacts who have clinical rubella. Rashes first appear 14–17 days after natural exposure to infected cases, with a mean incubation period of 16 days.[4] This is preceded by postauricular lymphadenopathy 1–8 days earlier. The rash usually persists 1–4 days (Figure 9-1). Virus is detected in the blood from 3–

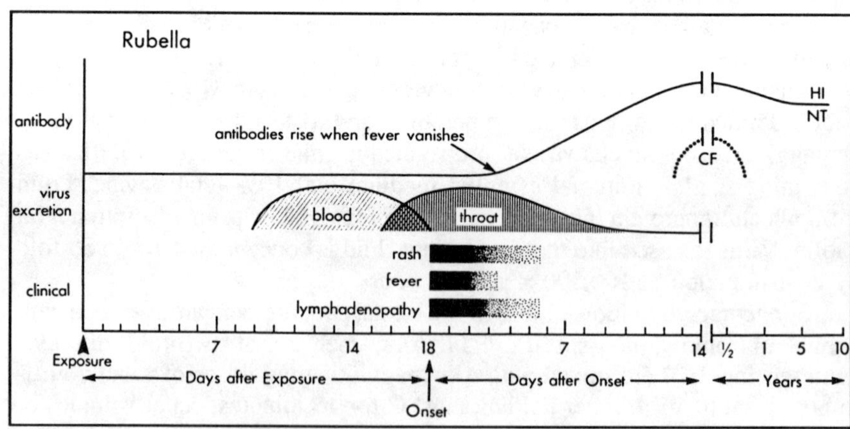

Figure 9-1: Time course of rubella infection. Reproduced with permission from McLean DM, 1980. Virology in Health Care, Williams and Wilkins, Baltimore, p. 140.

6 days before to the day of onset of rash[7], at peak titers of 10^2. Virus is found in the pharynx of naturally occurring or experimentally induced rubella regularly from 2–5 days before to 2–4 days after onset of rash[7,27] at peak titers of 10^3, but pharyngeal excretion may persist at least 9[27] to 21[7] days.

Rubella virus infection during the first trimester of pregnancy crosses the placenta and infects the fetus. Virus has been recovered from the heart, brain, lung, liver, other viscera, and eye[18] of infants under 1 month who died with the congenital rubella syndrome. Pathological findings have included myocardial necrosis, patent ductus arteriosus and interstitial pneumonia.[26] Rubella virus is excreted from the throat during the initial 20 weeks of life[1,13,15,24,25] and infrequently up to age 12 months.[24] Virus has also been isolated from the throats of normal infants born to mothers who contracted rubella during the first trimester or immediately before delivery.[1] Virus appears in the urine during the first 8 weeks of life[13] and in feces up to second week of life.[25] Virus is found in conjunctival swabs[1] or eyes[18] of infants with congenital cataracts during the initial few weeks of life, or from the eye or lens for 18 months[25] to 3 years.[17] Virus has been found in the cerebrospinal fluid (CSF) up to 1 year of age[25] and in leukocytes of peripheral blood up to 6 months.[12]

Rubella antibodies in infants with CRS are carried mainly in the IgM component during the first 6 months of life,[3] but by the first birthday antibodies are mainly in the IgG fraction. The antibody titer in the child equals or exceeds that of the mother[2,15] and may increase during the first few months of life, in contrast to the decline of antibody to undetectable levels between 6 and 15 months in normal children.[24]

SYMPTOMATOLOGY

RUBELLA

Rubella presents with a fine intense macular ("peach bloom") rash over the face and trunk, accompanied regularly by mild fever and characteristic enlargement of the postauricular or suboccipital lymph nodes.[32] The incubation period is about 18 days. Fever subsides after 1–2 days and the rash fades after 3–4 days without staining of the skin. In some rubella epidemics[4,27] one third or more of virologically confirmed rubella cases showed no rash, but all had enlarged lymph nodes.

Complications of rubella include arthritis and encephalitis. Arthritis characteristically affects the fingers, wrists, elbows, knees or ankles of 1–2% females between 15 and 55 years of age, within 6 days before onset of rash to 4 days after onset, but young children may also contract arthritis.[22] Swelling and pain in the joints may persist for a few days to 3 weeks. Rubella arthritis has also affected 10% subjects aged 13–33 years who received live attenuated HPV 77 duck embryo rubella vaccine 9–22 days previously and symptoms persisted 1–8 days.[29] Occasionally arthritis has affected recipients of RA 27/3 vaccine, which in one woman relapsed during the succeeding 3-1/2 years.[30]

Encephalitis is a rare complication, affecting 5–21 per 100,000 cases of rubella.[5]

CONGENITAL RUBELLA SYNDROME

Congenital rubella syndrome describes the clinical features of newborn infants born to mothers who contracted rubella infections during the first trimester of pregnancy. Clinical features of laboratory confirmed cases in four North American centers after the 1963–64 rubella epidemic are summarized in Table 9-1.[13,15,24,25] They comprise: (1) *cardiac anomalies,* especially patent

TABLE 9-1
**CLINICAL FEATURES OF THE CONGENITAL RUBELLA SYNDROME IN
FOUR CENTERS DURING 1964–1965[a]**

	Percentage Involvement			
Sign	*Houston* 25 cases[b]	*Memphis* 17 cases[c]	*Philadelphia* 21 cases[d]	*Toronto* 7 cases[e]
Ocular defects	50	72	76	86
Cardiac anomalies	70	100	67	86
Thrombocytopenic purpura	80	42	43	57
Birthweight below 2500 g	80	72	57	71
Hepatomegaly	70	24	33	43
Bone changes	70	6	33	43
Rubella in first trimester	76	68		86
Rubella exposure	8	12		14[f]
Rubella virus in throat	63	96	95	71

a Deafness was not recorded in the above series, but significant hearing loss was detected in 19–37% of school-age children in Britain[28] and Australia.[23]
b Rudolph et al. (1965) JAMA 191:843.[25]
c Korones et al. (1965) J Pediatr 67:166.[13]
d Plotkin et al. (1965) J Pediatr 67:182.[24]
e McLean et al. (1966) Can Med Assoc J 95:1174.[15]
f The mother of this patient received gammaglobulin within 24 hours after her husband developed rubella.

ductus arteriosus; (iii) *deafness,* although not recorded in the four North American series due to technical difficulties with its assessment in infants, was encountered initially in 26% of infants in an Australian study,[23] increasing to 37% at 4–8 years of age, and significant loss of hearing was found in 19%

of British children[28] aged 8–11 years; (iv) *thrombocytopenic purpura* giving the appearance of a blueberry muffin, with platelet counts depressed to 10,000–30,000 per mm³, returning to normal spontaneously after 2–3 weeks; (v) *birth weight below 2500 grams despite a normal gestational age;* (vi) *hepatomegaly,* sometimes accompanied by splenomegaly; (vii) *radiological changes* in the metaphyses of long bones, giving the appearance of a celery stalk. Although mental retardation[15] was noted in 14% of cases and delay in development of motor activity was observed in 4% of infants,[23] the distribution of intelligence quotients among offspring of maternal rubella did not differ from the offspring of non-infected pregnancies.[28]

Clinically typical rubella during the first-trimester was noted in 68–86% mothers, but no rash was observed in 8–14 pregnant contacts of clinical cases. In some instances where immune serum globulin (human) was administered to pregnant women following rubella contact during the first trimester, babies were born with CRS.[15,24]

The category of congenital anomaly arising from intrauterine rubella infection was related to the gestational age of occurrence of clinical rubella in the mother.[23,24,28] Cataracts and cardiac anomalies occurred following maternal rubella during the initial 8 weeks of gestation, but deafness was commonly associated with rubella at 5–15 weeks, and multiple anomalies were encountered only with rubella before the 9th gestational week. No major anomalies were found following maternal rubella later than 16 weeks gestation, although embryonic pigmentary retinopathy has been observed after onset of rubella as late as the 20th gestational week.

REFERENCES

[1]Banatvala JE, Horstmann DM, Payne MC, Gluck L: Rubella syndrome and thrombocytopenic purpura in newborn infants. Clinical and virological observations. New Eng J Med 273:474, 1965.

[2]Banatvala JE, Kennedy EA, Best JM: Clinical virology: a year's experience. Brit Med J 2:609, 1967.

[3]Bellanti JA, Artenstein MS, Olson LC, Buescher EL, Luhrs CE, Milstead KL: Congenital rubella. Clinicopathologic, virologic and immunologic studies. Am J Dis Child 110:464, 1965.

[4]Brody JA, Sever JL, McAlister R, Schiff GM, Cutting R: Rubella epidemic on St. Paul Island in the Pribilofs, 1963. I. Epidemiologic, clinical and serologic findings. JAMA 191:619, 1965.

[5]Centers for Disease Control: Encephalitis Surveillance Annual Summary 1978, issued May 1981.

[6]Centers for Disease Control: Rubella and Congenital Rubella - United States, 1983. MMWR 33:237, 1984.

[7]Green RH, Balsamo MR, Giles JP, Krugman S, Mirick GS: Studies on the natural history and prevention of rubella. Am J Dis Child 110:348, 1965.

[8]Gregg NM: Congenital cataract following German measles in the mother. Trans Ophthalmol Soc Aust 3:35, 1941.

[9]Hill AB, Doll R, Galloway TM, Hughes JPW: Virus disease in pregnancy and congenital defects. Brit J Prev Soc Med 12:1, 1958.

[10]Hinman AR, Bart KJ, Orenstein WA, Preblud SR: Rational strategy for rubella vaccination. Lancet 1:39, 1983.

[11]Ingalls TH, Babbott FL Jr, Hampson KW, Gordon JE: Rubella: its epidemiology and teratology. Am J Med Sci 239:363, 1960.

[12]Jack I, Grutzner J: Cellular viremia in babies infected with rubella virus before birth. Brit Med J 1:289, 1969.

[13]Korones SB, Ainger LE, Monif GRF, Roane J, Sever JL, Fuste F: Congenital rubella syndrome: new clinical aspects with recovery of virus from affected infants. J Pediat 67:166, 1965.

[14]Kurtz JB, Mortimer PP, Mortimer PR, Morgan-Capner P, Shafi MS, White GBB: Rubella antibody measured by radial haemolysis. Characteristics and performance of a single screening method for use in diagnostic laboratories. J Hyg (Camb) 84:213, 1980.

[15]McLean DM, McNaughton GA, Givan KF, Best JM, Smith PA, Coleman MA: Rubella virus infections during pregnancy, Toronto 1963–66. Can Med Ass J 95:1174, 1966.

[16]Matthews REF: Classification and nomenclature of viruses. Intervirology 17:1, 1982.

[17] Menser M, Harley JD, Hertzberg R, Dorman DC, Murphy AM: Persistence of virus in lens for three years after prenatal rubella. Lancet 2:387, 1967.

[18]Monif GRF, Avery GB, Korones SB, Sever JL: Postmortem isolation of rubella virus from three children with rubella-syndrome defects. Lancet 1:723, 1965.

[19]O'Shea S, Best JM, Banatvala JE, Marshall WC, Dudgeon JA: Persistence of rubella antibody 8–18 years after vaccination. Brit Med J 288:1043, 1984.

[20]Parkman PD, Meyer HM, Artenstein MS: Recovery of rubella virus from army recruits. Proc Soc Exp Biol Med 111:225, 1962.

[21]Parkman, PD, Meyer HM, Kirschstein RL, Hopps HE: Attenuated rubella virus. I. Development and laboratory characterization. New Eng J Med 275:569, 1966.

[22]Phillips CA, Behbehani AM, Johnson LW, Melnick JL: Isolation of rubella virus: an epidemic characterized by rash and arthritis. JAMA 191:615, 1965.

[23]Pitt D, Keir EH: Results of rubella in pregnancy. Med J Aust 2:647 and 739, 1965.

[24]Plotkin SA, Cochran W, Lindquist J, Cockran G, Schaffer D, Scheie H, Furukawa T: Congenital rubella syndrome in late infancy. JAMA 200:435, 1967.

[25]Rudolph AJ, Yow MD, Phillips CA, Desmond MM, Blattner RJ, Melnick JL: Transplacental rubella infection in newly born infants. JAMA 191:843, 1965.

[26]Selzer G: Virus isolation, inclusion bodies and chromosomes in a rubella-infected human embryo. Lancet 2:336, 1963.

[27]Sever JL, Brody JA, Schiff GM, McAlister R, Cutting R: Rubella epidemic on St. Paul Island in the Pribilofs, 1963. II. Clinical and laboratory findings for the intensive study population. JAMA 191:624, 1965.

[28]Sheridan MD: Final report of a prospective study of children whose mothers had rubella in early pregnancy. Brit Med J 2:536, 1964.

[29]Swartz TA, Klingberg W, Goldwasser RA, Klingberg MA, Goldblum N, Hilleman MR: Clinical manifestations, according to age, among females given HPV-77 duck rubella vaccine. Am J Epidemiol 94:246, 1971.

[30]Tingle AJ, Pot CH, Chanter JK: Prolonged arthritis, viraemia, hypogammaglobulinaemia, and failed seroconversion following rubella immunization. Lancet 1:1475, 1984.

[31]Wesselhoeft C: In Modern Practice in Infectious Fevers, Rubella and Congenital Defects. I. Rubella, ed. HS Banks, Butterworth, London, 1951, p. 521.

[32]Young SEJ, Ramsay AM: The diagnosis of rubella. Brit Med J 2:1295, 1963.

CHAPTER 10

ARTHROPOD-BORNE VIRUSES

TOGAVIRIDAE, BUNYAVIRIDAE, RHABDOVIRIDAE

*AR*thropod-*BO*rne viruses (Arboviruses) are "...viruses maintained in nature principally, or to an important extent, through biological transmission between susceptible vertebrate hosts by hematophagous (blood-feeding) arthropods (mosquitoes, ticks, sandflies) or through transovarian and possibly venereal transmission in arthropods; they multiply and produce viremia in the vertebrates, multiply in the tissues of arthropods, and are passed on to new vertebrates (humans, other mammals, birds) by the bites of arthropods after a period of extrinsic incubation.[46] This definition provides a functional or ecological basis for consideration as a whole, the large and diverse collection of 532 catalogued virus serotypes within 67 antigenic groups (serogroups), as of 31 December 1989,[2] which are actually or presumably maintained in nature by biological cycles of transmission between vertebrate reservoirs and arthropod vectors. Among this functional collection of 532 arboviruses, 440 serotypes within 60 serogroups are classified into 5 principal families: Togaviridae (28 serotypes), Flaviviridae (68 serotypes), Bunyaviridae (232 serotypes), Rhabdoviridae (49 serotypes) and Reoviridae (63 serotypes). The remaining 92 serotypes are within 9 families (Table 10-1). Although many Rhabdoviridae members are transmitted by arthropods, an important member, rabies virus, clearly is not arthropod-borne. Orbivirus is the sole genus within the family Reoviridae (chapter 7) which contains arthropod-borne serotypes. Some non-arthropod-borne viruses are prevalent in the same geographic regions as arboviruses and these traditionally are studied by arbovirologists. They include agents such as Lassa and Machupo viruses within the Arenaviridae, which are probably transmitted in nature by contamination of fomites by urine of rodents, and other agents such as Marburg virus (Filoviridae) (chapter 11).

HISTORICAL

Yellow fever virus was the first arbovirus to be studied in the laboratory.

TABLE 10-1

ANTIGENIC GROUPS OF 532 VIRUSES REGISTERED TO 31 DECEMBER 1989*

Virus Family and Genus	Antigenic Group	Abbreviation	No. Viruses	Registered in Group	Percent
Arenaviridae					
Arenavirus	Tacaribe	TCR		11	2.1
	Quaranfil	QRF		2	0.4
	Ungrouped			1	0.2
Bunyaviridae					
Bunyavirus				131	24.6
Bunyamwera	Anopheles A	ANA	5		
Supergroup	Anopheles B	ANB	2		
	Bunyamera	BUN	25		
	Bwamba	BWA	2		
	C	C	12		
	California	CAL	13		
	Capim	CAP	8		
	Gamboa	GAM	3		
	Guama	GMA	12		
	Koongol	KOO	2		
	Minatitlan	MNT	2		
	Olifantsvlei	OLI	5		
	Patois	PAT	7		
	Simbu	SIM	21		
	Tete	TETE	5		
	Turlock	TUR	4		
	Unassigned	SBU	3		
Nairovirus				24	4.5
	CHF-Congo	CHF-CON		4	
	Dera Ghazi Khan	DGK		5	
	Hughes	HUG		4	
	Nairobi sheep disease	NSD		3	
	Qalyub	QYB		3	
	Sakhalin	SAK		5	
Phlebovirus	Phlebotomus fever	PHL		38	7.2
Uukuvirus	Uukuniemi	UUK		6	1.1
Hantavirus	Hantaan	HTN		4	0.8
"Bunyavirus-like"	Bakau	BAK		5	0.9
(Unassigned,	Bhanja	BHA		3	0.6
probable or poss-	Kaisodi	KSO		3	0.6
ible members)	Mapputta	MAP		4	0.8
	Matariya	MTY		3	0.6
	Nyando	NDO		1	0.2
	Resistencia	RTA		3	0.6
	Tanga	TAN		2	0.4
	Thiafora	TFA		2	0.4
	Upolu	UPO		2	0.4
	Yogue	YOG		1	0.2
	Ungrouped			22	6.1
Reoviridae					
Orbivirus	African horse sickness	AHS		1	0.2
	Bluetongue	BLU		1	0.2
	Changuinola	CGL		12	2.3

TABLE 10-1 (Continued)
ANTIGENIC GROUPS OF 532 VIRUSES REGISTERED TO 31 DECEMBER 1989*

Virus Family and Genus	Antigenic Group	Abbreviation	No. Viruses	Registered in Group	Percent
	Chogar Gorge	CG		2	0.4
	Colorado tick fever	CTF		2	0.4
	Corriparta	COR		3	0.6
	Epizootic hemorrhagic dis.	EHD		2	0.4
	Eubenangee	EUB		3	0.6
	Ieri			3	0.6
	Kemerovo	KEM		18	3.4
	Palyam	PAL		9	1.7
	Umatilla	UMA		3	0.6
	Wallal	WAL		1	0.2
	Warrego	WAR		1	0.2
	Wongorr	WGR		2	0.4
	Ungrouped			8	1.5
Unassigned	Ungrouped			6	0.9
Rhabdoviridae					
Vesiculovirus	Vesicular stomatitis	VSV		17	3.2
Lyssavirus	Rabies			16	3.0
Unassigned or	Hart Park	HP		5	0.9
possible members	Kern Canyon	KC		3	0.6
	Le Dantec	LD		2	0.4
	Sawgrass	SAW		3	0.6
	Timbo	TIM		3	0.6
	Ungrouped			17	3.2
Filoviridae					
Filovirus	Marburg	MBG		2	0.4
Togaviridae					
Alphavirus	A	A		28	5.3
Possible members	Ungrouped			1	0.2
Flaviviridae					
Flavivirus	B	B		64	13.1
Possible members	Ungrouped			2	0.4
Coronaviridae					
Coronavirus	Ungrouped			2	0.4
Herpesviridae	Ungrouped			1	0.2
African Swine Fever	Ungrouped			1	0.2
Nodaviridae					
Nodavirus	Ungrouped			1	0.2
Orthomyxoviridae	Thogoto	THO		1	0.2
	Ungrouped			1	0.2
Paramyxoviridae					
Paramyxovirus	Ungrouped			2	0.4
	Salanga			1	0.2
Poxviridae	Ungrouped			3	0.6
Unclassified	Nyamanini	NYM		1	0.2
	Somone	SOM		1	0.2
	Ungrouped			6	1.3
Total:				532	

*Berge TO (ed): US DHEW Pub No (CDC) 75-8301 updated to 31 Dec 31 1983.[2]

It was first isolated in 1927, by inoculation of rhesus monkeys, with the blood of an African man named Asibi living near Accra, Ghana who contracted yellow fever.[37] Adaptation of yellow fever virus to mice in 1930[40] provided a convenient technique for large-scale investigations of yellow fever epidemiology, and its subsequent adaptation to growth in chick embryo tissue culture led to development of the highly successful 17D strain of live yellow fever vaccine in 1937.[42] Without these laboratory tests however, the Reed Commission of 1900 had shown that yellow fever was transmitted from human to human by bites of *Aedes aegypti* mosquitoes after an extrinsic incubation period of 12 days, and that yellow fever could be transmitted experimentally by subcutaneous injection of blood from a patient during the first or second day of fever.[37] Through rigorous application of sanitary measures to control mosquitoes, the spread of yellow fever had been halted in Havana and Panama by 1902. Effective mosquito abatement also rendered possible the completion of the Panama Canal in 1914, which hitherto had been stalled through enormous loss of life from yellow fever among workers before adequate mosquito control at construction sites.

Epidemiological evidence in Brazil and Colombia during the early 1930's pointed conclusively towards the maintenance of yellow fever away from urban areas through a "jungle" or "sylvan" natural cycle of infection involving monkeys as vertebrate reservoirs, forest canopy mosquitoes especially *Haemagogus spegazzinii* as arthropod vectors. Human infections were acquired tangentially to this cycle, for example after bites by forest canopy mosquitoes which were brought to ground level during tree felling for road construction or establishment of new farms. Sponsorship of virus laboratories by the Rockefeller Foundation in Trinidad during 1953, and Belem, Brazil in 1954, where suckling mice were used as a more sensitive virus detection system, resulted in the isolation of numerous arboviruses in addition to yellow fever from humans, other vertebrates and mosquitoes. Meanwhile in tropical regions of Africa, many arbovirus serotypes in addition to yellow fever had been isolated from human, vertebrate and arthropod specimens since the initial isolation of Bwamba virus in 1937.[35]

Western equine encephalomyelitis (WEE) virus was first arbovirus serotype clearly associated with epidemic encephalitis in North America. It was initially isolated from the brains of horses during an epidemic affecting both humans and horses in the San Joaquin Valley, California in 1930.[24] Antigenically distinct eastern equine encephalomyelitis (EEE) virus was first isolated from brains of horses in New Jersey during 1933[39] and from humans in Massachusetts during 1938.[44] St. Louis encephalitis (SLE) virus was first isolated from brains of patients who died with encephalitis in St. Louis and other midwestern communities during 1933.[43] Isolation of Japanese B encephalitis (JBE) virus (Nakayama strain) from CSF of a child who died with encephalitis in Japan during 1935[19] and Murray Valley encephalitis (MVE) from the brain of a fatal case of encephalitis in southeastern Australia in 1951[14] demonstrated the world wide prevalence of arboviruses causing encephalitis.

The term "arthropod-borne virus encephalitis" was first applied in 1943 following epidemiological investigations of SLE and WEE viruses in California and Washington State during the early 1940's.[16] Subsequently the term "arthropod-borne virus," abbreviated to ARBO virus in 1962[38] came into general usage to include all viruses which were transmitted biologically in nature by cycles involving both blood-sucking arthropods and vertebrates which develop viremic infections, irrespective of whether they induced encephalitis in humans or other vertebrates.

Widespread application of hemagglutination inhibition (HI) tests[5] in 1954 revealed for the first time antigenic cross-relationships between arboviruses with widely different epidemiological patterns such as mosquito-borne Japanese B encephalitis in Oriental regions, yellow fever in tropical Africa and South America, and tick-borne encephalitis (TBE) of northern Asia and Europe. However the above agents were antigenically distinct from EEE and WEE viruses which, together with Semliki Forest and other agents, comprised a different serogroup. Extensive use of tissue cultures for propagation of a wide range of arboviruses by 1958,[4] provided the basis for current advances in our understanding of their morphology and molecular virology, which offer additional criteria for classification into families and genera. Adaptation of the plaque reduction neutralization test (PRNT) in 1979[17] to a wide range of arboviruses provided serological criteria in addition to the HI tests for the classification of arboviruses into the current 67 serogroups, within 5 principal families containing 10 named genera, as of 31 December 1989.[2]

BIOLOGICAL ATTRIBUTES

Arboviruses share many common biological attributes, despite their diverse morphological, serological and epidemiological characteristics (Table 10-2).

1. All arboviruses multiply after intracerebral injection of suckling mice aged less than 48 hours, inducing encephalitis which terminates fatally 1 day (EEE) to about 10–14 days (dengue-3) subsequently. Brains of moribund mice usually contain the highest titers of infections virus except for the group C arboviruses where maximum concentrations are found in the liver. Many arboviruses multiply and induce fatal encephalitis in suckling mice after intraperitoneal inoculation. Some arboviruses such as MVE and snowshoe hare (SSH) viruses induce fatal encephalitis after intracerebral

TABLE 10-2
CHARACTERISTIC PROPERTIES OF ARBOVIRUSES*

Nucleic acid	(+)ss RNA	(+)ss RNA	(−)ss RNA	(−)ss RNA	ds RNA
Morphology	Enveloped virions, principally within five families				
Family	Togaviridae	Flaviviridae	Bunyaviridae	Rhabdoviridae	Reoviridae
Symmetry	Cubic	Cubic	Helical	Bullet-shaped	Cubic (double shell)
total diameter (nm)	60–65	40–50	90–100	170 x 70	65–80
Serotypes	28	68	232	49	63
Action of diethyl ether or sodium deoxycholate	Inactivates infectivity				
Laboratory test systems	Suckling mice (all viruses); weaned mice (some viruses) - encephalitis. Tissue cultures: continuous BHK or VERO (most viruses) - cytopathic effects and plaques; primary chick embryo (EEE, WEE), hamster kidney (some viruses).				
Diluent for infectivity titration	Bovalbumin 0.75% or fetal calf serum 20%.				
Diluent for hemagglutinin	0.15 M borate saline, pH 9.0				
Conditions for hemagglutinin	pH 6.0–7.0 and 4–37° C (specific pH and temp. for each serotype)				
Multiplication in mosquitoes	Most arboviruses				
Multiplication in ticks	Tick-borne flaviviruses; Colorado, Congo, Kaisodi serogroups				
Multiplication in sandflies	Phlebovirus				

*Adapted from McLean DM, 1980 "Virology in Health Care," Williams and Wilkins, Baltimore, p. 161.

injection of weaned mice aged 3–4 weeks; relatively few arboviruses induce encephalitis following intraperitoneal inoculation of weaned mice.

2. Most arboviruses multiply in continuous polyploid tissue cultures of baby hamster kidney (BHK)[18] and grivet monkey kidney (VERO),[17] inducing cytopathic effects when maintained in fluid media, and plaques under agarose overlay.

3. Many arboviruses multiply in insect cells in continuous culture, for example Singh's tissue culture line derived from larval *Aedes albopictus,*[33] usually without induction of cytopathic effect.

4. Arthropod-borne viruses multiply in mosquitoes after intrathoracic injection, attaining high titers in salivary glands, and viral antigen is detected in salivary glands by immunofluorescence and immunoenzyme techniques[22] or in head-squash preparations by immunofluorescence.[1,20]

5. Dilutions of arboviruses for infectivity titrations and neutralization tests should always be performed in buffered saline solutions containing added protein such as 0.75% bovalbumin or 20% fetal calf serum (which are devoid of inhibitors of virus infectivity). This prevents rapid loss of infectivity which occurs over a few minutes at room temperature 22° C when arboviruses are suspended in saline only.

6. Infectivity of all arboviruses is inactivated, or at least a 100-fold decline of infectivity is observed, after exposure to diethyl ether overnight at 4° C or after treatment with 1:1000 sodium deoxycholate.

7. Infectivity is preserved virtually intact for at least 2 years after storage frozen at –70° C and indefinitely (20 years or more) after lyophilization.

8. Following acetone-extraction of suspensions in sucrose of arbovirus-infected suckling mouse brains, in order to remove lipid inhibitors, most arboviruses induce hemagglutination of erythrocytes of geese or newly hatched chickens under defined conditions of temperature and pH (see chapter 3). Hemagglutination is inhibited by antiviral antibodies to the same serotype or other arboviruses within the same serogroup, after extraction of sera with acetone or kaolin to remove non-specific lipid inhibitors.

9. Complement fixing antigens for all arboviruses are prepared by acetone extraction of infected suckling mouse brains suspended in sucrose.

10. Neutralization tests in mice require inoculation of undiluted sera with serial dilutions of virus, and the antibody titer is expressed as the neutralization index. Neutralization tests in tissue culture are best performed by the plaque reduction technique, where serial dilutions of serum are mixed with 100 plaque forming units of virus, and the antibody titer is expressed as the highest serum dilution which exerts a 90% reduction of the plaque count.

CLASSIFICATION

Electron microscopic observations of purified preparations of arboviruses has facilitated their classification into families and genera according to size and shape of virus particles. Serological investigations by HI and PRNT techniques provide the basis for classification into serogroups within genera, but as yet 8% of named arboviruses within families and 9% unclassified agents have not been assigned to any antigenic group.

Togaviridae (alphavirus) comprise 28 serotypes with spherical virus particles with total diameters 60–65nm and envelopes tightly applied to spherical capsids 25–35nm diameter with icosahedral symmetry[23] (Table 10-2). Surface projections are demonstrable in most togaviruses. Viruses contain a single molecule of positive sense ss RNA with molecules weight 4 X 10^6, 3–4 polypeptides, one or more of which are glycosylated and virus-specific glycopeptides within the lipoprotein envelope, whose lipids are cell-derived. Flaviviridae (Flavivirus) resemble Alphavirus particles morphologically, but show smaller diameters 40–50nm.

Alphavirus particles typically have total diameters approaching 70 nm. Currently there are 28 alphavirus serotypes, all within serogroup A, and they include the important encephalitis-inducing agents EEE and WEE viruses (Table 10-3). Flavivirus particles usually measure 40–50nm diameter (Figure 10-1). Currently there are 68 flavivirus serotypes including yellow fever, dengue, SLE and MVE viruses which are mosquito-borne, plus TBE and Powassan viruses which are tick-borne.

Bunyaviridae comprise 232 serotypes with spherical, oval enveloped particles 90–100 nm total diameter with glycoprotein surface projections, 3 ribonucleocapsids composed of circular long helical strands 2–2.5 nm diameter.[23] Viruses contain 3 molecules of negative sense ss RNA (large, medium, small L, M, S), with molecular weights 3-5, 1-2 and 0.4 – 0.8 x 10^6 respectively, several proteins and lipid within the envelope. Bunyaviridae contain 5 genera: Bunyavirus, Nairovirus, Phlebovirus, Uukuvirus, Hantavirus, plus an additional 28 serotypes which are termed "Bunyavirus-like."

Bunyavirus genus contains 131 serotypes within the Bunyamwera Super-group which is subdivided into 17 serogroups. Most viruses are mosquito-borne. Important human pathogens are included in the California (CAL) (Figure 10-2) and Simbu serogroups. Nairovirus genus contains 24 serotypes within 6 serogroups and includes the human pathogens Crimean hemorrhagic fever and Congo viruses. Many viruses are tick-borne. Phlebovirus genus contains 38 serotypes within one serogroup (Phlebotomus) and includes the human pathogens Rift Valley fever and sandfly fever viruses. Most viruses are sandfly-borne. Uukuvirus genus contains 6 serotypes within one serogroup (Uukuniemi). Most viruses are tick-borne.

Reoviridae contain 63 serotypes of the genus Orbovirus, which are classified within 15 serogroups. Orbivirus particles are naked double-shelled virions containing ss RNA, with total diameters 65–80 nm and the inner shell has 32 morphological units showing circular surface configurations.[23] Viruses are transmitted by ticks, mosquitoes or sandflies, according to the particular serogroup.

Rhabdoviridae contain 49 serotypes with bullet-shaped enveloped virions (Figure 10-3) 130–380nm x 50–95nm total diameter with pro-teinaceous surface projections, and one molecule of negative sense ss RNA in a helical nucleocapsid.[23] Rhabdoviridae contain 2 genera: (a) Vesiculo-

TABLE 10-3
CLINICAL SYNDROMES ASSOCIATED WITH SELECTED ARBOVIRUSES*

Syndrome	Serogroup	Causative Arbovirus serotype	Geographic Distribution
Encephalitis or Aseptic meningitis	A	Venezuelan equine encephalitis	Central and South America
		western equine encephalomyelitis	Western Canada and USA, Caribbean
	B (mosq. borne)	Japanese B encephalitis	Orient (Japan to Malaysia)
		Murray Valley encephalitis	Australia
		St. Louis encephalitis	Canada, USA, Central America
	B (tick-borne)	Louping ill	Scotland, Northern Ireland
		Powassan	Canada, Northern USA
		tickborne encephalitis	Central and northern Europe, Siberia
	CAL	La Crosse	USA
		snowshoe hare	Canada
Yellow Fever	B	yellow fever	Tropical Africa, Caribbean, tropical South America
Dengue	A	chikungunya	East Africa, India, Southeast Asia
	B	dengue (4 types)	Entire Tropical Zone
Hemorrhagic Fever	A	chikungunya	East Africa, India, Southeast Asia
	B (mosq)	dengue (4 types)	India, Philippines, Southeast Asia, Oceania, Caribbean
	B (tick)	Kyasanur Forest disease	India
		Omsk hemorrhagic fever	Siberia
	CHF-CON (tick)	Congo	Central and southern Africa
Undifferentiated tropical fever	A	chikungunya	East Africa, India, Southeast Asia
		Ross River	Australia, Oceania
	B	Ilheus	Caribbean, South America
		West Nile	Central and northern Africa
	PHL (mosq borne)	Rift Valley fever	Northern, eastern and southern Africa
	PHL sandfly-borne	Punta Toro	Central America
		sandfly fever-Naples	Mediterranean
	SIM	Oropouche	Caribbean, South America

*McLean DM, 1983 "Imported Arbovirus Infections" in Recent Advances in Clinical Virology 3, ed AP Waterson, Churchill Livingstone, Edinburgh, p. 240.

virus contains 17 serotypes within the vesicular stomatitis virus (VSV) serogroup, most of which are transmitted by sandflies or mosquitoes; (b) Lyssavirus contains 16 serotypes which are antigenically related to but distinct from rabies virus which is not arthropod-borne (see p. 176). An additional 16 serotypes, net yet assigned to a species, are classified within 5 serogroups and a further 17 serotypes are as yet ungrouped.

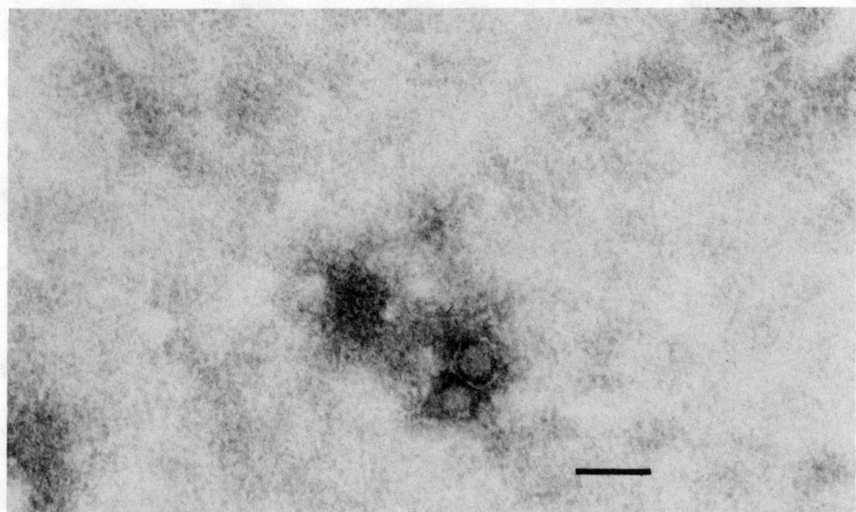

Figure 10-1: Powassan virus strain LB (X120,120). Negatively stained preparation after propagation in suckling mouse brain.

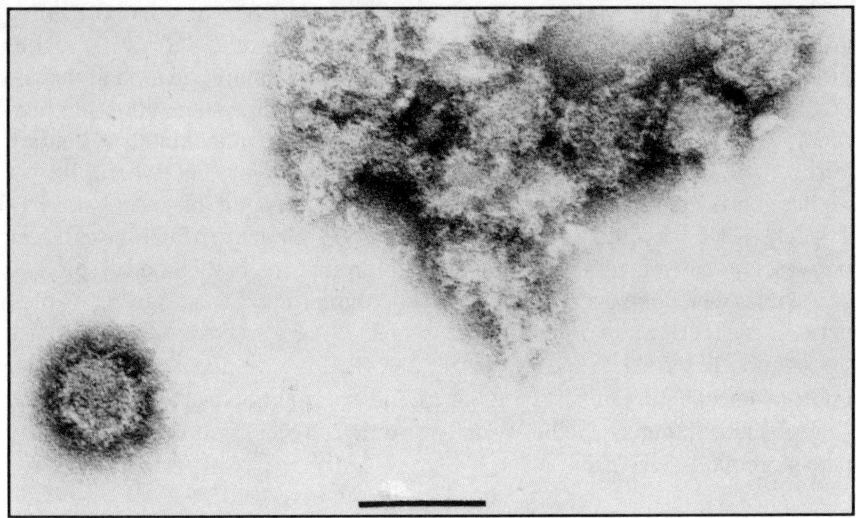

Figure 10-2: Snowshoe hare virus strain 78-Y-133 (X193,050). Negatively stained preparation after propagation in BHK cultures and purification by ultracentrifugation on a sucrose density gradient.

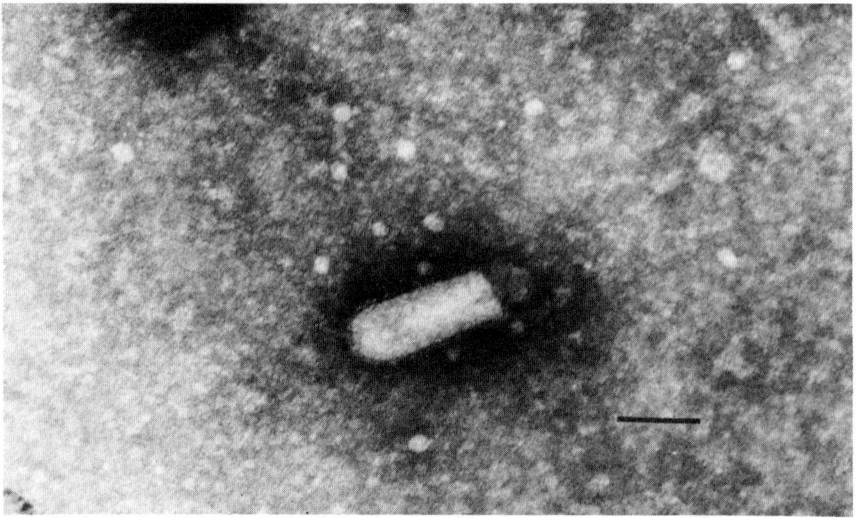

Figure 10-3: Vesicular stomatitis virus (X129,360).

PATHOGENESIS

Virus enters the vertebrate host naturally by the bite of a blood-feeding arthropod, or experimentally by subcutaneous injections. Shortly thereafter virus enters the blood vascular system, without initial multiplication at the site of entry. Virus multiplies readily in the blood vascular system, attaining high titers in the blood within 2 days in birds and 3–4 days in mammals (viremia). Virus thereby gains access to the central nervous system where further replication occurs, giving rise to symptoms of meningitis or encephalitis 1–2 weeks after the initial infection (Figure 4-5). Brains of fatal cases show perivascular cuffing with mononuclear cells around cerebral blood vessels, and glial knots which are accumulations of microglia (macrophages of the central nervous system), around necrotic neurones.

Antibodies are detected by HI, NT and ELISA tests about one week after onset of encephalitis in surviving cases and these antibodies persist lifelong. Complement fixing antibodies usually appear 2–3 weeks after onset and they persist about 1–3 years.

SYMPTOMATOLOGY

Arbovirus infections may induce encephalitis or aseptic meningitis, yellow fever (hepatic involvement), dengue, other undifferentiated tropical fevers with or without hemorrhagic manifestations, or involvement of joints (arthritis) (Table 10-3). Many arbovirus infections however are subclinical (asymptomatic), and are diagnosed only by induction of antibody subsequently. Some general principles apply to arbovirus infections: (i) a high proportion of subclinical infections to clinical illnesses; (ii) many different serotypes may induce the same syndrome; (iii) most arboviruses are localized to a particular continent or geographic zone, except dengue which is prevalent world wide throughout the tropics.

ENCEPHALITIS

Typical symptoms comprise the sudden onset of fever and headache, followed by neck stiffness, nausea or vomiting, drowsiness and disorientation frequently deteriorating into stupor and coma.[21,47] Some patients may present with convulsions. Rigidity or weakness of the limbs may occur, together with absent or irregular deep tendon reflexes and upgoing plantar reflexes. The incubation period is usually 1–2 weeks. Symptoms may reach the peak of their severity 2–5 days after onset, after which patients may die, or the fever and other symptoms abate during the next 1–2 weeks. Cerebrospinal fluid cell count usually is elevated beyond 100/mm³, with a predominance of lymphocytes, but the sugar and protein levels remain normal. The peripheral blood leukocyte count usually does not exceed 8000/mm³, and shows a predominance of lymphocytes. During many outbreaks of encephalitis, for example in Manitoba Canada during summer 1981,[12] about 50% of cases exhibited fever and mild neck stiffness, without stupor or spasticity i.e., they developed aseptic meningitis without encephalitis. It is important to distinguish arbovirus infections both from enteroviral aseptic meningitis which may occur concomitantly, and from encephalitis due to measles, rubella, chickenpox or herpes simplex, by appropriate laboratory tests.

YELLOW FEVER

Patients suddenly develop headache and fever, accompanied by myalgia, nausea, vomiting, apprehension and injected conjunctivae, after an incubation period of 3–6 days.[26,36] Convulsions may herald the onset of yellow fever in children. Jaundice may appear on the third day of illness, sometimes accompanied by hematemesis and melena, epistaxis and bleeding gums. Albuminuria and oliguria may also begin suddenly during the first week of illness. In severe cases, death may occur 3 days or more after onset of illness, and midzonal necrosis is observed in the liver. The mortality rate from all cases of yellow fever is 5–10%. Mild cases may develop fever, headache and myalgia only, and it is important to distinguish these cases from dengue or other tropical arbovirus infections by isolation of virus from the blood or appropriate serological tests. Severe cases of yellow fever must be distinguished from hepatitis A, hepatitis B, leptospirosis, borreliosis or malaria by detailed laboratory investigations.

DENGUE

Patients suddenly develop fever and severe frontal headache, accompanied by retro-ocular pain, myalgia, pain in the back and limbs ("break-bone fever"), perversion of taste and lymphadenopathy, in the absence of persisting respiratory symptoms.[7,30] A maculopapular rash lasting 2–7 days may affect two-thirds of the patients, and pruritus about half the patients. Fever may persist 3–5 days, and it may show a remission followed by a relapse ("saddleback fever") in about half the patients. Leukopenia with relative lymphocytosis is a constant finding. Complete recovery is the rule after typical dengue. Any of the 4 serotypes of dengue virus (Flavivirus) have induced clinical dengue, but the same syndrome has been encountered after chikungunya (Alphavirus) infections.[10]

HEMORRHAGIC FEVERS

In Southeast Asia since 1958, and in islands of the Southwest Pacific since 1971, hemorrhagic manifestations including purpura, epistaxis, hematuria and gastrointestinal bleeding, which are accompanied by varying degrees of shock, have been observed in association with typical symptoms of dengue.[15,25] Both children and adults are affected, but in Southeast Asia the incidence of severe and fatal cases is highest among children 3–7 years of age. Thrombocytopenia with platelet counts below $100,000/mm^3$ is found in about two-thirds of cases, persisting 1–2 weeks, but counts have been as low as $10,000–16,000/mm^3$ 4–6 days after onset. The case fatality rate from hemorrhagic dengue is 4–12%.

Although hemorrhagic dengue usually follows infection by one or more dengue serotypes, similar clinical manifestations have been observed after infection with chikungunya[31] and Kyasanur Forest disease virus[45] in India, Omsk hemorrhagic fever[8] in Siberia and by Congo virus[28] in South Africa. Non-arthropod-borne Lassa virus also induces severe hemorrhagic disease.[13]

UNDIFFERENTIATED TROPICAL FEVERS

These may exhibit some clinical features resembling dengue. They may arise after infection with the alphavirus Ross River,[11] the flaviviruses Ilheus[41] and West Nile,[3] the phleboviruses Rift Valley fever,[6] sandfly fever[33] and Punta Toro,[32] and the bunyavirus Oropouche.[27] Ross River virus infections are frequently associated with polyarthritis,[9] particularly affecting the wrists and metacarpophalangeal joints.[29]

REFERENCES

[1]Beaty BJ, Thompson WH: Emergence of La Crosse Virus from endemic foci. Fluorescent antibody studies of overwintered *Aedes triseriatus*. Am J Trop Med Hyg 24:685, 1975.

[2]Berge TO (ed): International Catalogue of Arboviruses including certain other Viruses of Vertebrates. Ed 2. U.S. Dept of Health, Education and Welfare Publ No. (CDC) 75-8301, 1975, with updatings by Subcommittee on Information Exchange to 31 Dec. 1989.

[3]Bernkoff H, Levine S, Nerson R: Isolation of West Nile Virus in Israel. J Infect Dis 93:207, 1953.

[4]Buckley SM: Propagation, cytopathogenicity and hemagglutination - hemadsorption of some arthropod-borne viruses in tissue culture. Ann NY Acad Sci 81:172, 1959.

[5]Casals J, Brown LV: Hemagglutination with arthropod-borne viruses. J Exp Med 99:429, 1954.

[6]Centers for Disease Control: Rift Valley fever - Egypt. MMWR 29:178, 1980.

[7]Centers for Disease Control: Imported dengue type 4 - Florida. MMWR 30:622, 1982.

[8]Chumakov MP: Terapert Arch 2:68, 1948. Data have been assembled in the English language. In: Berge TO (ed): US DHEW Publ No (CDC) 75-8301, 1975.

[9]Clarke JA, Marshall ID, Gard G: Annually recurrent epidemic polyarthritis and Ross River virus activity in a coastal area of New South Wales. I. Occurrence of the disease. Am J Trop Med Hyg 22:543, 1973.

[10]Deller JJ, Russell PK: Chikungunya disease. Am J Trop Med Hyg 17:107, 1968.

[11]Doherty RL, Carley JG, Best JC: Isolation of Ross River virus from man. Med J Aust 1:1083, 1972.

[12]Eadie JA, Friesen B: Epidemiological study of western equine encephalitis - Manitoba 1981. Manitoba Ministry of Health Publ. Dec. 1982, p. 142.

[13]Emond RTD, Bannister B, Southee TJ, Bowen ETW: A case of Lassa Fever: clinical and virological findings. Brit Med J 285:1001, 1982.

[14]French EL: Murray valley encephalitis: isolation and characterization of the aetiological agent. Med J Aust 1:100, 1952.

[15]Halstead SB, Voulgaropoulos E, Tien NH, Udomsadki S: Dengue hemorrhagic fever in South Vietnam: report of the 1963 outbreak. Am J Trop Med Hyg 14:819, 1965.

[16]Hammon W McD, Reeves WC, Gray M: Mosquito vectors and inapparent animal reservoirs of St. Louis and western equine encephalitis viruses. Am J Pub Health 33:201, 1943.

[17]Hunt AR, Calisher CH: Relationships of Bunyamwera group viruses by neutralization. Am J Trop Med Hyg 28:740, 1979.

[18]Karabatsos N, Buckley SM: Susceptibility of the baby hamster kidney cell line (BHK 21) to infection with arboviruses. Am J Trop Med Hyg 16:99, 1967.

[19]Kashara S et al: Kitasato Arch Exp Med 13:48, 1936.

[20]Kuberski TT, Rosen L: A simple technique for the detection of dengue antigen in mosquitoes by immunofluorescence. Am J Trop Med Hyg 26:533, 1977.

[21]McLean DM, Donohue WL: Powassan virus: Isolation of virus from a fatal case of encephalitis. Can Med Ass J 80:708, 1959.

[22]McLean DM, Grass PN, Judd BD, Stolz KJ: Bunyavirus development in arctic and *Aedes aegypti* mosquitoes as revealed by glucose oxidase staining and immunofluorescence. Arch Virol 62:313, 1979.

[23]Matthews REF: Classification and nomenclature of viruses. Intervirology 17:1, 1982.

[24]Meyer KF, Haring CM, Howitt B: The etiology of epizootic encephalomyelitis in horses in the San Joaquin Valley, 1930. Science 74:227, 1931.

[25]Moreau JP, Rosen L, Saugrain L, Lagraulet J: An epidemic of dengue on Tahiti associated with hemorrhagic manifestations. Am J Trop Med Hyg 22:237, 1973.

[26]Pinheiro FP, Travassos da Rosa APA, Morales MAP, Neto JCA, Camargo S, Filgueras JP: An epidemic of yellow fever in central Brazil 1972–1973. I. Epidemiological studies. Am J Trop Med Hyg 27:125, 1978.

[27]Pinheiro FP, Travassos da Rosa APA, Travassos da Rosa JFS, Ishak R, Freitas RB, Gomes MLC, Le Duc JW, Olivia OFP: Oropouche virus. I. A review of clinical, epidemiological and ecological findings. Am J Trop Med Hyg 30:149, 1981.

[28]Public Health Laboratory Service. A case of Congo/Crimean hemorrhagic fever in South Africa. Communicable Disease Report 81/19, 1983, p. 3.

[29]Rosen L, Gubler DJ, Bennett PH: Epidemic polyarthritis (Ross River) virus infection in the Cook Islands. Am J Trop Med Hyg 30:1294, 1981.

[30]Russell PK, Buescher EL, McCown JM, Ordonez J: Recovery of dengue viruses from patients during epidemics in Puerto Rico and East Pakistan. Am J Trop Med Hyg 15:573, 1966.

[31]Sarkar JK, Pavri KM, Chaterjee SN, Shakravarty SK, Anderson CR: Virological and serological studies in cases of hemorrhagic fever in Calcutta. Material collected by the Calcutta School of Tropical Medicine. Indian J Med Res 52:684, 1964.

[32]Sather GE: Punta Toro (PT) Strain 4021A. Am J Trop Med Hyg Supp 19:1103, 1970.

[33]Schmidt JR, Schmidt ML, Said MI: Phlebotomus fever in Egypt. Isolation of phlebotomus fever viruses from *Phlebotomus papatasi*. Am J Trop Med Hyg 20:483, 1971.

[34]Singh KRP, Paul SD: Multiplication of arboviruses in cell lines derived from *Aedes albopictus* and *Aedes aegypti*. Curr Sci (India) 37:65, 1968.

[35]Smithburn KC, Mahaffy AF, Paul JH: Bwamba fever and its causative virus. Am J Trop Med 21:75, 1941.

[36]Spence L, Downs WG, Boyd C, Aitken THG: Description of human yellow fever cases seen in Trinidad in 1959. West Indian Med J 9:273, 1960.

[37]Strode GK: Yellow Fever. McGraw Hill, New York, 1951.

[38]Subcommittee of International Nomenclature Committee. Virology 21:516, 1963.

[39]Ten Broeck C, Merrill MH: A serological difference between eastern and western equine encephalomyelitis virus. Proc Soc Exp Biol Med 31:217, 1933.

[40]Theiler M: Studies on the action of yellow fever in mice. Am J Trop Med 24:249, 1930.

[41]Theiler M, Downs WG: The Arthropod-Borne Viruses of Vertebrates. An account of The Rockefeller Foundation Virus Program 1951–1970. Yale University Press, New Haven, 1973.

[42]Theiler M, Smith HH: Use of yellow fever virus modified by in vitro cultivation for human immunization. J Exp Med 65:787, 1937.

[43]Webster LT, Fite GL: A virus encountered in the study of material from cases of encephalitis in the St. Louis and Kansas City epidemics of 1933. Science 78:463, 1933.

[44]Webster LT, Wright FH: Recovery of eastern equine encephalomyelitis virus from brain tissue of human cases of encephalitis in Massachusetts. Science 88:305, 1938.

[45]Work TH: Russian spring-summer virus in India. Kyasanur Forest disease. Progr Med Virol 1:248, 1958.

[46]World Health Organization: Arboviruses and Human Disease. Techn Rep Ser No 369, 1985.

[47]Zweighaft RM, Rasmussen C, Brobnitsky A, Lashof JC: St. Louis encephalitis: the Chicago experience. Am J Trop Med Hyg 28:114, 1979.

CHAPTER 11

RABIES AND SELECTED NON-ARTHROPOD-BORNE AGENTS INVESTIGATED BY ARBOVIROLOGISTS

Rabies virus (Rhabdoviridae family), Lassa, Machupo and Junin viruses (Arenaviridae family) and Marburg serogroup viruses (Filoviridae family) are encountered during field and laboratory investigations by arbovirologists, yet clearly these viruses are not transmitted biologically by arthropods. Generally their biological properties resemble those of arthropod-borne viruses (see p. 161), but additional attributes are noted under each serotype.

RABIES

BIOLOGICAL PROPERTIES

Rabies virus particles show the bullet-shaped morphology typical of the Rhabdoviridae. Rabies virus is assigned to the Lyssavirus genus which contains 2 serologically related viruses: Kotonkan virus isolated from *Culicoids sp.* in Nigeria which is probably arthropod-borne and Lagos bat virus isolated from bats which is not arthropod-borne.

Rabies virus is pathogenic for humans plus most domestic and wild animals, inducing encephalitis. Usually animals develop great excitability, unprovoked biting or snapping activity, and increased salivation ("furious rabies"), which may be followed by depression and paralysis ("dumb rabies") before terminating fatally about 7–10 days later. Mice develop fatal encephalitis 11–14 days after intracerebral injection with brain or saliva from an infected human case.[5] All these animals excrete rabies in the saliva several days before death (street virus). However after numerous brain-to-brain passages in rabbits, sheep or other domestic mammals, the incubation period becomes shortened to 6–10 days and virus is not excreted in the saliva (fixed virus).

Rabies virus propagates readily in a variety of tissue cultures including hamster kidney, continuous spinner cultures of polyploid baby hamster kidney (BHK 21/S) from which hemagglutinin has been prepared[3] and continuous human diploid cells (W1–38).[8] Excellent antibody responses have followed intramuscular and intradermal administration of rabies vaccine prepared after propagation of fixed rabies virus in human continuous diploid cells and inactivation by ß-propiolactone[2,6] with antibody levels substantially higher than those attained after administration of the previously licensed duck embryo vaccine for pre-exposure immunization. Current experience in Kenya has shown complete protection against death from rabies following post-exposure administration of 6 doses of human diploid cell vaccine.[7]

PATHOGENESIS

Rabies virus may reach the central nervous system either by propagation along nerve pathways, or by the blood-borne route, after salivary contamination of wounds by bites of rabid animals which excrete substantial quantities of rabies virus in saliva. Virus replicates in the central nervous system inducing encephalitis. The neurones, especially in Ammon's horn of the hippocampus, show acidophilic cytoplasmic inclusions (Negri bodies) which are typical of rabies infection (Figure 11-1), and the presence of rabies antigen is demon-

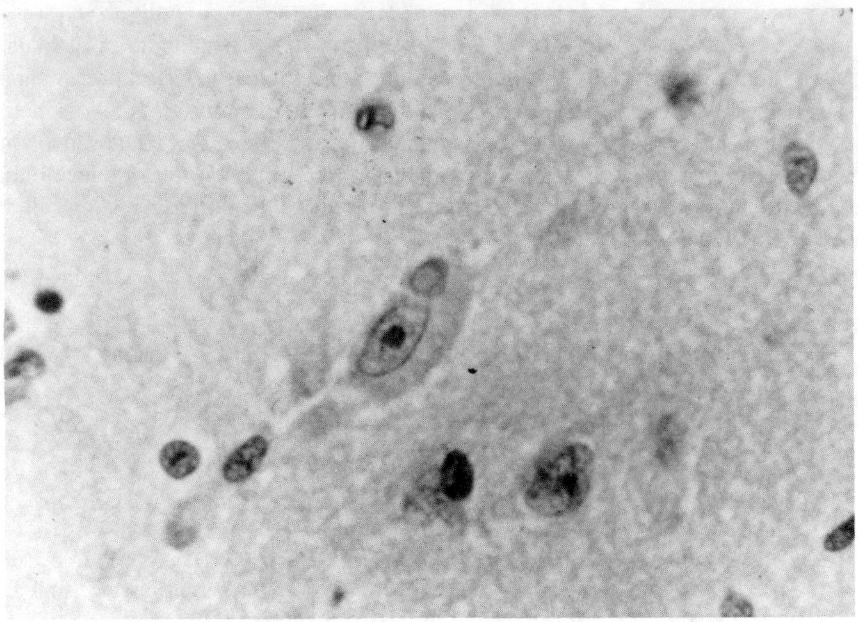

Figure 11-1: Rabies: Negri body in cytoplasm of neurone within Ammon's horn of the hippocampus of a boy aged 8 years. Reproduced with permission from McLean DM, 1980. Virology in Health Care, Williams and Wilkins, Baltimore, p. 131.

strated readily by immunofluorescence. Rabies virus also reaches the submandibular salivary glands where it proliferates and is excreted in the saliva.

SYMPTOMATOLOGY

The incubation period in humans is usually 3–8 weeks after the bite by a rabid animal, but it may range from 19 days to 6 months or more. Early symptoms include undue anxiety and overactivity, or there may be muscular weakness. Children may exhibit mental confusion, shrill voice or cry, and excessive limb movement, while adults may remain alert despite excessive and sometimes violent, uncontrolled limb movements. Usually there is excessive salivation accompanied by inability to swallow fluids (hydrophobia). The neck remains supple, CSF shows normal levels of glucose and protein, and few lymphocytes. The case fatality rate is virtually 100%.

Rabies has caused fatal infections in two recipients of corneal transplants from donors in whom rabies was not recognized clinically at the time of their deaths. An Idaho resident developed numbness, dysarthria, disorientation of handwriting, unsteadiness of gait progressing to quadriplegia, profound dysphagia, respiratory distress and coma which terminated fatally. Symptoms began 4-1/2 weeks after receiving a corneal transplant from a donor in Idaho who died after a rapidly progressive acute neurological deterioration, which subsequently was confirmed virologically to be due to rabies virus.[4] A resident of southern France died with rabies 41 days after receiving a corneal transplant from a donor who contracted a fatal neurological illness due to rabies about 2 months after moving to France from Egypt where the donor had been bitten by a dog which died.[1]

REFERENCES - RABIES

[1]Centers for Disease Control: Human-to-human transmission of rabies via corneal transplant - France. MMWR 29:25, 1980.

[2]Hafkin B, Hattwick MAW, Smith JS, Alls ME, Yager PA, Corey L, Hoke CH, Baer GM: A comparison of a W1–38 vaccine and duck embryo vaccine for preexposure rabies prophylaxis. Am J Epidemiol 107:439, 1978.

[3]Halonen PE, Murphy FA, Fields BN, Reese DR: Hemagglutinin of rabies and some other bullet-shaped viruses. Proc Soc Exp Biol Med 127:1037, 1968.

[4]Houff SA, Burton RC, Wilson RW, Henson TE, London WT, Baer GM, Anderson LJ, Winkler WG, Madden DL, Sever JL: Human-to-human transmission of rabies virus by corneal transplant. New Eng J Med 300:603, 1979.

[5]McLean DM, Krause VW, Wilson WM, Hawke WA: Rabies following skunk bite. Can Med Ass J 82:315, 1960.

[6]Nicholson KG, Prestage H, Cole PJ, Turner GS, Bauer SP: Multisite intradermal antirabies vaccination. Lancet 1:915, 1981.

[7]Rees P, Mathiu J, Timms G: Post-exposure rabies vaccination. Lancet 1:1469, 1984.
[8]Witkor TJ, Fernandes MV, Koprowski H: Cultivation of rabies virus in human diploid cell strain WI-38. J Immunol 93:353, 1964.

ARENAVIRIDAE

Arenaviridae comprise 11 serotypes within the Tacaribe serogroup (Table 10-1), including 3 important human pathogens: Lassa, Machupo and Junin.

LASSA virus was first isolated from the blood of a patient with a severe, prostrating febrile illness at Jos, Nigeria (10° N, 8° E) in February 1969.[1] Characteristic clinical features include severe constitutional upset with high fever, anorexia, nausea, vomiting, pharyngitis with petechiae or ulcers, abdominal pain and hypotension, with a case fatality rate of 40% or higher, both at Jos, Nigeria[3] and at Zorzor, Liberia in 1972.[6] Medical and nursing attendants and laboratory workers have contracted severe or fatal infections after working with patients.[3,5] Development of Lassa fever in a patient at a major teaching hospital in London, England shortly after arrival by air from Jos, Nigeria in early 1982[2] created an infection hazard involving hundreds of health care personnel. Fortunately no secondary cases occurred and the patient recovered from this hemorrhagic fever following a protracted convalescence.

Lassa virus has been isolated from the blood, throat washings and urine of patients. It is excreted in urine of rodents. Natural transmission of virus occurs by contact of abraded skin or mucosal surfaces with fomites contaminated by urine of infected rodents or through contact with discharges of infected patients.

MACHUPO virus was first isolated from the spleen of a child who contracted fatal hemorrhagic fever at San Joaquin, Bolivia (13° S, 64° W) in May 1963, during an extensive epidemic.[4] Transmission to humans occurs by contact with fomites contaminated by urine excreted by infected *Calomys callosus* rodents.

JUNIN virus was first isolated from the blood of a man with hemorrhagic fever near Junin, Argentina (34° S, 60° W) in June 1958.[7] It has since been isolated from several species of domestic and wild rodents in Argentina, and human cases continue to occur.

REFERENCES - ARENAVIRIDAE

[1]Buckley SM, Casals J: Lassa fever, a new virus disease of man from West Africa.

III. Isolation and characterization of the virus. Am J Trop Med Hyg 19:680, 1970.

[2]Cooper CB, Grandsen WR, Webster M, King M, O'Mahony M, Young S, Banatvala JE: A case of Lassa fever: experience at St. Thomas's Hospital: Brit Med J 285:1003, 1982.

[3]Frame JD, Baldwin JM, Gocke DJ, Troup JM: Lassa fever, a virus disease of man from West Africa. I. Clinical description and pathological findings. Am J Trop Med Hyg 19:670, 1970.

[4]Johnson KM, Wiebenga NH, Mackenzie RB, Kuns ML, Zauroso NM, Shelokov A, Webb PA, Justines G, Beye HK: Virus isolations from human cases of hemorrhagic fever in Bolivia. Proc Soc Exp Biol Med 118:113, 1965.

[5]Leifer E, Gocke DJ, Bourne H: Lassa fever, a new virus disease of man from West Africa. II. Report of a laboratory-acquired infection treated with plasma from a person recently recovered from the disease. Am J Trop Med Hyg 19:677, 1970.

[6]Mertens PE, Patton R, Baum JJ, Monath TP: Clinical presentation of Lassa fever cases during the hospital epidemic at Zorzor, Liberia, March–April 1972. Am J Trop Med Hyg 22:780, 1973.

[7]Parodi AS, Greenway DJ, Rugiero HR, Frigerio M, de la Barrera JM, Mettler N, Garzon F, Boxoca M, de Guerrero L, Nota N: Sobre la etiologia del brote epidemico de Junin. Dia Med 30:2300, 1958.

FILOVIRIDAE

MARBURG virus was first isolated from the blood of man aged 40 years who developed a febrile illness with rash, hemorrhagic manifestations and mental confusion at Marburg-Am-Lahn, West Germany in August 1967.[6] Among 31 cases, 7 died. The disease occurred largely among workers who handled viscera from African green monkeys imported from Uganda during preparation of tissue cultures. Marburg disease affected 2 Kenya residents in 1980,[7] one of whom died. The virus particle shows rhabdovirus-like morphology. A slight degree of antigenic overlap has been demonstrated by indirect immunofluorescence between Marburg and Ebola virus,[3] which together comprise the Marburg serogroup (Filoviridae family).

EBOLA virus was first isolated from the serum of a woman who developed severe hemorrhagic fever in a tropical rain forest at Yambuku, Equateur Province, Zaire (3° N, 22° E) in September 1976,[5] and from blood of another patient in Southern Sudan at the same time.[1] These virions showed rhabdovirus morphology resembling Marburg virus. Although the Zaire and Sudan strains were related antigenically,[3] they were serologically distinct from Marburg virus. Oligonucleotide mapping has confirmed the existence of two distinct subtypes of Ebola virus.[2] The taxonomic term Filoviridae was proposed to group Ebola and Marburg viruses.[4]

REFERENCES - FILOVIRIDAE

[1]Bowen ETW, Platt GS, Lloyd G, Baskerville A, Harris WJ, Vella EE: Viral haemorrhagic fever in southern Sudan and northern Zaire: Preliminary studies on the aetiological agent. Lancet 1:571, 1977.

[2]Cox NJ, McCormick JB, Johnson KM, Kiley MP: Evidence for two subtypes of Ebola virus based on oligonucleotide mapping of RNA. J Infect Dis 147:272, 1983.

[3]Johnson KM, Webb PA, Lange JV, Murphy FA: Isolation and partial characterization of a new virus causing acute haemorrhagic fever in Zaire. Lancet 1:569, 1977.

[4]Kiley MP, Bowen ETW, Eddy GA, Isaacson M, Johnson KM, McCormick JB, Murphy FA, Pattyn SR, Peters D, Prozesky OW, Regnery RL, Simpson DIH, Slenczka W, Sureau P, van der Groen G, Webb PA, Wulff H: Filoviridae: taxonomic home for Marburg and Ebola viruses. Intervirology 18:24, 1982.

[5]Pattyn S, Jacob W, van der Groen G, Piot P, Courteille G: Isolation of Marburg-like virus from a case of haemorrhagic fever in Zaire. Lancet 1:573, 1977.

[6]Siegert R, Shu HL, Slenczka W, Peters D, Muller G: Zur Atiologic einer unbekannten, van Affen ausgegangenen, menschlichen Infektionskrankheit. Deutsch Med Wochenschr 92:2341, 1967.

[7]Smith DH, Johnson BK, Isaacson M, Swanafoel R, Johnson KM, Kiley M, Bagshawe A, Siongok T, Keruga WK: Marburg-virus disease in Kenya. Lancet 1:816, 1982.

HERPESVIRIDAE

CLASSIFICATION

Herpesviridae include several enveloped DNA containing viruses with icosahedral symmetry which induce vesicular eruptions or generalized infections. Human pathogens are classified within three subfamilies.[22,28]

HERPES SIMPLEX VIRUS GROUP

ALPHAHERPESVIRINAE, including: Human (alpha) herpesvirus 1 (herpes simplex virus type 1): facial vesicles; Human (alpha) herpesvirus 2 (herpes simplex virus type 2): genital vesicles; Human (alpha) herpesvirus 3 (varicella-zoster): chickenpox, herpes zoster.

CYTOMEGALOVIRUS GROUP

BETAHERPESVIRINAE, including: Human (beta) herpesvirus 5 (human cytomegalovirus): congenital anomalies, fevers.

LYMPHOPROLIFERATIVE VIRUS GROUP

GAMMAHERPESVIRINAE, including: Human (gamma) herpesvirus 4 (Epstein-Barr virus): mononucleosis; Human herpesvirus 6: rashes.

Also included within the Alphaherpesvirinae subfamily as a probable member is cercopithecoid herpesvirus 1 (B), formerly termed B virus or *Herpesvirus simiae*. This causes a vesicular disease of monkeys which occasionally has caused fatal encephalitis in human patients who were bitten by infected monkeys or exposed to virus-contaminated tissue cultures.

HISTORICAL

The name herpes is derived from the Greek *herpes, herpetos*, which denotes a creeping, crawling creature, from the spreading nature of herpetic lesions on the face. Herpes simplex virus was first isolated in 1912, and again in 1919[12] by induction of keratitis in rabbits following inoculation with material from human herpetic keratitis and from vesicles on the lips. Mice were first used for titration of herpes simplex virus in 1932.[31] By 1939, chorioallantoic inoculation of chick embryos was used for quantitation of herpesvirus,[2] and by 1962 this was superseded by plaque assays in tissue culture.[30] Antigenic differences between strains of herpesvirus inducing facial or oral vesicles (type 1) and genital vesicles (type 2) were first recognized in 1967.[6] An association was first described between herpesvirus 2 and carcinoma of the cervix uteri in 1969.[27] Demonstration of the antiviral effectiveness of the synthetic compound Idoxuridine[17] in 1961 against herpetic keratitis paved the way for the currently prescribed acycloguanosine (Acyclovir, Zovirax) for treatment of genital herpes,[4,25] following the 1979 report of its therapeutic effectiveness in herpetic corneal ulcers.[15]

Varicella-Zoster (chickenpox) virus was first isolated in 1953 by inoculation of primary tissue cultures of human embryonic skin-muscle and human foreskin fibroblasts.[33] Antigenic identity between varicella and herpes zoster viruses was first demonstrated in 1954 by immunofluorescence tests in tissue cultures,[34] but both these agents were shown to be antigenically distinct from herpes simplex virus.

Human cytomegalovirus (CMV) isolations were first reported independently by three groups during 1956–57 employing tissue cultures of human uterine wall,[32] human adenoid tissue[29] and human embryonic skin-muscle.[35] Although the virus was named initially for the enlarged cells containing intranuclear and often intracytoplasmic inclusions (cytomegalia) which were induced by it in mentally retarded infants who died with "salivary gland disease," it has also been associated with microcephaly and mental retardation in surviving infants who were born to mothers who acquired new recrudescent CMV infections during pregnancy.[11]

Epstein-Barr (EB) virus was first identified in 1965 as a herpes-like agent in tissue cultures of Burkitt's lymphomas[7] and it was first clearly attributed to be the causative agent of infectious mononucleosis in 1967.[5]

BIOLOGICAL ATTRIBUTES

FEATURES IN COMMON

Herpesviridae virions are enveloped particles with total diameters 120–200 nm and each contains one molecule of linear dS DNA with molecular weight $80 - 150 \times 10^6$ plus more than 20 structural polypeptides with molecular weights ranging from 12,000 to more than 220,000.[22] Of the 4 structural components within the virion, the core consists of a fibrillar spool on which the DNA is wrapped. The ends of the fibers are anchored to the underside of the capsid shell. The core is surrounded by the capsid 100–110nm diameter which is composed of 162 capsomers arranged as an icosahedron with 150 hexameric and 12 pentameric capsomers. The capsomers are hexagonal in cross section and contain a hole running half-way down the long axis. The tegument surrounding the capsid consists of globular material which is frequently asymmetrically distributed and may be variable in amount. The envelope, a bilayer membrane surrounding the tegument, has surface projections. The intact envelope is impermeable to negative stain. Viral DNA replication occurs within the nucleus of susceptible cells and forms immature nucleocapsids which acquire envelopes by budding through the nuclear membrane, and these infective virus particles are released by transport to the surface of cells through the modified endoplasmic reticulum.

Although herpesviruses have been isolated from many vertebrate hosts, often a particular herpesvirus is infectious for one vertebrate species exclusively. For example cytomegalovirus propagates only in human tissues and mouse cytomegalovirus in mouse tissues exclusively. On the contrary, human herpesvirus 1 (simplex) grows in mice, rabbits and chick embryos in addition to diploid and polyploid tissue cultures of human cells. However it has been recovered in nature exclusively from human infections.

FEATURES OF EACH SEROTYPE

HERPES SIMPLEX TYPES 1 AND 2

(Human [alpha] herpesvirus 1 and 2). Both serotypes induce cytopathic effects—enlarged nuclei and shrunken cytoplasm, often appearing as grape-like clusters containing multinucleate syncytial mass—after inoculation of tissue cultures. Virus is transferred between cells through intercellular bridges but it is also liberated extracellularly into the tissue culture medium. For isolation of virus from vesicle fluid or scrapings from patients, the best tissue culture systems are monolayers of human diploid fibroblasts prepared either from foreskins of newborn babies locally, or from established cell lines MRC-5 or WI-38 which are derived from human embryo lung. Continuous polyploid human cell lines such as HeLa and HEp-2, and rabbit kidney cells RK-13 also develop cytopathic effects within 2 days after inoculation of herpesviruses. Suckling mice (aged less than 48 hours) develop fatal encephalitis 2–5 days after intracerebral inoculation with herpesviruses. Pocks develop on chorioallantoic membranes of chick embryos within 3 days after inoculation. Tissue culture cells infected with herpesviruses show intranuclear inclusions. Antigenic differences between herpesvirus 1 and herpesvirus 2 were first demonstrated by kinetic neutralization tests in tissue culture. Currently, serotyping of fresh isolates in tissue culture, or virus in infected cells from vesicle fluid or patients, is often achieved by direct immunofluorescence using fluorescein-conjugated antisera against each serotype.[21]

VARICELLA-ZOSTER (VZ) VIRUS

(Chickenpox or human [alpha] herpesvirus 3). With difficulty this virus is isolated from vesicle fluid of patients by inoculation of tissue cultures of primary human amnion or foreskin fibroblasts, or continuous human diploid cells. Cytopathic effects resembling those of herpesvirus 1 may appear after 5–7 days incubation. Although the tissue culture supernatant fluid contains complement fixing antigen, serial passage of virus from culture to culture requires transfer of infected tissue culture cells as well as supernatant fluid. Virus isolates in tissue culture or unpassaged virus in scrapings from vesicles is usually serotyped using varicella antiserum in an anticomplement im-munofluorescence test.[20] This test is necessary to circumvent non-specific binding of the Fc component of antibody to cells infected with varicella or cytomegalovirus.

CYTOMEGALOVIRUS (CMV)

(Human [beta] herpesvirus 5). This virus is isolated from freshly collected (not frozen) urine, other secretions or tissues obtained at biopsy, by inoculation of primary human foreskin fibroblasts or continuous human diploid cells in which it induces herpesvirus-like cytopathic effects after 1–4 weeks incuba-tion. Serial passage of CMV in tissue cultures is aided by transfer of cells in addition to supernatant fluid. Serotyping of virus isolates is accomplished by the anticomplement immunofluorescence (ACIF) test.

EPSTEIN-BARR (EBV) VIRUS

(Human [gamma] herpesvirus 4). This virus is isolated from throat secretions with considerable difficulty by inoculation of freshly prepared cultures of human umbilical cord leukocytes or leukocytes from normal adult humans or marmosets after pretreatment with phytohemagglutinin and placing on feeder layers of human placental cells.[23] Lymphoblastoid transformation is induced by EBV and observed after 2–5 weeks incubation, appearing as cell aggregates in an acid supernatant fluid. The presence of EBV-associated antigen is revealed in 0.8–1.2% human and 3.2–10% marmoset cells trans-formed by EBV by indirect immunofluorescence. Antigen is also detected in suspensions containing 5×10^7 cells/ml by complement fixation using antibody-positive human sera.[10,23] Convalescent phase sera from mononu-cleosis patients completely inhibited EBV-induced lymphoblastoid transfor-mation.

Several antigenic components have been found within the EBV particle. Antibodies to each component are now detected routinely by immunofluorescence.[8] Lymphoblastoid cell lines derived from patients with Burkitt's lymphoma provide the source of cells containing the several antigens of EBV. Cells of the P3HR-1 subline of EB3 cells provide a rich source of viral capsid antigen (VCA). Cells of the Raji line, following superinfection with EBV 2–3 days previously, are employed for tests for antibody to the early antigen (anti-EA). Raji cells alone, which are devoid of EA or VCA, are used in tests for antibody to the Epstein Barr virus-associated nuclear antigen (EBNA). Antibodies to EA and VCA are detected by indirect immunofluorescence, anti-EBNA is detected by anticomplement immunofluorescence.

PATHOGENESIS

HERPESVIRUS 1 AND 2 gain access to the proliferating layer of cells in the epidermis, or the oral or genital mucous membranes, through minute abrasions or by direct mucosal contact. Viruses multiply at the site of entry, inducing liquefactive necrosis of epithelial cells resulting in formation of vesicles. Usually virus remains localized to the site of implantation, but this stimulates production of neutralizing antibody which is followed by retrogression of the vesicles and scabbing. The viruses become latent within the epithelium and may be reactivated with production of fresh vesicles at the same site after external or internal stimuli. Occasionally herpesvirus 1 may enter the blood stream of children or adults, localize in the central nervous system and induce aseptic meningitis or encephalitis. In newborn infants, herpesvirus 2 which enters through minute skin abrasions by passage through the mother's infected birth canal, may rapidly enter the blood stream and multiply in a variety of viscera, inducing generalized disease which terminates fatally in about 50% of cases.

VARICELLA-ZOSTER virus enters the new host presumably by inhalation of droplets from the throat of a virus excreter. Viremia occurs about 1 week later, thus conveying virus to all parts of the body including the skin where vesicles appear in the epidermis 14–18 days after exposure to a known case. Virus replication occurs in the respiratory tract, and droplets are infectious for 2 days before to 4 days after onset of rash. Complement fixing antibodies are detected in the blood 2–3 weeks after onset of rash and persist 1 year or more (Figure 12-1).

CYTOMEGALOVIRUS may enter the fetus transplacentally from the mother who becomes infected at any time during pregnancy.[11] Virus multiplication occurs extensively in the lung, liver, kidney and brain, giving rise to gross congenital anomalies in the infant such as microcephaly and mental retardation. The risk of infants developing congenital CMV infection was 3

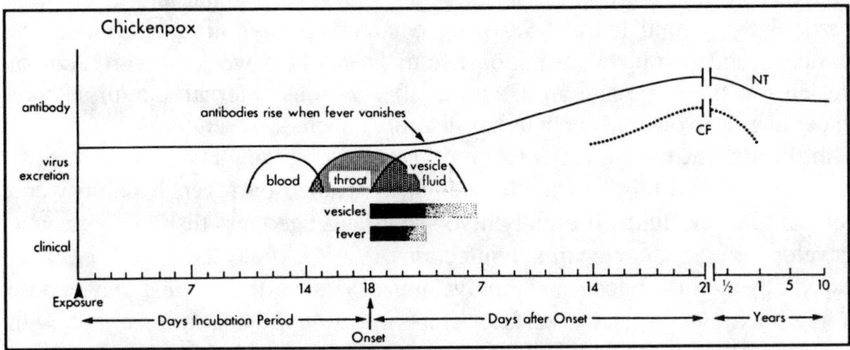

Figure 12-1: Time course of chickenpox infection. Reproduced with permission from McLean DM, 1980. Virology in Health Care, Williams and Wilkins, Baltimore, p. 218.

per 1000 in a large series in London, England.[26] Of infected infants, 7% showed serious anomalies, 33% exhibited minor or transient problems, and 60% had no detectable abnormality. Virus has been detected in urine as long as 26 months.[19] Urine contains large cells with eosinophilic intranuclear or cytoplasmic inclusions.

Cytomegalovirus may also be transmitted by blood transfusions, inducing a mononucleosis-like febrile illness with a negative Paul-Bunnell test,[16] and by renal homografts inducing pneumonia.[9]

EPSTEIN-BARR virus probably gains access to a new host by salivary transfer from a virus excreter during intimate mucosal contact such as kissing. The incubation period of infectious mononucleosis is 2–7 weeks, and virus is excreted in the throat 8–176 days after onset of symptoms.[23] Virus transfer may also occur during blood transfusions, especially in open heart surgery where 8% of patients subsequently developed mononucleosis.[14]

SYMPTOMATOLOGY

HERPES SIMPLEX TYPES 1 AND 2

This is characterized by a vesicular eruption affecting either: (i) mainly the face or upper trunk, due principally to herpesvirus 1; or (ii) mainly the genital area, due regularly to herpesvirus 2.[24,37] Localized or generalized infections of newborn infants are usually due to herpesvirus 2.[24,37] Vesicles 1 mm diameter frequently coalesce into raised lesions 1–2 cm across, particularly at certain mucocutaneous junctions such as lips in type 1 infections, whilst at the vaginal introitus the vesicles in type 2 infections frequently remain discrete. Vesicular eruptions are often accompanied by pain and tenderness, particularly genital herpes. Scabbing occurs 1–3 days after appearance of vesicles, and complete resolution occurs in about a week. Recurrences of vesicles at the same site are common after various external stimuli such as excessive heat or cold, or internal disorders such as fever.

Gingivostomatitis is a vesicular eruption involving the gums, buccal mucosa and anterior two-thirds of the tongue, accompanied by fever, irritability and refusal to drink fluids. It usually involves infants aged less than one year who develop primary herpesvirus 1 infections. Vesicles may become confluent, especially over the buccal and gingival mucosa, and after bursting they expose a raw, extremely tender surface. Superinfection is common, either with *Candida sp.* giving yellowish plaques ("thrush") or with fusospirochaetes to induce a smelly blackened appearance to the mucosa ("noma"). Vesicles may also appear on the lips.

Vesicles on Lips and the immediately adjacent facial skin are common in older children and adults. Virus is detected in swabs or scrapings of vesicles only within the initial 2–3 days after eruption. Virus is not found on the lips or in saliva when lesions are absent i.e., the virus becomes latent. However virus is recovered readily during recurrence of vesicles, despite the presence of neutralizing antibody in patients' sera.

Skin Vesicles may appear elsewhere as a result of predisposing factors. (i) Eczema herpeticum is an eruption of herpesvirus vesicles over areas where the skin epithelium is denuded by thermal burns or the Stevens-Johnson syndrome. (ii) Herpetic whitlows may develop on the fingers of health care personnel who care for tracheotomy stomas which are infected with herpesvirus.

Conjunctivitis and Keratitis are important ophthalmological complications. Involvement of the cornea (keratitis) may be superficial, which resolves without scarring, or it may include the stroma which may lead to corneal scarring and opacity formation. Cataracts, iridocyclitis and panuveitis have been attributed to herpesvirus infections.

Encephalitis due to herpesvirus is a severe but rare complication, involving 77 cases with 31 deaths in 1978.[3] Several days after the appearance of an herpetic vesicle, the patient develops high fever, clouding of consciousness, disorientation, and may convulse or show spastic weakness of limbs.

Genital Herpes. Males develop extremely painful pinpoint vesicles 1 mm diameter on the shaft of the penis. Females develop most painful 1 mm vesicles over the vulva and/or perineum, sometimes accompanied by pain on voiding of urine. vesicles may sometimes be observed on the cervix uteri.

Neonatal Herpes. Newborn babies usually acquire herpesvirus infections while passing through the infected birth canals of their mothers. Within a few days of birth, infants develop extensive vesicular eruptions over the presenting part during the birth process (usually the face), accompanied by high fever, refusal to feed, and irritability or extreme lassitude. The case fatality rate is about 50%. Post mortem, vesicular lesions are observed diffusely throughout the liver and other viscera, and the cerebral neurones and meninges are usually involved also. Characteristically herpesvirus 2 is isolated from the skin vesicles, liver and brain.

VARICELLA-ZOSTER

Chickenpox has an incubation period of 14–18 days. Vesicles 2–3 mm diameter surrounded by red areolas 1–2 mm diameter appear over the face, trunk and proximal parts of the limbs, but rarely involve the palms of the hands and soles of the feet. Successive crops of vesicles appear over a period of 4 days. Fever usually abates after the initial 2 days. Vesicles burst after 1–2 days and become covered with scabs which separate within 7 days. Patients are infectious by throat secretions and droplets for about 2 days before to 4 days after onset of vesicles. Children develop remarkably few complications, except an occasional case of croup; adults may develop varicella pneumonitis. The incidence of encephalitis appearing 1–3 weeks after chickenpox is 22.8–55.8 per 100,000.[3] During 1978, chickenpox encephalitis involved 40 patients in USA with 3 deaths.

Herpes Zoster is an eruption of vesicles 1–5 mm diameter occurring along dermatomes (cutaneous distribution of sensory nerve endings connected with a particular segment of the spinal cord and its corresponding dorsal root ganglion). Characteristically the eruption is unilateral e.g., involving the left 8th thoracic segment. Usually fever and varying degrees of pain accompany the vesicular eruption which persists 1 week or longer. Herpes zoster characteristically involves immunosuppressed patients e.g., those with leukemia, but it may also affect immunologically competent subjects, particularly middle aged or elderly persons who have recently experienced severe emotional trauma. In the latter category of patient, herpes zoster arises from recrudescence of latent VZ virus which caused chickenpox many years previously. Occasionally herpes zoster comprises the only clinical manifestation of VZ virus infection in a child. During 1978, varicella-zoster encephalitis involved 17 cases with 13 deaths.[3]

CYTOMEGALOVIRUS

Newborn babies acquire CMV infections from their mothers who contract either primary infections or recrudescences of infection at some stage during gestation.[11] Characteristic stigmata are microcephaly, mental retardation, hepatosplenomegaly, jaundice, and thrombocytopenia which may terminate fatally within a few weeks of life.[35,36] Some infants survive for several years with varying degrees of mental retardation. Other infants may live and develop normally with no clinical stigmata of CMV infection. Pneumonitis and chorioretinitis have also been described.

Adults infected with CMV may present symptoms clinically indistinguishable from acute mononucleosis[18] but the Paul-Bunnell test remains negative in contrast to mononucleosis induced by EBV where the Paul-Bunnell test is uniformly positive. CMV has induced a mononucleosis-like condition after blood transfusion.[16] CMV frequently induces opportunistic infections in immunosuppressed patients, causing pneumonia which may relapse clinically.[9]

MONONUCLEOSIS

Commonly called "glandular fever" usually arises after EBV infections. Characteristically it affects adolescents and young adults. The incubation period is 2–7 weeks, followed by onset of fever, malaise and yellow exudate on the fauces and enlargement of the lymph nodes in the neck, axillae and groins. Sometimes the spleen and liver may be enlarged, but there is no characteristic skin rash. Almost uniformly the peripheral blood smear shows 10% or more atypical monocytes among the leukocytes whose total count may be within the normal range. Symptoms persist 4–20 days after which convalescence may be slow. The Paul-Bunnell test ("heterophil" agglutination of sheep erythrocytes by patients' serum diluted 1:32 or higher after incubation at 37° C) is positive in cases of mononucleosis induced by EBV (about 85% of total cases of the mononucleosis syndrome) but negative in cases of CMV-induced mononucleosis.

The commonest cause of mononucleosis is infection by EBV.[13] It appears that mononucleosis is spread by close personal contact, permitting direct juxtaposition of buccal mucosal surfaces, as in kissing.

In tropical Africa, the clinical manifestation of EBV infection among the native population is Burkitt's lymphoma.[11]

REFERENCES

[1]Burkitt DP: Determining the climatic limitations of a children's cancer common in Africa. Brit Med J 2:1019, 1962.

[2]Burnet FM, Lush D: Studies on experimental herpes infection in mice, using the chorio-allantoic technique. J Path Bact 49:241, 1939.

[3]Centers for Disease Control: Encephalitis Surveillance. Annual Summary 1978, Issued May 1981.

[4]Corey L, Nahmias AJ, Guinan ME, Benedetti JK, Critchlow CW, Holmes KK: A trial of topical Acyclovir in genital herpes simplex virus infections. New Eng J Med 306:1313, 1982.

[5]Diehl V, Henle G, Henle W, Kohn G: Demonstration of a herpes group virus in cultures of peripheral leukocytes from patients with infectious mononucleosis. J Virol 2:663, 1968.

[6]Dowdle WR, Nahmias AJ, Harwell RW, Pauls FP: Association of antigenic type of *Herpesvirus hominis* with site of viral recovery. J Immunol 99:974, 1967.

[7]Epstein MA, Barr YM, Achong BG: Studies with Burkitt's lymphoma. Wistar Inst Symp Monogr 4:69, 1965.

[8]Fleisher G, Henle W, Henle G, Lennette ET, Biggar RJ: Primary infection with Epstein-Barr virus in infants in the United States: clinical and serologic observations. J Infect Dis 139:553, 1979.

[9]Friedman HM, Grossman RA, Plotkin SA, Perloff LJ, Barker CF: Relapse of pneumonia caused by cytomegalovirus in two recipients of renal transplants. J Infect Dis 139:465, 1979.

[10]Gerber P: EB Herpesvirus: In Manual of Clinical Microbiology 3rd ed., EH Lennette, Editor, American Society for Microbiology, Washington DC, 1980, p. 807.

[11]Griffiths PD: Congenital cytomegalovirus infection. In Recent Advances in Clinical Virology 3, ed AP Waterson, Churchill Livingstone, Edinburgh, 1983, p. 57.

[12]Gruter W (1912): Cited in Lowenstein A. Aetiologische Untersuchungen uber den fieberhaften Herpes. Muench Med Wochenschr 66:769, 1919.

[13]Henle G, Henle W, Diehl V: Relation of Burkitt's tumor-associated herpes-type virus to infectious mononucleosis. Proc Nat Acad Sc USA 59:94, 1968.

[14]Henle W, Henle G, Scriba M, Joyner CR, Harrison FS Jr, von Essen R, Paloheimo J, Klemola E: Antibody responses to Epstein-Barr virus and cytomegaloviruses after open-heart and other surgery. New Eng J Med 282:1068, 1970.

[15]Jones BR, Costar JD, Fison PN, Thompson GN, Cobo LM, Falcon MG: Efficacy of Acycloguanosine (Wellcome 248U) against herpes-simplex corneal ulcers. Lancet 1:243, 1979.

[16]Kaariainen L, Klemola E, Paloheimo J: Rise of cytomegalovirus antibodies in an infectious mononucleosis-like syndrome after transfusion. Brit Med J 2:1270, 1966.

[17]Kaufman HE: Clinical cure of herpes simplex keratitis by 5-iodo-2'-deoxyuridine. Proc Soc Exp Biol Med 109:251, 1962.

[18]Klemola E, Kaariainen L: Cytomegalovirus as a possible cause of disease resembling infectious mononucleosis. Brit Med J 2:1099, 1965.

[19]Kluge RC, Wicksman RS, Weller TH: Cytomegalic inclusion disease of the newborn: report of a case with persistent viremia. Pediatrics 25:35, 1960.

[20]McLean DM: Immunological Investigation of Human Virus Diseases. Churchill Livingstone, Edinburgh, 1982.

[21]McLean DM, Wong KK: Same-day Diagnosis of Human Virus Infections. CRC Press, Boca Raton, FL, 1984.

[22]Matthews REF: Classification and nomenclature of viruses. Intervirology 17:1, 1982.

[23]Miller G, Niederman JC, Andrews L: Prolonged oropharyngeal excretion of Epstein-Barr virus after infectious mononucleosis. New Eng J Med 288:229, 1973.

[24]Nahmias AJ, Roizman B: Infection with herpes simplex viruses 1 and 2. New Eng

J Med 289:667, 719, 781, 1973.

[25]Nilsen AE, Aasen T, Halsos AM, Kinge BR, Tjotta EAL, Wikstrom K, Fiddian AP: Efficacy of oral Acyclovir in the treatment of initial and recurrent genital herpes. Lancet 2:571, 1982.

[26]Peckham CS, Chin KS, Coleman JC, Henderson K, Hurley R, Preece PM: Cytomegalovirus infection in pregnancy: preliminary findings from a prospective study. Lancet 1:1352, 1983.

[27]Rawls WE, Tompkins WAF, Melnick JL: The association of *Herpesvirus* type 2 and carcinoma of the uterine cervix. Am J Epidemiol 89:547, 1969.

[28]Roizman B, Carmichael LE, Deinhardt F, de-The G, Nahmias AJ, Plowright W, Rapp F, Sheldrick P, Takahashi M, Wolf K: Herpesviridae: Definition, provisional nomenclature, and taxonomy. Intervirology 16:201, 1981.

[29]Rowe WP, Hartley JW, Waterman S, Turner HC, Huebner RJ: Cytopathogenic agent resembling human salivary gland virus recovered from tissue cultures of human adenoids. Proc Soc Exp Biol Med 92:418, 1956.

[30]Russell WC: A sensitive and precise plaque assay for herpes virus. Nature 195: 1028, 1962.

[31]Saddington ES: Cultivation of herpes virus and use of the mouse in its titration. Proc Soc Exp Biol Med 29:1012, 1932.

[32]Smith MG: Propagation in tissue cultures of a cytopathogenic virus from human salivary gland virus (SGV) disease. Proc Soc Exp Biol Med 92:424, 1956.

[33]Weller TH: Serial propagation in vitro of agents producing inclusion bodies derived from varicella and herpes zoster. Proc Soc Exp Biol Med 83:340, 1953.

[34]Weller TH, Coons AH: Fluorescent antibody studies with agents of varicella and herpes zoster propagated in vitro. Proc Soc Exp Biol Med 86:789, 1954.

[35]Weller TH, Macaulay JC, Craig JM, Wirth P: Isolation of intranuclear inclusion producing agents from infants with illnesses resembling cytomegalic inclusion disease. Proc Soc Exp Biol Med 94:4, 1957.

[36]Weller TH, Hanshaw JB: Virologic and clinical observations on cytomegalic inclusion disease. New Eng J Med 266:1233, 1962.

[37]Wolontis S, Jeansson S: Correlation of herpes simplex virus types 1 and 2 with clinical features of infection. J Infect Dis 135:28, 1977.

CHAPTER 13

ADENOVIRIDAE

Adenoviridae include 41 serotypes within the genus Mastadenovirus, a few of which have caused respiratory infections in humans.[21] Also included within the genus Mastadenovirus are numerous serotypes infecting cattle, pigs, sheep, horses, dogs, goats and mice. A second genus, Aviadenovirus contains many serotypes which infect domestic chickens, turkeys, geese, pheasants and ducks.

HISTORICAL

Adenoviruses were first isolated from the throats of military recruits at Fort Leonard Wood, Missouri who developed undifferentiated acute respiratory disease or primary atypical pneumonia during winter 1952–53[14] by inoculation of human tracheal cultures, and subsequently cytopathic effects were observed after passage to continuous human polyploid cells, HeLa. The prototype strain RI-67 was serotyped subsequently as adenovirus 4.[25] Almost simultaneously in Washington, DC and Maryland during 1953, adenovirus types 1, 2 and 5 were isolated from children with hypertrophied tonsils and adenoids when explant cultures of these tissues exhibited spontaneous degeneration after prolonged culture.[26] Adenovirus 3 was first isolated from nasal washings of an adult male volunteer in a common cold project in Maryland during 1953.[27] During summer 1954 this serotype caused a large outbreak of pharyngoconjunctival fever among bathers at several swimming pools in Washington, DC and suburbs.[2] In Glasgow, Scotland during 1960, adenovirus 3 was isolated during a family outbreak of gastroenteritis.[10] Adenovirus 7 was first isolated from the throat washing of a military recruit with pharyngitis during an outbreak of acute respiratory disease at Fort Ord, California in 1954,[3] and this serotype was isolated from cases of swimming pool conjunctivitis in Toronto, Canada during 1955[23] and Kansas during 1973.[6] Adenovirus 14 was first isolated from the throat washings of a military recruit with acute respiratory illness in the Netherlands during 1955.[31] Adenovirus 8 was first isolated from the eye swab of a patient with epidemic keratoconjunctivitis ("shipyard eye") in California during 1955,[15] and subsequently from cases of keratoconjunctivitis in Florida during 1975[33] and Georgia during

1977.[9] Keratoconjunctivitis has also been attributed to infection with adenovirus 19 in Nashville, Tennessee during 1973.[13] Electron microscopic examination of feces from infantile gastroenteritis in Great Britain during 1974 revealed for the first time adenovirus virions in 12% of Birmingham patients[5] and 3% of Glasgow patients.[19] However it was difficult or not feasible to isolate these enteric adenoviruses using standard laboratory tissue culture techniques. During an outbreak of infantile gastroenteritis in Sapporo, Japan in 1982[7] enteric adenoviruses were visualized in feces from 8 of 11 patients and these were typed as adenovirus 40 by DNA-DNA homology tests.

BIOLOGICAL ATTRIBUTES

Adenovirus virions are non-enveloped particles 70–90nm diameter with icosahedral symmetry, their genomes comprise single linear molecules of ds DNA with molecular weight $20–25 \times 10^6$ for mammalian strains or $28–30 \times 10^6$ for avian strains, and each virion contains at least 10 polypeptides.[21] Their infectivity is retained after treatment with sodium deoxycholate or diethyl ether. Each particle contains 252 capsomers, 8–9nm diameter including 12 vertex capsomers (or penton bases) which carry one (mammalian) or two (avian) glycoprotein filamentous projections (or fibers) of different length, and 240 nonvertex capsomers (or hexons) which are different from penton bases and fibers.

Antigens at the surface of the virions are mainly species-specific: hexon for neutralization, fiber for hemagglutination and hemagglutination inhibition. Soluble antigens are surplus products of capsid proteins; free hexon acts mainly as a genus-specific antigen which is shared by most mammalian strains but these differ from the hexon antigen common to avian strains.

Adenoviruses multiply readily in continuous tissue cultures of human diploid cells such as locally prepared foreskin fibroblasts or standard cell lines MRC-5 or WI-38, and in human polyploid cells such as HeLa, HEp-2 or KB. After several days incubation, characteristic cytopathic effects appear, including acidophilic intranuclear inclusions, crenation of cell edges and an acid reaction to the supernatant fluid. Plaque formation occurs after incubation for 10–21 days. Some strains of adenovirus also multiply in primary tissue cultures of human amnion or human tracheal epithelium or human embryo kidney. Enteric adenoviruses do not propagate readily in the above standard tissue culture system. However, multiplication has been demonstrated by observation of immunofluorescent foci in 293 cells[30] after incubation for several days following inoculation of enteric adenoviruses. The 293 cell line comprises adenovirus 5 transformed human embryo kidney cells.

Non-cultural techniques involving DNA-DNA hybridization have been applied recently to detect both cultivable adenoviruses in nasopharyngeal aspirates within 20 hours after their collection from children with acute respiratory infections[32] and non-cultivable enteric adenoviruses from infants with acute gastroenteritis.[7] Enteric adenoviruses are serotypes 40 and 41.

At least 41 species (serotypes) of human adenovirus have been catalogued to 1983.[1] Each serotype is identified by the serotype-specific neutralization test. Many serotypes agglutinate grivet monkey erythrocytes at pH 7 and 37° C, thus providing a rapid means of serotype identification. Soluble complement fixing antigen released into tissue culture supernatant fluid after growth of adenovirus in tissue culture is common to most mammalian serotypes and provides a convenient means of distinguishing adenoviruses from other cytopathic agents. Recently DNA-DNA homology tests have been employed successfully to serotype enteric adenoviruses without propagation in tissue culture. On the basis of several biochemical, biological, immunological and structural characteristics, the 41 currently recognized human adenovirus serotypes have been classified into 6 subgenera (subgroups A–F).

Adenoviruses are not pathogenic for any of the commonly available laboratory animals. However adenovirus types 12, 18 and 31 have induced tumors after inoculation of newborn hamsters and rats.

PATHOGENESIS

Adenoviruses enter new hosts by inhalation of virus-laden droplets expelled during sneezing or coughing by adenovirus-infected patients, or by direct mechanical contact with the conjunctiva during rubbing of the eyes by infected fingers or fomites. Viruses multiply in the epithelium of the nasopharynx or conjunctiva inducing catarrhal inflammation as manifested by sore throat or reddened injected conjunctivae after an incubation period of 5–8 days. Blood-borne infections are rare, but occasionally these are followed by rubella-like rash[12] or meningoencephalitis.[16] Occasional fatal cases of pneumonia have been observed among children, sometimes from remote subarctic areas, following infection with adenovirus type 3[24] or 7.[4] The lungs showed necrotizing patchy alveolar fibropurulent exudate plus necrotizing bronchitis and bronchiolitis and some cells showed intranuclear and some intracytoplasmic inclusion bodies.

SYMPTOMATOLOGY

Clinical manifestations of adenovirus infections include pharyngoconjunctival fever, acute respiratory disease which occasionally is complicated by whooping-cough-like disease or fatal pneumonia in infants, epidemic kerato-conjunctivitis, gastroenteritis, cystitis.

PHARYNGOCONJUNCTIONAL FEVER fever due to infection with adenovirus type 3, 4 or 7 has been frequently been associated with swimming pools.[2,6,8,20,23] Symptoms comprise fever, headache, lassitude and sore throat, accompanied by conjunctivitis without myalgia or retro-orbital pain, following an incubation period of 5–8 days.

ACUTE RESPIRATORY DISEASE. In MILITARY RECRUITS, fever, malaise, headache, cough and sore throat with or without cervical lymph-adenopathy, occur after an incubation period of 5–6 days. Adenovirus types, 3, 4, 7, 14 and 21 have usually been implicated as causative agents. Additional symptoms include bronchitis and a form of primary atypical pneumonia.

In **INFANTS AND YOUNG CHILDREN,** adenovirus types 3[24] and 7[4] in Canada, and type 21[17] in New Zealand have been isolated from nasopharyngeal, tracheal or lung aspirates of patients with severe bronchopneumonia or bronchiolitis which affected clusters of natives more commonly then Caucasians. Case fatality rates were as high as 23%,[4] with necrotizing bronchitis and bronchiolitis, patchy alveolar fibrinopurulent exudate and hyaline membrane formation in fatal cases. Chronic cough and repeated chest infections persisted in 30–60% of survivors. A pertussis-like syndrome has also been attributed to adenovirus infection.[29]

NOSOCOMIAL INFECTIONS have recently been attributed to adenovirus 7b.[28] Severe respiratory distress progressing to pneumonia affected 5 infants or children already hospitalized at a Childrens Hospital, following admission of the index case for tracheal incubation for croup during August 1980. The index case and 3 other patients died within the succeeding 3 weeks. Pharyngoconjunctival fever was first reported among hospital employees 7 days after admission of the index case and eventually 300 of 383 (78%) hospital employees developed mild pharyngoconjunctival fever during the subsequent month, 11 of whom shed adenovirus 7b in throat cultures and another 7 showed rising CF antibody titers. A statistically significant higher proportion of employees working in units with adenovirus-positive patients had laboratory-confirmed adenovirus infections, thus indicating nosocomial spread of virus.

KERATOCONJUNCTIVITIS, usually due to adenovirus 8 infection,[9,15] exhibits redness of the conjunctiva followed by small superficial opacities of the cornea 4–14 days after onset. Symptoms may persist 2–4 weeks, accompanied by periorbital edema and preauricular lymphadenopathy. Frequently these outbreaks are associated with attendance at ophthalmological offices or clinics where sterilization of intraocular instruments after each use on individual patients is inadequate. Spread of epidemic keratoconjunctivitis due to adenovirus 8 among refugees at a camp in Florida during summer 1975[33] was attributed to the shared use of wet towels to mop the sweated brows of many children, together with lack of handwashing routines.

CYSTITIS. Acute hemorrhagic cystitis was associated regularly with isolation of adenovirus 11 from urine of patients at Sendai, Japan.[22] Symptoms included sudden onset of non-bacterial hematuria and dysuria.

GASTROENTERITIS. Gastroenteritis of infants and young children is manifested by expulsion of as many as 10 loose watery green stools per day, accompanied frequently by vomiting. Although the onset frequently is sudden, acute gastroenteritis may appear after a protracted period of expulsion of loose (but not green-coloured) stools. Fever is uncommon, and dehydration frequently is minimal, with less than 25% hospitalized patients in Vancouver, Canada requiring intravenous administration of fluids and electrolytes for correction of imbalances. The incubation period is 2–3 days, and loose watery stools persist usually for 2–4 days, but the watery diarrhea often ceases within one day after withholding of oral feeding and commencement of intravenous fluid infusions. Since the disease is readily transmissible by fecally contaminated hands or fomites, it is important to nurse hospitalized patients in units designed for enteric isolation procedures.

Adenoviruses, which are visualized readily by electron microscopy[18] are detected in a small but significant proportion of children with gastroenteritis in many Temperature Zone communities, especially during cooler months of most years. In Vancouver, Canada between 1976 and 1981, 5.9% of 1000 children revealed enteric adenoviruses,[18] whilst in Birmingham, England during 1974 adenoviruses were encountered in 12% of gastroenteritis patients.[5] By contrast, cultivable adenoviruses have been detected most infrequently in family outbreaks of acute gastroenteritis,[10] or intussusception as a complication of gastroenteritis.[11] During an institutional outbreak of gastroenteritis in Sapporo, Japan in 1982, adenovirus 40 was identified as the causative agent by DNA-DNA homology without propagation in tissue culture[7]; elsewhere adenovirus types 40 and 41 have been implicated.

REFERENCES

[1] American Type Culture Collection. Catalogue of Strains II, 4th ed., 1983.
[2] Bell JA, Rowe WP, Engler JI, Parrott RH, Huebner RJ: Pharyngo-conjunctival fever.

Epidemiologic studies of a recently recognized disease entity. JAMA 157:1083, 1955.

[3]Berge TO, England B, Mauris C, Shuey HE, Lennette EH: Etiology of acute respiratory disease among service personnel at Fort Ord, California. Am J Hyg 62:283, 1955.

[4]Brown RS, Nogrady MB, Spence L, Wiglesworth FW: An outbreak of adenovirus type 7 infection in children in Montreal. Can Med Ass J 108:436, 1973.

[5]Bryden AS, Davies H, Hadley RE, Flewett TH, Morris CA, Oliver P: Rotavirus enteritis in the West Midlands during 1974. Lancet 2:241, 1975.

[6]Caldwell GG, Lindsey NJ, Wulff H, Donnelly DD, Bohl FN: Epidemic of adenovirus 7 acute conjunctivitis in swimmers. Am J Epidemiol 99:230, 1974.

[7]Chiba S, Nakata S, Nakamura I, Taniguchi K, Urasawa S, Fujinaga K, Nakao T: Outbreak of infantile gastroenteritis due to type 40 adenovirus. Lancet 2:954, 1983.

[8]D'Angelo LJ, Hierholzer JC, Keenlyside RA, Anderson LJ, Martone WJ: Pharyngoconjunctival fever caused by adenovirus type 4: report of a swimming pool-related outbreak with recovery of virus from pool water. J Infect Dis 140:42, 1979.

[9]D'Angelo LJ, Hierholzer JC, Holman RC, Smith DJ: Epidemic keratoconjunctivitis caused by adenovirus type 8: epidemiologic and laboratory aspects of a large outbreak. Am J Epidemiol 113:44, 1981.

[10]Duncan IBR, Hutchison JGP: Type 3 adenovirus infection with gastrointestinal symptoms. Lancet 1:530, 1961.

[11]Gardner PS, McGregor CB, Dick K: Association between diarrhoea and adenovirus type 7. Brit Med J 1:91, 1960.

[12]Gutekunst RR, Heggie AD: Viremia and viruria in adenovirus infections. Detection in patients with rubella or rubelliform illness. New Eng J Med 264:374, 1961.

[13]Guyer B, O'Day DM, Hierholzer JC, Schaffner W: Epidemic keratoconjunctivitis. A community outbreak of mixed adenovirus type 8 and type 19 infection. J Infect Dis 132:142, 1975.

[14]Hilleman MR, Werner JH: Recovery of a new agent from patients with acute respiratory illness. Proc Soc Exp Biol Med 85:183, 1954.

[15]Jawetz E, Kimura S, Nicholas AN, Thygeson P, Hanna L: New type of APC virus from epidemic keratoconjunctivitis. Science 122:1190, 1955.

[16]Kelsey DS: Adenovirus meningoencephalitis. Pediatrics 61:291, 1978.

[17]Lang WR, Howden CW, Laws J, Burton JF: Bronchopneumonia with serious sequelae in children with evidence of adenovirus type 21 infection. Brit Med J 1:73, 1969.

[18]McLean DM, Wong KK: Same-day diagnosis of human virus infection. CRC Press, Boca Raton, FL, 1984.

[19]Madeley CR, Cosgrove BP, Bell EJ, Fallon RJ: Stool viruses in babies in Glasgow. I. Hospital admissions with diarrhoea. J Hyg 78:261, 1977.

[20]Martone WJ, Hierholzer JC, Keenlyside RA, Fraser DW, D'Angelo LJ, Winkler WJ: An outbreak of adenovirus type 3 disease at a private recreation center

swimming pool. Am J Epidemiol 111:229, 1980.

[21]Matthews REF: Classification and nomenclature of viruses. Intervirology 17:1, 1982.

[22]Numazaki Y, Kumasaka T, Yano N, Yamanaka M, Miyazawa T, Takai S, Ishida N: Further study on acute hemorrhagic cystitis due to adenovirus type 11. New Eng J Med 289:344, 1973.

[23]Ormsby HL, Aitchison WS: The role of the swimming pool in the transmission of pharyngeal-conjunctival fever. Can Med Ass J 73:864, 1955.

[24]Parker WL, Wilt JC, Stackiw W: Adenovirus infections. Can J Pub Health 52:246, 1961.

[25]Pereira HG, Huebner RJ, Ginsberg HS, van der Veen J: A short description of the adenovirus group. Virology 20:613, 1963.

[26]Rowe WP, Huebner RJ, Gilmore LK, Parrott RH, Ward TG: Isolation of a cytopathogenic agent from human adenoids undergoing spontaneous degeneration in tissue culture. Proc Soc Exp Biol Med 84:570, 1953.

[27]Rowe WP, Huebner RJ, Hartley JW, Ward TG, Parrott RH: Studies of the adenoidal-pharyngeal-conjunctival (APC) group of viruses. Am J Hyg 61:197, 1955.

[28]Straube RC, Thompson MA, van Dyke RB, Wadell G, Connor JD, Wingard D, Spector SA: Adenovirus type 7b in a children's hospital. J Infect Dis 147:814, 1983.

[29]Sturdy PM, Court SDM, Gardner PS: Viruses and whooping cough. Lancet 2:978, 1971.

[30]Takiff HE, Straus SE, Garon CF: Propagation and in vitro studies of previously noncultivable enteral adenoviruses in 293 cells. Lancet 2:832, 1981.

[31]Van der Veen J, Kok G: Isolation and typing of adenoviruses recovered from military recruits with acute respiratory disease in the Netherlands. Am J Hyg 65:119, 1957.

[32]Virtanen M, Palva A, Laaksonen M, Halonen P, Soderlund H, Ranki M: Novel test for rapid diagnosis: detection of adenovirus in nasopharyngeal mucus aspirates by means of nucleic-acid sandwich hybridization. Lancet 1:381, 1983.

[33]Zweighaft RM, Hierholzer JC, Bryan JA: Epidemic keratoconjunctivitis at a Vietnamese refugee camp in Florida. Am J Epidemiol 106:399, 1977.

CHAPTER 14

POXVIRIDAE

Poxviridae contain 6 genera (subgroups) of viruses which characteristically induce vesicular lesions in the respective mammalian or avian hosts (Table 14-1).

TABLE 14-1

Genus (subgroup)	International name	Vertebrate host definitive	additional
Vaccinia	Orthopoxvirus	human	bovine, rabbit
Orf	Parapoxvirus	sheep	human
Fowlpox	Avipoxvirus	chickens	
Sheep pox	Capripoxvirus	sheep	
Myxoma	Leporipoxvirus	rabbits	
Swinepox	Suipoxvirus	swine	

Vaccinia is the sole member of the Orthopoxvirus genus which is a human pathogen, following the world-wide extinction of smallpox in October 1977.

HISTORICAL

Smallpox (variola) has been prevalent since antiquity, especially in Asia, and its outbreaks have been documented regularly during the past 4 centuries in Europe, Africa and the Americas. A benign form of smallpox (alastrim) was first recognized in Britain, Western Europe and the Americas about 2 centuries ago. Active immunization was initially attempted by scarification of skin of fresh subjects with vesicle fluid from mild cases of smallpox (variolation), but following the publication of Jenner's treatise in 1798, inoculation of vesicle fluid from cows with cowpox (vaccination) superseded variolation. Although this agent, vaccinia virus, presumably derived from cowpox, was initially maintained from arm to arm transfer among humans, during the past century vaccinia virus has been propagated by intradermal inoculation of calves, sheep or rabbits.

The last-known case of naturally acquired smallpox occurred in Somalia in October 1977.[2] Since smallpox can only be transmitted from human to human, and there is no known extrahuman reservoir, this disease can now be considered to be eradicated from the world. This remarkable public health victory was achieved following an intensive program of global eradication which was sponsored by the World Health Organization commencing in January 1967. Routine vaccination against smallpox is no longer required for international travel, manufacture of vaccinia stocks has been terminated, and the practice of vaccination has ceased through public health bans on distribution of remaining supplies of vaccinia virus.

BIOLOGICAL ATTRIBUTES

Poxvirus virions are enveloped brick-shaped or ovoid particles 300–450nm x 170–250nm which contain single molecules of ds DNA with molecular weight 85–240 x 10^6 and more than 30 structural proteins plus several viral enzymes.[3] The viral envelope contains lipid and tubular protein structures, and it encloses one or two lateral bodies and a core which contains the genome. Viruses multiply in the cytoplasm of susceptible cells with production of acidophilic inclusion bodies (Guarnieri bodies). Viruses of the Orthopoxvirus genus produce a lipoprotein hemagglutinin for erythrocytes of selected chickens and geese, this 65 nm particle is separate from the virus particle. About 10 major antigens occur within the virion, one of which cross-reacts with most poxviruses of vertebrates.

Vaccinia virus, the type species of Orthopoxvirus, propagates readily in a variety of human diploid and polyploid cells, and in primary monkey kidney tissue cultures, inducing cytopathic effects. Pocks 2–3mm diameter, which are sometimes hemorrhagic, are produced on chorioallantoic membranes after 2–3 days incubation at 35–37° C. Saline extracts of infected chorioallantoic membranes provide a rich source of vaccinia hemagglutinin which agglutinates chicken or goose erythrocytes after incubation for 1/2 hour at 23 or 37° C in unbuffered saline. Hemagglutination is inhibited by antibodies to vaccinia virus by other members of the Orthopoxvirus genus including cowpox, ectromelia (mousepox), monkeypox, rabbitpox, and variola.

On account of antigenic cross-reactions between vaccinia and variola, antibodies induced as a consequence of intradermal administration of vaccinia virus into humans during the past century has halted the growth of variola virus after natural exposure to subjects with smallpox and this has resulted in the elimination of smallpox worldwide.

PATHOGENESIS

Vaccinia virus is usually introduced into the human host by intradermal injection or scarification. Virus multiplies in the epithelium and dermis, inducing a large vesicle 1cm diameter 4–7 days later, and a scab forms 3–4 days subsequently. Mild constitutional upsets occur at the time of vesicle formation. Antibodies detected by HI or neutralization appear within one week after vesicle formation and they persist at diminishing titers for several years. Complement fixing antibodies appear 2–3 weeks after vesicle formation and persist 1–3 years.

Although no longer prevalent, the pathogenesis of smallpox (variola) is mentioned briefly. Variola virus usually entered susceptible humans by inhalation of virus-laden droplets from infected humans. After initial replication, possibly in lymphoid or other internal tissues, viremia developed a few days before the onset of rash, thus distributing virus to the skin over the entire body surface including palms and soles, where it induced formation of vesicles. Lesions usually appeared on the pharyngeal mucosa, thus providing a source of infected droplets during coughing. Antibodies were detected by HI shortly after defervescence.

SYMPTOMATOLOGY

Vaccinia lesions are large 1cm diameter vesicles surrounded by erythema extending an additional 0.5–1cm which appear at the site of intradermal implantation of vaccinia virus. When the skin is broken by scratching soon after vaccination, the hands may transfer virus mechanically to other abraded areas where vesicles develop subsequently, as in Figure 14-1. Vaccinia virions may be observed by electron microscopic examination of the site of secondary viral implantation. Virus may also be implanted on the perineum or vagina, causing a painful vesicular eruption, or on the eyelids during scratching the eyes, inducing gross swelling of the eyelids, which often show vesicles around the eyelashes. This is accompanied by reddening and injection of the conjunctiva (blepharoconjunctivitis), but the cornea usually remains non-involved. In subjects with extensive atopic eczema, vesicle formation may occur extensively over eczematous areas (eczema vaccinatum). Occasionally blood-borne spread of infection results in vesicles distributed over the entire body surface (generalized vaccinia). Post-vaccinal encephalitis is a rare complication, which affected about 1:100,000 vaccinia recipients in New York during a massive vaccination campaign in 1947.[1]

REFERENCES

[1]Greenberg M: Complications of vaccination against smallpox. Am J Dis Child 76:492, 1948.

[2]Henderson DA: The saga of smallpox eradication: an end and a beginning. Can J Pub Health 70:21, 1979.
[3]Matthews REF: Classification and nomenclature of viruses. Intervirology 17:1, 1982.

CHAPTER 15

HEPADNAVIRIDAE

Hepadnaviridae family contains one genus Hepadnavirus which includes the human pathogen hepatitis B virus (HBV). Hepatitis induced by HBV infection is manifested clinically by appearance of jaundice 60 days or more after exposure, in contrast to infections by hepatitis A virus (HAV) which induce jaundice 15–40 days after exposure (Chapter 7). Recently HBV has named hepadnavirus 1 and HAV enterovirus 72.[21]

HISTORICAL

Hepatitis was recognized as an increasingly important complication of blood transfusion[2,23] or following administration of pooled adult human plasma for measles prophylaxis[20] during the 1930's. Hepatitis developed in some volunteers who received yellow fever vaccine stabilized by addition of human serum in 1937[9] and among military personnel in 1942,[10] some 2–4 months after injection of vaccine, but this complication was eliminated following removal of human serum from subsequent batches of vaccine. Similar histopathological features were observed in liver samples collected by a needle aspiration biopsy technique[15] which was developed in 1938, both in patients who presented with hepatitis 2 or more months after parenteral administration of blood or its products, and in those who developed hepatitis about 4 weeks after ingestion of contaminated food or water. These pathological and epidemiological findings gave rise to the terms hepatitis A (erstwhile "infectious hepatitis" or "catarrhal jaundice") which denoted the short incubation disease and hepatitis B (formerly "serum hepatitis" or "homologous serum jaundice") which referred to disease with a long incubation period.

At Willowbrook State School, New York, simultaneous prevalence of two hepatitis serotypes, HAV and HBV, was reported during 1967.[16] These studies confirmed earlier observations that no cross immunity exists between HAV and HBV. Most of our present concepts of the pathogenesis, infective periods, epidemiology, and seroprophylaxis have been established firmly through human volunteer studies at Willowbrook State School between 1956 and 1971,[17] in the absence of any convenient laboratory system for isolation of the causative viruses.

The Dane particle, a 42–44 nm double-shelled particle[8] with an electron-dense core 27 nm diameter containing DNA and a surface which disrupts easily to furnish the 20–22 nm surface antigen, was first described in electron micrographs of sera from patients with hepatitis B in 1970, and is now generally believed to be the infectious HBV particle. The surface antigen was first reported in the serum of an Australian aborigine in 1965[3] and was termed "Australia antigen" until superseded in 1974[7] by its designation as hepatitis B surface antigen (HBsAg). Application of the radioimmunoassay (RIA) technique[20] to detection of HBsAg and its antibody (anti-HBs) in patients sera in 1970 provided for the first time a practicable and highly sensitive laboratory method for epidemiological and clinical investigations of hepatitis B which was superseded in 1972 by the more convenient solid phase RIA technique.[19] Enzyme immunoassay (ELISA) which was adapted to the hepatitis B system in 1976[31] provided an equally convenient and sensitive technique as RIA for detection of hepatitis B antigens and their respective antibodies.

A vaccine consisting of formalin-inactivated highly purified HBsAg particles was first developed in 1978[13] from sera of chronic HBsAg carriers. This procedure was devised to overcome the technical inability to propagate HBV in any convenient tissue culture system. Following the 1980 report[28] that this HBV vaccine showed a 92% efficacy in reduction of the HBV attack rate in a high-risk population in eastern USA, hepatitis B vaccine became available commercially during 1982 for HBV prophylaxis.

Delta antigen (HDAg) was first detected in 1977 by immunofluorescence in hepatocyte nuclei of patients chronically infected with HBV.[26] Delta antigen and RNA are organized as internal components within a coat of HBsAg.[4] In addition to its worldwide prevalence in HBsAg carriers, HDV has been implicated in a recent outbreak of severe hepatitis in Venezuela.[11]

Post-transfusion hepatitis, with incubation periods ranging from 14 to 170 days (average 40 days), has been documented regularly through the years, following infusion of substantial quantities of blood, usually from commercial sources. Results reported in 1974 of a prospective study of 204 cardiovascular surgery patients who received an average of 18 units of HBsAg-negative blood showed a hepatitis attack rate of 25% in the absence of laboratory evidence of HAV or HBV infection.[24] This syndrome is termed non-A non-B (NANB) hepatitis. Although NANB hepatitis is transmissible to chimpanzees by parenteral inoculation of human plasma or its fractions, current evidence points towards the coexistence of two or more etiological agents.[5] Hepatitis affecting 447 patients at a Montreal, Canada hospital between 1970 and 1979 included 25% HAV infections, 62% HBV infections and 13% had NANB hepatitis.[25] Some NANB agents are now termed Hepatitis C virus (HCV).

BIOLOGICAL ATTRIBUTES

Currently no convenient tissue culture system is available for isolation and propagation of HBV. Detailed characterization of the molecular and antigenic properties of HBV and its subunits has been obtained using purified material from human blood or liver. Chimpanzees are the sole laboratory animal to which HBV infection has been transmitted successfully by parenteral injection.[1]

Hepadnaviridae particles, of which HBV is the only human pathogen, show the following common characteristics:[21] (i) the complete virion is a double shelled particle 40–50 nm with a core 27 nm diameter and there are incomplete forms comprising 22 nm spheres and filaments; (ii) circular viral dsDNA with length corresponding to 3200 base pairs and containing a single-stranded region; (iii) virion DNA polymerase that repairs the single-stranded region in the DNA; (iv) polypeptide covalently attached to the 5' end of the long DNA strand; (vi) characteristic virion polypeptides; (vii) sharing of some DNA and virion polypeptide homology; (viii) protein kinase activity in the virion core; (ix) liver tropism; (x) persistent infection with large amounts of incomplete viral forms continuously in the blood; (xi) infection is associated with hepatitis, hepatocellular carcinoma, and immune-complex-mediated extrahepatic tissue injury.

Sera from patients with hepatitis B contain 3 morphologically distinct particles:[22,30] (i) double-shelled 42 nm Dane particles which are believed to be HBV virions which contain outer shells surrounding electron-dense cores 27 nm diameter (HBcAg). Cores are observed optimally in hepatocytes of chimpanzees dying of HBV infection;[14] (ii) spherical 20–22 nm particles represent the surface antigen (HBsAg) of the Dane particle; (iii) filaments 20 nm diameter X 300–400 nm long represent aggregates of surface antigen. The e antigen (HBeAg) is associated with the core. The nomenclature of hepatitis B antigens and their respective antibodies is shown in Table 15-1.

PATHOGENESIS

Hepatitis B virus typically enters a susceptible host by parenteral injection of blood or plasma fractions from asymptomatic humans with HBV infections. This may arise through direct infusion of HBV positive blood, plasma, antihemophilic globulin or platelets, or during procedures such as dental surgery or ear-piercing where instruments contaminated by viremic blood may pierce the intact skin of the operator. Immune serum globulin

TABLE 15-1
NOMENCLATURE OF ANTIGENS WITH ANTIBODIES
ASSOCIATED WITH HEPATITIS B[a]

Abbreviation	Description
HBsAg	Antigen found on the surface of the Dane particle and on the unattached 20 nm particles.
HBcAg	Antigen found within the core of the Dane particle.
Dane particle	The double-shelled 42 nm particle believed to be the etiological agent of hepatitis B.
HBV	Abbreviation for hepatitis B virus (distinct from hepatitis A virus, HAV and non-A, non-B hepatitis).
HbsAg/adr	Hepatitis B surface antigen manifesting the group determinant a, and subtype determinants d or y, r or w. Currently there are four well defined subtypes adr, ayr, adw, ayw.
HBeAg	Associated with the core of the Dane particle.
anti-HBs	Antibody to hepatitis B surface antigen.
anti-HBc	Antibody to hepatitis B core antigen.
anti-HBe	Antibody to hepatitis B e antigen.

[a]Adapted from Morbidity and Mortality Weekly Report, 23:29, 1974.[7]

(gammaglobulin) does not transmit HBV because this agent is eliminated during chemical fractionation of the product. Since HBsAG has been detected in saliva and semen[12] transmission of HBV by intimate mucosal contact, as in sexual intercourse, becomes possible, especially among homosexuals.[6,28] Viral replication occurs extensively in the liver and presumably in the reticuloendothelial system as shown by prolonged HBs antigenemia,[18] and virus is excreted in the feces, urine, bile, saliva and semen. When mothers contract HBV infection during the third trimester of pregnancy, infection has been transmitted transplacentally to their offspring.[27]

Biochemical abnormalities of liver function are first detected during the incubation period, 2 weeks or more before onset of jaundice which typically becomes obvious after an incubation period of 60 days or more. Abnormalities comprise raised levels of alanine aminotransferase (ALT) (formerly serum glutamic pyruvic transaminase, normal 6–35 units/ml), and aspartate aminotransferase (AST) (formerly serum glutamic oxalacetic transaminase, normal 15–40 units/ml). Transaminase levels may remain elevated for 2 months or more after onset of jaundice. These biochemical determinations provide the best single piece of laboratory evidence of abnormal function of liver cells.

Histological evidence of damage to liver cells is found in biopsy or autopsy specimens. Characteristic early findings are cloudy swelling and fatty change, progressing to necrosis of liver parenchyma cells surrounding the central veins of liver lobules (centrilobular necrosis). Although recovery usually occurs with complete restitution of normal liver architecture, in cases of chronic or relapsing hepatitis there is an accumulation of fibrous tissue leading eventually to disruption of liver lobules into nodules of liver cells which often exhibit fatty changes due to chronic impairment of function.

Detection of serological markers during a typical attack of hepatitis B infection followed by recovery[18] is illustrated diagrammatically in Figure 15-1. The incubation period to onset of jaundice is about 2 months and jaundice

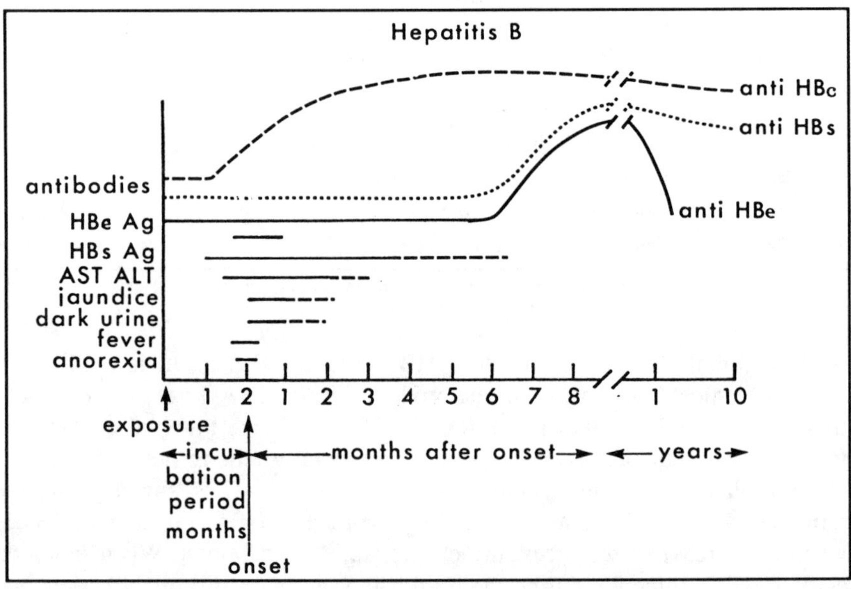

Figure 15-1: Time course of hepatitis B infection. Reproduced with permission from McLean DM, 1982. Immunological Investigation of Human Virus Diseases, Churchill Livingstone, Edinburgh, p. 65.

accompanied by dark urine may persist 1 month or more. Abnormal elevation of ALT and AST are found 2 weeks before to 2 months or more after onset of jaundice. Hepatitis B surface antigen may be detected 1 month before to 3 months or more after onset of jaundice; HBe Ag may be found after HBsAg is first detected and it persists for shorter periods than HBsAg except in chronic carriers where both antigens may persist for several years.[18] Antibodies are initially detected against the core antigen (anti HBc) shortly before onset of jaundice and anti HBc persists for many years; anti HBs usually appears one month or more after disappearance of HBsAg from serum and persists indefinitely; anti HBe appears after HBeAg becomes undetectable and anti HBe disappears after 1–2 years.

SYMPTOMATOLOGY

The incubation period ranges from 50 to 160 days, with an average somewhat greater than 60 days. The onset is insidious, characterized by increasing degrees of anorexia and nausea for 1–2 weeks before onset of jaundice. Fever may occur with development of jaundice. Yellow staining of sclerae and skin is usually accompanied by dark urine (due to excretion of bilirulin and urobilin) and pale feces due to lack of bile pigment. Enlargement and/or tenderness of the liver may be detected at onset of jaundice. Symptoms may persist with decreasing intensity for several weeks. Elevations of blood levels of ALT and AST may be detected 2 weeks before to 2 or more months after onset of jaundice, and these abnormalities may be detected in the absence of jaundice (anicteric hepatitis). Although recovery occurs slowly over many weeks, some patients may develop relapsing bouts of hepatitis which proceed eventually to cirrhosis of the liver.

Clinical diagnosis of hepatitis B depends substantially on its epidemiological characteristics (Table 15-2). Although symptoms of HBV infection resemble those of HAV, HBV disease has a longer incubation period and symptoms persist significantly longer than in HAV disease. Furthermore HBV infection is transmitted naturally by blood or by intimate mucosal contact, so that groups of subjects at high risk to HBV infection include: (i) health care personnel who are phlebotomists or members of renal dialysis teams where frequent venepunctures continually provides opportunity for needle-stick exposures; (ii) biochemical laboratory personnel who fail to observe the precaution of avoiding pipetting by mouth; (iii) dental teams who work with patients from high-risk groups such as immigrants from Southeast Asia where HBV prevalence may exceed 10% in contrast to 0.5% or less for most residents of North America and Europe; (iv) homosexuals with many partners.

REFERENCES

[1] Barker LF, Maynard JE, Purcell RH, Hoofnagle JH, Berquist KR, London WT, Gerety RJ, Krushak DH: Hepatitis B infection in chimpanzees: titration of subtypes. J Infect Dis 132:451, 1975.

[2] Beeson PB: Jaundice occurring one to four months after transfusion of blood or plasma. Report of 7 cases. JAMA 121:1332, 1943.

TABLE 15-2
EPIDEMIOLOGICAL FEATURES OF HEPATITIS

Feature	Hepatitis A	Hepatitis B	Hepatitis Non-A, Non-B[a]
Former synonyms	Infectious hepatitis Catarrhal jaundice	Serum hepatitis Homologous serum jaundice	Post-transfusion hepatitis
Incubation period	15–40 days (avg. 30)	50–160 days (avg. 60+)	14–170 days (avg. 40)
Onset	Acute	Insidious or acute	Insidious
Symptomatology	Anorexia, nausea, temperature 38° C, jaundice, dark urine, pale feces.	Same as hepatitis A	Same as hepatitis A
Duration of illness	1–3 weeks	variable, often 3 weeks	variable
Method of spread	Fecal-oral	Blood contamina- tion, injection equipment of mucous membranes	Blood transfusion
Seasonal incidence	Autumn, winter	Year round	Year round
Communicability	15 days before to 10 days after onset of jaundice	Intermittent but often 2 weeks before to 1–3 months after onset of jaundice.	Many weeks after onset
Prophylaxis	Pooled human IgG	titered lots of human IgG	Titered lots of human IgG
Electron microscopy of serum	27-nm particle	22-nm surface antigen 27-nm core antigen 42-nm Dane particle	

[a]Distinguished from hepatitis B since 1974.

[3]Blumberg BS, Gerstley BJ, Hungerford DA, London WT, Sutnick AI: A serum antigen (Australia antigen) in Down's syndrome, leukemia and hepatitis. Ann Int
Med 66:924, 1967.

[4]Bonino F, Hoyer BH, Shik W-K, Rizzetto M, Purcell RH, Gerin JL: Delta hepatitis
agent: structural and antigenic properties of the delta-associated particle. Infection
and Immunity 43:1000, 1984.

[5]Bradley DW, Maynard JE, Popper H, Cook EH, Ebert JW, McCaustland KA, Schable CA, Fields HA: Posttransfusion non-A, non-B hepatitis: physiochemical properties of two distinct agents. J Infect Dis 148:254, 1983.

[6]Coleman JC, Thornton A, Zuckerman AJ: Homosexual hepatitis. J Infection 1:61, 1979.

[7]Committee on Viral Hepatitis of the National Research Council - National Academy of Sciences. Nomenclature of antigens associated with viral hepatitis type B. MMWR 23:29, 1974.

[8]Dane DS, Cameron CH, Briggs M: Virus-like particles in serum of patients with Australia-antigen-associated hepatitis. Lancet 1:695, 1970.

[9]Findlay GM, MacCallum FO: Note on acute hepatitis and yellow fever immunization. Trans R Soc Trop Med Hyg 31:297, 1937.

[10]Fox JP, Manso C, Penna HA, Para M: Observations on occurrence of icterus in Brazil following vaccination against yellow fever. Am J Hyg 36:68, 1942.

[11]Hadler S, Anzola E, Ponzetta A, de Monzon M, Rivera D, Mondolfi A, Bracho A, Gerber M, Thung S, Maynard JE, Popper H, Purcell RH: An epidemic of severe hepatitis due to delta virus infection in Yucpa Indians in Venezuela. Proceedings of 56th Annual Meeting of the American Epidemiological Society, Tucson, Arizona, 24 March 1983.

[12]Heathcote J, Cameron CH, Dane DS: Hepatitis-B antigen in saliva and semen. Lancet 1:71, 1974.

[13]Hilleman MR, Bertland AU, Buynak EB et al: Clinical laboratory studies of HBsAg vaccine. In Vyas G, Cohen SN, Schmid N. Eds. Viral Hepatitis. Franklin Institute Press, Philadelphia, 1978, p. 525.

[14]Hoofnagle JH, Gerety RJ, Barker LF: Antibody to hepatitis B core in man. Lancet 2:869, 1973.

[15]Iversen P, Roholm K: On aspiration biopsy of the liver with remarks on its diagnostic significance. Acta Med Scand 102:1, 1939.

[16]Krugman S, Giles JP, Hammond J: Infectious hepatitis. Evidence for two distinctive clinical, epidemiological and immunological types of infection. JAMA 200:365, 1967.

[17]Krugman S, Giles JP: The natural history of viral hepatitis. Can Med Ass J 106:442, 1972.

[18]Krugman S, Overby LR, Mushahwar KW, Ling C-M, Frozner GG, Deinhardt F: Viral hepatitis B. Studies on natural history and prevention re-examined. JAMA 300:101, 1979.

[19]Ling CM, Overby LR: Prevalence of hepatitis B virus antigen as revealed by direct radioimmune assay with ^{125}I-antibody. J Immunol 109:834, 1972.

[20]McNalty AS: Great Britain Ministry of Health. Report of Chief Medical Officer, Annual Report, London 1937.

[21]Melnick JL: Classification of Hepatitis A as Enterovirus type 72 and Hepatitis B virus as Hepadnavirus type 1. Intervirology 18:105, 1982.

[22]Melnick JL, Dreesman GR, Hollinger FB: Approaching the control of viral hepatitis type B. J Infect Dis 133:210, 1976.

[23]Morgan HV, Williamson DAJ: Jaundice following administration of human blood products. Brit Med J 1:750, 1943.

[24]Prince AM, Brotman B, Grady GF, Kuhns WJ, Hazzi C, Levine RW, Millian SJ: Long-incubation post-transfusion hepatitis without serological evidence of exposure to hepatitis-B virus. Lancet 2:241, 1974.

[25]Richer G, Chen Y-Y, Huet P-M: Incidence of hepatitis non-A, non-B compared with types A and B in hospital patients. Can Med Ass J 127:384, 1982.

[26]Rizzeto M, Canese MG, Arico S, Crivelli O, Bonino F, Trepo CG, Verme G: Immunofluorescence detection of a new antigen-antibody system (δ/anti δ) associated to the hepatitis B virus in the liver and in the serum of HBsAg carriers. Gut 18:997, 1977.

[27]Schweitzer IL, Dunn AEG, Peters RL, Spears RL: Viral hepatitis B in neonates and infants. Am J Med 55:762, 1973.

[28]Szmuness W, Stevens CE, Harley EJ, Zang EA, Oleszko WR, William DC, Sadovsky R, Morrison JM, Kellner A: Hepatitis B vaccine. Demonstration of efficacy in a controlled clinical trial in a high-risk population in the United States. New Eng J Med 303:833, 1980.

[29]Walsh JH, Yalow R, Berson SA: Detection of Australia antigen and antibody by means of radioimmunoassay techniques. J Infect Dis 130:383, 1970.

[30]Waterson AP: Infectious particles in hepatitis. Ann Rev Med 27:23, 1976.

[31]Wolters G, Kuijpers LPC, Kacaki J, Schuurs AHWM: Enzyme-linked immunosorbent assay for hepatitis B surface antigen. J Infect Dis 136 (Supp):311, 1977.

CHAPTER 16

RETROVIRIDAE

Retroviridae comprise a wide range of enveloped virions 80–110nm diameter which contain ssRNA and reverse transcriptase.[18]

HISTORICAL

Rous sarcoma virus was first described by Peyton Rous in 1910 as a transmissible agent by which solid malignant tumors (sarcomas) of domestic chickens were transmitted from bird to bird by cell-free filtrates.[27] This work followed the 1908 report by Ellerman and Bang of a filterable agent which transmitted chicken leukosis. Thus Rous sarcoma virus became the first retrovirus to be considered as the causative agent of a solid tumor. Mouse mammary adenocarcinoma was reported by Bittner in 1936[4] to be transmitted from mother to offspring by a virus in the milk, and Gross in 1951[15] first demonstrated the transmission of murine leukemia virus to newborn mice by injection of cell-free extracts from leukemic C3H mice. Isolation of human T-lymphotropic virus (HTLV) from a line of T-cells from an American patient with cutaneous T-cell leukemia/lymphoma by Gallo and associates in 1980[24,26] demonstrated for the first time the etiological relationship between a retrovirus and a human malignancy. Reports in 1983 of the isolation of HTLV from peripheral blood leukocytes of an American patient[12] with acquired immune deficiency syndrome (AIDS),[14] and from biopsy of a lymph node from a French patient[2] with lymphadenopathy who was at risk for AIDS, strongly suggested that retrovirus infections currently designated human immunodeficiency virus (HIV) types 1 and 2 were the etiological agents in AIDS.

BIOLOGICAL ATTRIBUTES

Retrovirus virions are spherical enveloped particles 80–100nm total diameter which show glycoprotein surface projections 8nm diameter.[18] The capsid is probably icosahedral which contains a possibly helical ribonucleoprotein. Thin sections of virus particles reveal an outer envelope, inner membrane (shell) and central nucleoid which is located acentrically in type

B Oncovirinae, and concentrically in type C Oncovirinae. The nucleic acid is an inverted dimer of linear positive-sense ssRNA with the two monomers held together at the 5' ends by hydrogen bonds, probably base pairing. Virions contain four internal non-glycosylated structural core *(gag)* proteins (p 24), two envelope *(env)* glycoproteins (gp 41) and reverse transcriptase *(pol)* (p 31). Virion proteins contain group-specific determinants, which are shared between members of a genus, and the internal *gag* protein is used to define subgenera e.g., mammalian type C oncoviruses. Type-specific envelope glycoproteins are involved in antibody neutralization.

After entry of retrovirus into a cell, viral replication starts with reverse transcription of virion RNA into DNA which becomes integrated into the chromosomal DNA of the host cell. This in turn is transcribed by cellular RNA polymerase II into virion RNA and m RNA. Several m RNA entities serve for the translation of *gag, pol* and *env* genes into their respective structural proteins, reverse transcriptase and envelope proteins, following which the daughter virions mature at the plasma membranes and are released from the cells by budding. Integration of viral DNA into host cell DNA appears to be a prerequisite for retrovirus replication. This explains the association of retroviruses particularly with leukemias, lymphomas, sarcomas and other tumors of mesodermal origin.

Retroviridae are classified into three subfamilies; Oncovirinae (RNA tumor virus group), Spumavirinae (foamy virus group of monkeys) and Lentivirinae (HIV and HTLV of humans and maedi/visna group of sheep). The Oncovirinae contain three genera - type B, type C, type D oncovirus. Type C oncovirus genus is subdivided into 3 subgenera: (i) mammalian type C oncoviruses which contain retroviruses pathogenic for mice (murine leuke-mia), cats, woolly monkeys and other mammals; (ii) avian type C oncoviruses which contain Rous sarcoma and other retroviruses pathogenic for birds; (iii) reptilian type C oncoviruses such as viper type C oncovirus. The Bittner virus associated with mouse mammary tumors is a species within the type B oncovirus genus. The Mason-Pfizer monkey virus is a species within the proposed type D retrovirus genus (Table 16-1).

Currently 4 serotypes of retrovirus have been associated with human infections: HTLV-I with adult T-cell lymphoma/leukemia,[24] HTLV-II with hairy T-cell leukemia,[16] and HIV-1 and -2 (formerly HTLV-III) with AIDS.[2,13]

Growth of HTLV in the laboratory became possible following the 1976 observation that a lymphokine T-cell growth factor[21] (interleukin-2) promoted the long-term growth of T-cells in tissue culture after they were previously activated with antigen, or mitogen such as phytohemagglutinin. However T-cells from some malignancies such as T-cell leukemia and cutaneous T-cell leukemia/lymphoma required no previous activation, but responded directly

TABLE 16-1
HUMAN IMMUNODEFICIENCY VIRUS (HIV) WITHIN THE RETROVIRIDAE FAMILY[18]

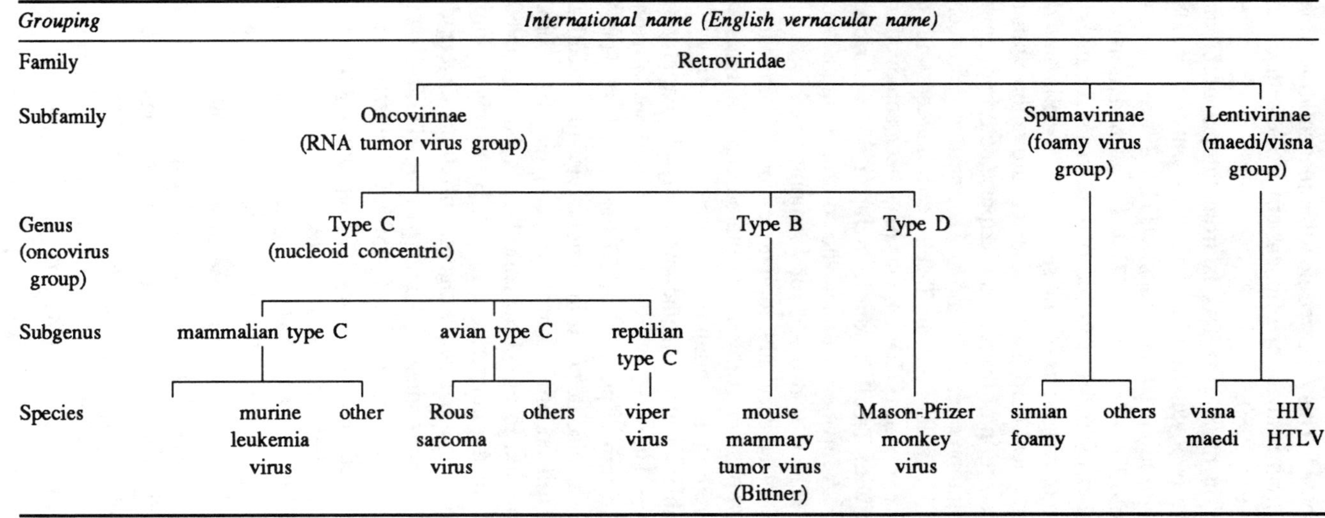

to T-cell growth factor.[23] This rendered possible the isolation of the prototype HTLV-I from a human resident of southeastern USA with cutaneous T-cell leukemia/lymphoma in 1980.[24]

By co-cultivation of normal T-cells from human umbilical cord with peripheral blood lymphocytes of a New York patient with AIDS which had previously been X-irradiated (6000 rads), HTLV-I was transmitted to the umbilical cord T-cells.[12] Evidence that HTLV-I virus had propagated in tissue cultures was revealed by (i) observation of retrovirus particles 100–150nm diameter in electron micrographs of thin sections of T-cells both directly from a patient and in umbilical cord T-cells after cocultivation with the patient's lymphocytes; (ii) detection of reverse transcriptase activity, core *gag* proteins p 24 by radioimmunoprecipitation and p 18 immunofluorescence, both in cultivated cells of the patient and in T-cells cocultivated with the patient's cells.[12] Antigenically similar HTLV isolates have been achieved from cultured T-cells of patients with T-cell leukemia in Japan,[20] the Caribbean,[19] Israel, Ecuador and USA.[26] A Japanese woman who contracted fatal T-cell leukemia/lymphoma carried HTLV-1 in blood for 17 months.[17]

Cells from a biopsied cervical lymph node from a French male homosexual patient, with lymphadenopathy and hematological findings antecedent to AIDS, were cultured in a medium containing T-cell growth factor plus antiserum to human interferon together with phytohemagglutinin. After 15 days of culture, the latter 12 of which were without phytohemagglutin, detection of reverse transcriptase revealed the growth of HTLV-III virus.[2] Virus propagation was also detected in lymphocytes of a healthy adult blood donor after 15 days of cocultivation of lymphocytes of the biopsied lymph node. Virus transmission to umbilical cord T-cells was achieved by transfer of cell-free extracts of the infected cocultures. By means of immunofluorescence and immunoprecipitin tests, antigenic differences were demonstrated between the core *gag* proteins. p24 and p18 of HTLV-III and HTLV-I. However typical retrovirus particles 120–150 nm diameter were observed in thin sections of infected cord lymphocytes. Employing similar cocultivation techniques, HIV (HTLV-III) strains were isolated from 2 French siblings with hemophilia B, one of whom had AIDS,[29] and also from a Zairian married couple, one of whom had AIDS and the other had prodromal features.[10] Antibodies to HIV were also found these in the patients' sera.

Cocultivation of HTLV-I-infected human T-cells with cells from continuous polyploid lines (indicator cells) from human carcinomas and sarcomas and from tissues of monkey, dog, cat, mink and rat induced formation of syncytia, usually after 18 hours incubation.[22] Syncytium formation correlated well with detection of immunofluorescence due to HTLV antigen, and it was specifically inhibited by mixture of antibody-containing human sera with HTLV-infected cell lines at the time of cocultivation with indicator cells. A human osteogenic sarcoma line HOS became an HTLV-producing subline 4 months after cocultivation with an X-irradiated virus-positive T-cell line derived from a patient,[8] but none of the other indicator cell lines permitted HTLV replication. This HOS/HTLV-I line: (i) expressed reverse transcriptase, (ii) revealed immunofluorescent foci after treatment both with HTLV-I antibody in human serum and monoclonal antibody to the core protein p19; (iii) induced syncytia in indicator rat XC cells; (iv) showed budding and mature retrovirus virions typical of HTLV in electron micrographs of thin sections of cells.

Pseudotypes, which are phenotypically mixed virions carrying the genome of one virus and the coat proteins of another, have provided a more convenient assay system for retroviruses and their antibodies than the cumbersome technique of syncytia formation. Recently a vesicular stomatitis - HTLV pseudotype was developed[9] by superinfection of HOS/HTLV-1 cells with vesicular stomatitis virus (VSV) Indiana serotype at a multiplicity of 10. Progency virus in the supernatant was harvested after 18 hours incubation. This was treated with an excess of anti-VSV serum. From an initial yield of about 9 log plaque forming units (PFU) virus, 4 log PFU unchanged VSV were neutralized by anti-VSV serum, but an additional 5 log PFU were neutralized only by anti-HTLV serum, not anti-VSV serum. This residual 5 log PFU represented the VSV-HTLV pseudotype composed of VSV genome (which conferred plaque forming capacity in human or mink cells) surrounded by a HTLV envelope (which reacted with antibody to HTLV). Thus plaque-reduction neutralizing antibody in patients sera were determined readily by inoculation of indicator mink cells and this correlated well with antibody determination by radioimmunoassay.[9]

Antibodies to HTLV have been detected fairly regularly in sera of virus-positive patients with AIDS, lymphadenopathy syndrome or T-cell leukemia/lymphoma using a variety of methods including immunofluorescence for membrane antigen,[2,11] ELISA[29] radioimmunoassay[7] and pseudotype neutralization.[9] Serological surveys[5] by radioimmunoassay or immunofluorescence have revealed HTLV-I antibody prevalence rates as high as 9–16% in normal Japanese residents of Shikoku and Kyushu islands where T-cell leukemia is endemic and 3–4% among Caribbean residents where this disease is prevalent. By ELISA tests, 59% of non-Hodgkin's lymphoma cases in Jamaica had anti HTLV-1 antibody.[6] Using a combination of all the currently available antibody-detection techniques,[28] anti-HTLV-I was found in less than 5% of 80 patients with lymphadenopathy syndrome possibly preceding AIDS and in none of 22 patients with AIDS, 85 hemophiliacs, or 940 normal blood donors in Great Britain, whilst anti-HTLV-II was detected in only 4% of 113 drug addicts. However anti-HTLV-III antibodies were demonstrated in 89–97% of

155 British patients with AIDS or prodromal lymphadenopathy[7] in contrast to 1.5% of 269 drug addicts and none of 1042 normal blood donors, thus strongly suggesting a causative relationship between HTLV-III and AIDS.

Electron microscopic examination of HTLV-I isolates in thin sections of lymphocytes co-cultivated with peripheral blood from American[12] Jamaican[19] or Japanese[20] patients with T-cell leukemia or AIDS and its preceding lymphadenopathy syndrome revealed spherical enveloped particles with total diameters 120–140nm whose crenated envelopes surround electron dense cores about 100nm diameter. Particles with similar dimensions have been observed budding from cell surfaces and extracellularly in lymphocyte cultures from French patients infected with HIV who had lymphadenopathy preceding AIDS[2] and hemophilia with AIDS.[29]

Thin sections of lymph nodes from 6 Australian men with persistent lymphadenopathy including one with AIDS revealed spherical particles 100–120nm total diameter with crenated outer coats and containing electron-dense nucleoids about 50nm diameter resembling retroviruses within follicular labyrinths.[1] Retrovirus virions 100–120nm with nucleoids 40–50nm have been observed extracellularly or budding from cell surfaces in biopsies of esophageal ulcers of 8 men in Vancouver, Canada[25] who had retrosternal pain unrelieved by food or antacids, lymphadenopathy and inverted T4/T8-lymphocyte ratios typical of the lymphadenopathy syndrome preceding AIDS (Figure 16-1). Some patients have yielded HIV isolates from peripheral leukocytes or shown HIV seroconversion; several have died with AIDS.

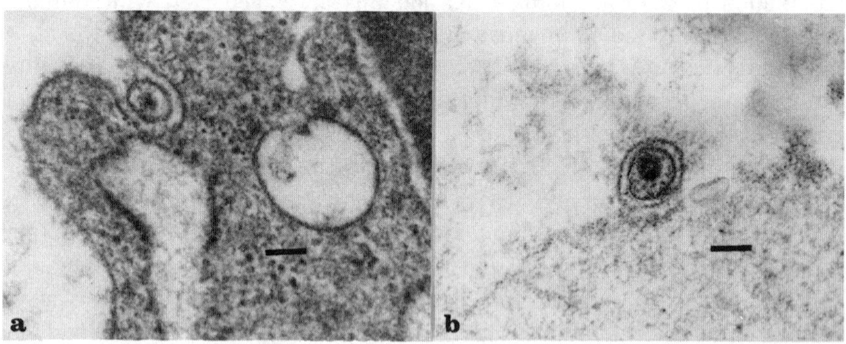

Figure 16-1: Retrovirus virions in thin section of biopsy from esophageal ulcer of patient with lymphadenopathy syndrome.[25] (X 59,400), uranyl acetate and lead citrate. Enveloped virions with total diameters 100–120 nm containing electron-dense nucleoids 50nm are observed: (a) adjacent to the cell surface, or (b) budding from the cell surface.

SUMMARY

Human retroviruses comprise at least 4 serotypes within the Lentivirinae group of the family Retroviridae. They are detected in peripheral blood lymphocytes or lymph node biopsies by co-cultivation with normal human cord blood T-cells in the presence of interleukin-2 and phytohemagglutinin and subsequent demonstration of reverse transcriptase activity and/or immunofluorescence after treatment with monoclonal antibodies to HIV or HTLV core protein p 24. Antibodies to the HIV envelope gp 41 and core p 24 appear 2–5 weeks after onset by ELISA or immunofluorescence. Anti gp 41 persists indefinitely, but anti p 24 becomes undetectable shortly before death if this should occur 2–8 years later. Antibody specificity is confirmed by western blot tests.

SYMPTOMATOLOGY

Clinical manifestations of human retrovirus infection arise from persistent virus growth in lymphoid tissues which eventually give rise to either: (i) adult T-cell leukemia/lymphoma (ATL) from extensive lymphocyte proliferation. This is due mainly to HTLV-I infection; or (ii) lymphadenopathy syndrome (LAS) which may progress into acquired immune deficiency syndrome (AIDS), where T-cell (and B-cell) functions are impaired severely. This follows infection usually with HIV-1, but less commonly with HIV-2.

ADULT T-CELL LEUKEMIA/LYMPHOMA. Among 11 virologically confirmed cases in USA, symptoms began abruptly with rapidly progressive symptoms, and a laboratory diagnosis was established after a median duration of 2 months from onset.[3] Presenting features usually comprised skin nodules, plaques, papules or erythroderma which became generalized within several weeks, and these were the sites of the initial biopsy which confirmed the diagnosis of malignant T-cells lymphoma. Malignant lymphocytes penetrated the dermis or formed focal aggregates in the epidermis. About 60% of patients presented with malaise, lethargy, weakness, nausea, confusion, polyuria and polydypsia accompanied by hypercalcemia, and malignant lymphoma cells were observed in biopsied lymph nodes. Circulating malignant lymphocytes were observed in 90% of patients at presentation and peripheral white cell counts ranged from 6700 to 14,500 (mean 42,600) per mm^3 with 15–94% (average 50%) lymphocytes. Liver enlargement affected about 50% patients, bilateral diffuse interstitial pulmonary infiltrates were observed in about 50% and lymphomatous meningitis was found in about 30%. Opportunistic infections with *Pneumocystis carinii* or *Candida* were common. Despite aggressive chemotherapy, the survival time ranged from 1 to 42 months (average 13 months).

ACQUIRED IMMUNODEFICIENCY SYNDROME (AIDS). The syndrome comprising *Pneumocystis carinii* pneumonia, extensive mucosal candidiasis, multiple viral infection and prolonged fever, cutaneous anergy, lymphopenia, with relative reduction of T4 helper T-cells and an increased percentage of T8 suppressor T-cells (inversion of the normally high T4/T8 ratio), was first described in 4 male homosexual patients in Los Angeles during 1981.[14] Kaposi's sarcoma subsequently affected 1 patient. During 1984, more than 3000 cases of AIDS have been reported throughout USA and AIDS patients have been diagnosed currently in most countries. Although AIDS characteristically involves young male homosexuals with numerous sexual partners, it has also affected monogamous males and females and it appears to have been transmitted both by blood transfusions and transplacentally. During 1989, 35,238 cases (14.1 per 100,000) were reported in USA. The incubation distribution (time from exposure to development of AIDS) currently averages 8–10 years. Clinical manifestations of AIDS were described by CDC according to stages (MMWR 35:334, 1986):

Stage I: mononucleosis-like syndrome 6–28 days after exposure with T4/T8<0.9 and HIV seroconversion after 2 weeks to 2 months.

Stage II: asymptomatic with high anti-core p 24 antibody with T4/T8>1.5.

Stage III: persistent generalized lymphadenopathy for 3 months often with T4/T8<0.9.

Stage IV: AIDS with severe immunosuppression, terminating fatally 1–10 years after exposure.

REFERENCES

[1]Armstrong JA, Horne R: Follicular dendritic cells and virus-like particles in AIDS-related lymphadenopathy. Lancet 2:370, 1984.

[2]Barre-Sinoussi F, Chermann JC, Rey F, Nugeyre MT, Charamet S, Gruest J, Dauguet C, Axler-Blin C, Vezinet-Brun F, Rouzioux CC, Rozenbaum W, Montagnier L: Isolation of a T-lymphotropic retrovirus from a patient at risk for acquired immune deficiency syndrome (AIDS). Science 220:868, 1983.

[3]Binn PA, Schechter GP, Jaffe E, Blayney D, Young RC, Matthews MT, Blattner W, Broder S, Robert-Guroff M, Gallo RC: Clinical course of retrovirus-associated adult T-cell lymphoma in the United States. New Eng J Med 309:257, 1983.

[4]Bittner JJ: Some possible effects of nursing on the mammary gland tumor incidence in mice. Science 84:162, 1936.

[5]Blattner WA, Blayney DW, Robert-Guroff M, Sarngadharam MG, Kalyanaraman VS, Sarin PS, Jaffe ES, Gallo RC: Epidemiology of human T-cell leukemia/lymphoma virus. J Infect Dis 147:406, 1983.

[6]Blattner WA, Gibbs WN, Saxinger C, Robert-Guroff M, Clark J, Lofters W, Hanchard

B, Campbell M, Gallo RC: Human T-cell leukemia/lymphoma virus-associated lymphoreticular neoplasm in Jamaica. Lancet 2:61, 1983.

[7]Cheingsong-Popov R, Weiss RA, Tedder RS, Shanson DC, Jeffries DJ, Ferns RB, Briggs EM, Weller IVD, Mitton S, Adler MW, Farthing C, Lawrence AG, Gazzard BG, Weber J, Harris JRW, Pinching AJ, Craske J, Barbara JAJ: Prevalence of antibody to human T-lymphotropic virus type III in AIDS and AIDS-risk patients in Britain. Lancet 2:477, 1984.

[8]Clapham P, Nagy K, Cheingsong-Popov R, Exley M, Weiss RA: Productive infection and cell-free transmission of human T-cell leukemia virus in a nonlymphoid cell line. Science 222:1125, 1983.

[9]Clapham P, Nagy K, Weiss RA: Pseudotypes of human T-cell leukemia virus types 1 and 2: neutralization by patients sera. Adult T-cell leukemia-lymphoma/ vesicular stomatitis virus; in Human T-cell Leukemia Viruses. 1984, ed. RC Gallo, M Essex, L Gross, Cold Spring Harbor Laboratory, NY.

[10]Ellrodt A, Barre-Sinoussi F, Le Bras P, Nugeyre MT, Palazzo L, Rey F, Brun-Vezinet F, Rouzioux C, Segard P, Caquet R, Montagnier L, Chermann JC: Isolations of human T-lymphotropic retrovirus (LAV) from Zairian married couple, one with AIDS, one with prodromes. Lancet 1:1383, 1984.

[11]Essex M, McLane MF, Lee TH, Falk L, Howe CWS, Mullins JI, Cabradilla C, Francis DP. Antibodies to cell membrane antigens associated with human T-cell leukemia virus in patients with AIDS. Science 220:859, 1983.

[12]Gallo RC, Sarin PS, Gelmann EP et al: Isolation of human T-cell leukemia virus in acquired immune deficiency syndrome (AIDS). Science 220:865, 1983.

[13]Gallo RC, Salahuddin SZ, Popovic M et al: Frequent detection and isolation of cytopathic retroviruses (HTLV-III), isolated from AIDS patients and donors at risk for AIDS. Science 224:500, 1984.

[14]Gottlieb MS, Schroff R, Schanker HM, Weisman JD, Fan PT, Wolf RA, Saxon A: *Pneumocystis carinii* pneumonia and mucosal candidiasis in previously healthy homosexual men. Evidence of a new acquired cellular immunodeficiency. New Eng J Med 305:1425, 1981.

[15]Gross L: Spontaneous leukemia developing in C3H mice following inoculation, in infancy, with AK-leukemic extracts or AK-embryos. Proc Soc Exp Biol Med 76:27, 1951.

[16]Kalyanaraman VS, Sarngadharan MG, Robert-Guroff M, Miyoski I, Blayney D, Golde D, Gallo RC: A new subtype of human T-cell leukemia virus (HTLV-II) associated with a T-cell variant of hairy cell leukemia. Science 218:571, 1982.

[17]Kobayashi M, Yoshimoto S, Fijishita M, Yano S, Niiya K, Kubonishi I, Taguchi H, Miyoski I: HTLV-positive T-cell lymphoma-leukemia in an AIDS patient. Lancet 1:1361, 1984.

[18]Matthews REF: Classification and nomenclature of viruses. Intervirology 17:1, 1982.

[19]Matutes E, Carrington D, Hedge U, Catovsky D: C-type particles in cells from T-cell lymphoma/leukaemia after 5–7 days culture. Lancet 2:335, 1983.

[20]Miyoshi I, Rubonishi I, Yoshimoto S, Agaki T, Ohtuski Y, Shiraishi Y, Nagata K, Hinuma Y: Type C virus particles in a cord T cell line derived by co-cultivating

normal human cord leukocytes and human leukaemic T cells. Nature 294:770, 1981.

[21]Morgan DA, Ruscetti FW, Gallo RC: Selective in vitro growth of T lymphocytes from normal human bone marrows. Science 193:1007, 1976.

[22]Nagy K, Clapham P, Cheingsong-Popov R, Weiss RA: Human T-cell leukemia virus type I: induction of syncytia and inhibition of patient's sera. Int J Cancer 32:321, 1983.

[23]Poiesz BJ, Ruscetti FW, Mier JW, Woods AM, Gallo RC: T-cell lines established from human T-lymphocytic neoplasias by direct response to T-cell growth factor. Proc Nat Acad Sci USA 77:6815, 1980.

[24]Poiesz BJ, Ruscetti FW, Gadzar AF, Binn PA, Minna JD, Gallo RC: Detection and isolation of type C retrovirus particles from fresh and cultured lymphocytes of a patient with cutaneous T-cell lymphoma. Proc Nat Acad Sc USA 77:7415, 1980.

[25]Rabeneck L, Boyko, WJ, McLean DM, McLeod WA, Wong KK: Unusual esophageal ulcers containing enveloped viral particles in homosexual males. Presented at 53rd Annual Meeting, Royal College of Physicians and Surgeons of Canada, Montreal, P.Q. 13 Sept. 1984.

[26]Reitz MS, Kalyanaraman VS, Robert-Guroff M, Popovic M, Sarngadharam MG, Sarin PS, Gallo RC: Human T-cell leukemia/lymphoma virus: the retrovirus of adult T-cell leukemia/lymphoma. J Infect Dis 147:399, 1983.

[27]Rous P: Transmission of a malignant new growth by means of a cell-free filtrate. JAMA 56:198, 1911.

[28]Tedder RS, Shanson DC, Jeffries DJ, Cheingsong-Popov R, Clapman P, Dalgleish A, Nagy K, Weiss RA: Low prevalence in UK of HTLV-I and HTLV-II infection in subject with AIDS, with extended lymphadenopathy, and at risk of AIDS. Lancet 2:125, 1984.

[29]Vilmer E, Barre-Sinoussi F, Rouzioux C, Gazengel C, Brun FV, Dauguet C, Fisher A, Manigne P, Chermann JC, Griscelli C, Montagnier L: Isolation of new lymphotropic retrovirus from two siblings with haemophilia B, one with AIDS. Lancet 1:753, 1984.

CHAPTER 17

RICKETTSIAE AND CHLAMYDIAE

Rickettsiae and chlamydiae are regarded taxonomically as two orders of bacteria, Rickettsiales and Chlamydiales,[2] but regularly they are investigated by virologists because they multiply exclusively inside living cells, although some rickettsiae are capable of metabolic activity independent of host cells. Thus current virology laboratory techniques are applied conveniently to the isolation and identification of these organisms and the conduct of relevant serological tests. Important human pathogens are assigned taxonomically to the 3 genera within the family Rickettsiaeceae (order Rickettsiales) and the single genus Chlamydia within the family Chlamydiaceae (order Chlamydiales).

BIOLOGICAL DISTINCTIVES

Rickettsiae are rod-shaped particles (elementary bodies) 300–500 nm x 800–2000 nm with trilaminar cell walls containing muramic acid (Table 17-1). They multiply by binary fission, usually within the cytoplasm, but some

TABLE 17-1
BIOLOGICAL DISTINCTION BETWEEN
RICKETTSIALES AND CHLAMYDIALES

Biological property	Rickettsiales	Chlamydiales
Particles (nm): elementary body	300–500 x 800–2000	200–400 (RNA:DNA=1)
reticulate body	None	600–1500 (RNA:DNA=3-4)
Muramic acid in cell walls in stoichiometric amounts	+	–
Oxidation of glutamate with net generation of ATP	+	–
Trilaminar cell wall	+	+
Arthropod vector	+	–
Extrahuman reservoir	+ (most species)	C. psittaci

Adapted from Bergey's Manual of Systematic Bacteriology, Williams and Wilkins, Baltimore, 1984.

species may also multiply within the nucleus. Some species exhibit oxidative metabolism of glutamate with production of adenosine triphosphate (ATP) independent of host cells.[2] Rickettsiae are normally transmitted naturally by bites of arthropod vectors (louse, flea, mite, tick) in which the rickettsia has undergone multiplication during a period of extrinsic incubation. Most rickettsiae are maintained in nature in vertebrate reservoirs apart from humans (rodents, ungulates) except for typhus *(Rickettsia prowazekii)* where the human is both reservoir and victim of the infection. Genera within the family Rickettsiaceae which are pathogenic for humans comprise *Rickettsia* with 8 species, *Rochalimaea* with 1 species and *Coxiella* with 1 species.

Chlamydiae exhibit round elementary bodies 200–400nm diameter with rigid trilaminar walls which do not contain muramic acid in stoichiometric amounts[2] (Table 17-1). Elementary bodies comprise the mature infectious form of the chlamydia. Replication occurs by binary fission within the cytoplasm of host cells, with the appearance of basophilic reticulate bodies 600–1500 nm as an intermediate stage before the emergence of daughter elementary bodies. The ratio RNA:DNA is 3–4 times higher in reticulate bodies than elementary bodies. Glutamate is not metabolized. Chlamydiae are not normally transmitted by arthropods in nature. Typically, *Chlamydia psittaci* is maintained in extrahuman vertebrate reservoirs, usually birds, in contrast to *C. trachomatis* which infects humans exclusively, except the mouse biovar (mouse pneumonitis) which infects mice solely. Both the two species of Chlamydia are human pathogens.

All Chlamydiae share a genus-specific heat-stable complement fixing (CF) group antigen associated with the lipopolysaccharide of the cell wall. Some strains produce hemagglutinin for rodent and fowl erythrocytes which is related to the group antigen. Cytoplasmic inclusions (basophil bodies with diameters about 10 microns) contain aggregates of *C. trachomatis* within a carbohydrate matrix which stains brownish blue with iodine, but carbohydrate is absent from *C. psittaci* inclusions (Table 17-2). Growth of *C. trachomatis* is inhibited by sulfadiazine, which indicates that folic acid synthesis is required for *C. trachomatis* replication, but the growth of *C. psittaci* is unaffected by sulfonamides. Within *C. trachomatis,* the trachoma biovar induces the eye disease, trachoma and inclusion conjunctivitis and genital infections (non-gonococcal urethritis), the lymphogranuloma venereum biovar is associated with the sexually-transmitted disease, lymphogranuloma venereum, and the mouse biovar induces pneumonitis in mice but it is not a human pathogen. Microimmunofluorescence tests employing as antigen the washed preparations of elementary bodies have demonstrated 12 serovars (A-K) for the trachoma biovar (endemic trachoma is associated with serovars A, B, Ba, C and genital or newborn infections with serovars D-K), plus 3 serovars (L1-L3) for the lymphogranuloma venereum biovar.

TABLE 17-2

DISTINCTION BETWEEN *CHLAMYDIA TRACHOMATIS* AND *C. PSITTACI*

Feature	C. trachomatis	C. psittaci
Vertebrate hosts	humans, mice	birds, mammals
Cytoplasmic inclusions	oval	variable
Glycogen in inclusions	+ (iodine stain)	−
Inhibition by sulfadiazine	+	−

Genus: Chlamydia (heat stable lipopolysaccharide CF antigen)

Species: C. trachomatis and C. psittaci (species-specific CF antigen).

Biovars of C. trachomatis:

trachoma (serovars A, B, Ba, C: trachoma; serovars D-K: non-gonococcal urethritis and neonatal conjunctivitis) (immunofluorescence).

lymphogranuloma venereum (serovar L1-L3) (immunofluorescence).

mouse (mouse pneumonitis) (single serotype).

LABORATORY CHARACTERISTICS

Both rickettsiae and chlamydiae are propagated readily in yolk sac endothelial cells following inoculation of the yolk sacs of embryonated eggs of about 8 days incubation. After 3–5 days incubation, the embryos become sluggish and die, and smears of their yolk sacs reveal inclusions (aggregations of elementary bodies) within the cytoplasm of endothelial cells. Inclusions are basophilic and they stain blue with Giemsa or red using Macchiavello or Gimenez stains. Care must be taken to ensure the absence of antibiotics such as streptomycin, tetracycline and sulfonamides from the inocula and also from food eaten by chickens which laid the embryonated eggs.

Rickettsiae multiply in tissue cultures of primary chick embryo fibroblasts and in continuous polyploid human (HeLa, HEp-2) or baby hamster kidney (BHK21) cells with production of basophilic cytoplasmic inclusions and cytopathic effects. *Chlamydia trachomatis* multiplies after centrifugation onto monolayer polyploid cultures of McCoy cells which are treated with cyclo-heximide at the time of inoculation, and inclusions which stain with iodine are observed in the cytoplasm after 24 hours incubation. *C. psittaci* multiplies in a variety of polyploid tissue cultures, but the basophilic inclusions do not stain with iodine. However, chlamydial antigens may be detected in the inclusions by immunofluorescence after treatment with respective antisera.

Washed suspensions containing high titers of rickettsial and chlamydial elementary bodies induce "toxic" effects, due to alteration in capillary permeability causing a shock-like state and death within a few hours following intravenous injection of mice. Toxic effects, which are associated with living rickettsial or chlamydial particles but not their multiplication, are inhibited by mixture of these organisms with their respective antisera before inoculation i.e., toxin neutralization.[1]

Rickettsiae are classified into antigenic groups according to their soluble CF antigen. However CF tests using washed preparations of whole rickettsiae as the particle CF antigen, or microimmunofluorescence (IF) or toxin neutralization tests are particularly useful for differentiation of rickettsial species, especially within the spotted fever group (Table 17-3). The Weil-Felix test in which several OX strains of Proteus are agglutinated by antisera to several rickettsiae, presumably due to sharing of surface carbohydrate antigens, is not longer reliable and it should not be used if other tests, preferably microimmunofluorescence, are available.

Chlamydiae are classified into two species according to the species-specific CF antigen which is revealed using antisera from which antibody to the common heat-stable chlamydial CF antigen has been removed by absorption with this boiled antigen. Microimmunofluorescence tests have demonstrated 12 serovars within the trachoma biovar of *C. trachomatis* and 3 serovars within the lymphogranuloma serovar, but there is a sole serotype of *C. psittaci.*

NATURAL CYCLES OF INFECTION

Rickettsiae are characteristically maintained in nature by a cycle of infection involving blood-feeding arthropod vectors (louse, flea, mite or tick) in which the organism multiplies, and non-human vertebrate reservoirs (rodents, sheep, cattle) in which the organism circulates in the blood for several days with or without induction of symptoms (Figure 17-1). Humans generally are infected tangentially to this natural cycle. Important exceptions to this general principle include: (i) epidemic typhus where humans comprise the sole natural reservoir and they may contract severe or fatal illnesses; (ii) Q-fever where infection is transmitted from infected sheep to humans either by direct contact with placenta or birth fluids, or pasture grasses contaminated by products of conception from infected sheep.

Chlamydiae, on the other hand, are not transmitted by arthropods. They are normally transmitted to humans by droplets, dust or fomites contaminated by discharges or viscera from infected birds as in psittacosis *(Chlamydia psittaci),* or by direct mucosal contact as in trachoma, inclusion conjunctivitis or non-gonococcal urethritis due to *Chlamydia trachomatis.*

SYMPTOMATOLOGY: RICKETTSIAE

RICKETTSIA PROWAZEKII (EPIDEMIC TYPHUS)

Patients suddenly develop high fever, chills, rigors and headache, followed a few days later by an intense maculopapular rash, sometimes becoming hemorrhagic, which covers the entire surface of the body. The incubation period is 6–15 days, and symptoms persist for 1–2 weeks. The case fatality rate ranges from 10–12% in young persons to exceed 60% in older subjects. Relapsing typhus (Brill's disease) shows less severe symptoms during the first attack, but recurrences may occur many years subsequently.

The disease is distributed world-wide, with pockets of infections in rural areas of Central and East Africa, Central and South America, and mountainous areas of Asia. Inadvertent infections have occurred occasionally among laboratory workers in USA, and 33 sporadic infections have been acquired in eastern USA between 1976 and 1984, often in close proximity to colonies of flying squirrels *(Glaucomys volans)*.[6]

Body lice *(Pediculus corporis)* comprise the natural vector and humans constitute the sole natural reservoir. Spread of disease is promoted by crowded insanitary conditions as in prisons and refugee camps.

Laboratory diagnosis is achieved by: (a) cultivation of rickettsiae from blood collected during the first week after onset of fever by inoculation of yolk sacs of fertile hen eggs; (b) demonstration of rising antibody titers during convalescence against the typhus-group-specific soluble CF antigen or by microimmunofluorescence. Treatment is by tetracycline or chloramphenicol.

RICKETTSIA TYPHI (MURINE TYPHUS)

Symptoms resemble those of epidemic typhus but they are less severe and the case fatality rate is below 0.5%. The disease is distributed worldwide. Pockets of infection in USA are found mainly in southeastern states and Texas, and human infections occur usually during summer. Murine typhus is maintained in nature by a cycle principally involving rat fleas *(Xenopsylla cheopis)* and domestic rats *(Rattus rattus* or *R. norvegicus)*, from which humans become infected tangentially (Figure 17-1). Laboratory workers may become infected by inhalation of aerosols or inadvertent needle stick.[4] Laboratory diagnosis is usually established by demonstration of rising antibody titers during convalescence to the soluble CF antigen supplemented by microimmunofluorescence.

RICKETTSIA RICKETTSII (ROCKY MOUNTAIN SPOTTED FEVER)

Symptoms begin suddenly with high fever, chills, severe headache, myalgia, followed 3 or more days later by a maculopapular rash which may eventually spread over the entire body. Progressive mental deterioration

TABLE 17-3

CLASSIFICATION AND EPIDEMIOLOGICAL CHARACTERISTICS OF RICKETTSIAE CAUSING HUMAN DISEASE[a]

| Rickettsia species | Clinical Entity | Antigenic Grouping[b] | | | | Weil-Felix Proteus Agglutination | Vector | | Reservoir | Geographic Distribution |
		Soluble CF group	Particle CF species	Micro IF species	Toxin NT species		Common species	Category		
R. prowazekii	Epidemic typhus; (Brill's disease = recrudescent typhus)	Typhus	+	+	+	OX19	Pediculus corporis	Body louse	Human	Ubiquitous
R. typhi (mooseri)	Murine (endemic) typhus		+	+	+	OX19	Xenopsylla cheopis	Rat flea	Rats	Ubiquitous
R. rickettsii	Rocky Mountain spotted fever	Spotted fever	+	+	+	OX19 or OX2	Dermacentor sp. Amblyomma sp. Riphicephalus sp.	Tick	Small rodents	North and South America
R. conorii	Boutonneuse fever South African tick typhus Kenya tick typhus Indian tick typhus		+	+	+	OX2 or OX19	Riphicephalus sp. Amblyomma sp. Haemaphysalis sp.	Tick	Small rodents	Africa, India
R. siberica	Siberican tick typhus		+	+	+	OX2 or OX19	Dermacentor sp. Haemaphysalis sp.	Tick	Small rodents	Northern Asia

TABLE 17-3 (Continued)

CLASSIFICATION AND EPIDEMIOLOGICAL CHARACTERISTICS OF RICKETTSIAE CAUSING HUMAN DISEASE[a]

| Rickettsia species | Clinical Entity | Antigenic Grouping[b] | | | | Weil-Felix Proteus Agglutina-tion | Vector | | Reservoir | Geographic Distribution |
		Soluble CF group	Particle CF species	Micro IF species	Toxin NT species		Common species	Category		
R. australis	Queensland tick typhus		+	+	0	None	Ixodes holocyclus	Tick	Small marsupials	Australia
R. akari	Rickettsial pox		+	+	0	None	Allodermanys-sus sp.	Gamasid mite	House mouse	USA, USSR
R. tsutsugamu-shi	Scrub typhus	Scrub typhus +	+	+	+	OXK	Trombicula akamushi	Trombiculid mite	Small rodents	Orient, tropical Australia
Rochalimaea quintana	Trench fever	Trench fever +	+	+	0	None	Pediculus corporis	Body louse	Human	Europe, Medi-terranean
Coxiella burnetii	Q fever	None	+	+	0	None	Dermacentor sp. Ixodes sp. Haemaphysalis sp.	Tick[c]	Sheep, cattle, small marsupials	Ubiquitous

[a]Adapted from BL Elisberg, and FM Bozeman, Diagnostic Procedures for Viral and Rickettsial Infections, Ed. 4, pp. 826–868, American Public Health Association, New York, 1969.
[b]CF, complement fixing; NT, neutralization; IF, immunofluorescence.
[c]May also be transmitted via the airborne or transplacental route without a tick vector.

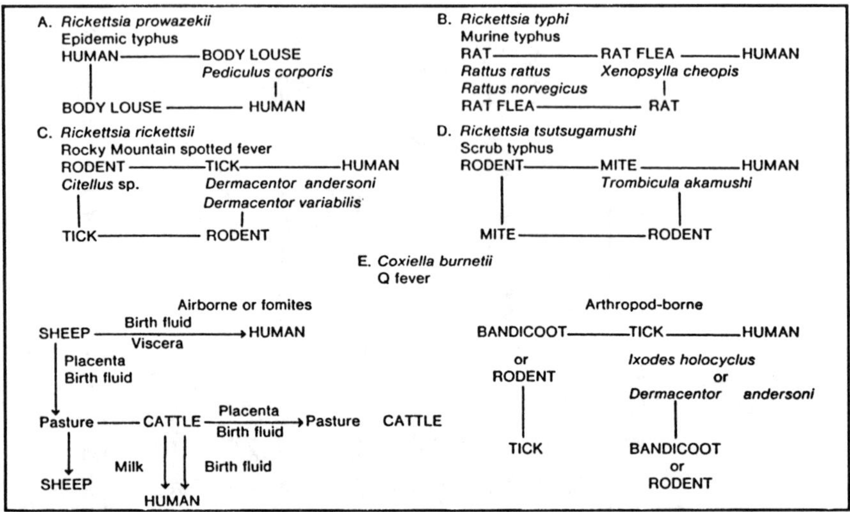

Figure 17-1: Natural cycles of the commoner rickettsiae. Reproduced with permission from McLean DM, 1980. Virology in Health Care, Williams and Wilkins, Baltimore, p. 250.

through stupor and coma may occur, accompanied in some cases by gastro-intestinal hemorrhage and pneumonia. The case fatality rate ranges from 4 to 8%. A history of recent tick bite may or may not be obtained.

Rocky Mountain spotted fever is distributed through North, Central and South America, but not on the other continents. In USA during recent years, most cases have occurred in eastern and southeastern states from Massachusetts to Texas and Oklahoma. Since 1970, less than 2% cases occurred in Pacific Northwestern States where the disease occurred commonly during the early 1900's. The disease occurs principally during spring and summer, particularly in suburban areas where partial regrowth of vegetation over previously deforested areas affords excellent natural habitats for ticks and rodents.

Hard ticks (*Dermacentor andersoni* west of the Continental Divide, *Dermacentor variabilis* elsewhere) are the principal natural vectors and wild rodents (particularly ground squirrels, *Citellus sp* in western USA) are the major natural reservoirs. Humans become infected tangentially to this cycle by tick bites.

Laboratory diagnosis is established by: (a) isolation of *R. rickettsii* from blood collected during the height of fever by intraperitoneal inoculation of male guinea pigs which develop fever accompanied by scrotal necrosis about 2 days later and they die shortly thereafter. High concentrations of rickettsiae are found in the tunica vaginalis, peritoneal fluid and spleen; they are visualized by Giemsa or Macchiavello stains, and they are confirmed serologically as *R. rickettsii* by microimmunofluorescence; (b) demonstrations of rising antibody titers during convalescence by complement fixation using the soluble (group) and particle (species-specific) antigens, or by microagglutination and microimmunofluorescence tests.

Treatment of *R. rickettsii* infections is achieved optimally by tetracycline which induces remission within 1–2 days,[7] but chloramphenicol is a satisfactory alternative antibiotic.

RICKETTSIA TSUTSUGAMUSHI (SCRUB TYPHUS)

Patients develop fever, headache and maculopapular rash after an incubation period of 6–21 days.[3] An eschar may be found at the site of biting by a mite. In untreated cases, fever may persist 1–2 weeks, and splenomegaly, pneumonia, myocarditis and neurological sequelae may appear. Although the case fatality rate among untreated patients may be 20–45%, treatment with tetracycline or chloramphenicol[7] has reduced this rate below 5%.

Scrub typhus is endemic throughout Pacific-Rim countries of the Orient from Siberia to the Southwest Pacific islands, including the Indian subcontinent. Infections may be imported into USA by tourists who contracted infections whilst visiting endemic foci in the Orient.[3] Trombiculid mites *(Trombicula akamushi)* are vectors and wild rodents are reservoirs.

Laboratory diagnosis is established by demonstration of rising antibody titers during convalescence, using CF or immunofluorescence tests. Three serotypes of *R. tsutsugamushi* are termed Gillian, Karp, Kato. Treatment is by tetracycline or chloramphenicol.

COXIELLA BURNETII (Q FEVER)

Patients develop fever, chills, sweating and severe headache after an incubation period of 7–17 days, and symptoms may persist for 10 days. Pneumonia may affect 52% adults and 14% may develop endocarditis.[5] The case fatality rate from Q fever is negligible, but endocarditis may show 30–50% mortality rate after protracted illness.

Q fever is distributed worldwide, particularly in sheep-raising areas. Natural transmission commonly occurs through contamination of pastures by rickettsia-laden placentas and birth fluids of infected sheep. Since Q fever elementary bodies are highly resistant to drying, Q fever may be spread by inhalation of dust or grass clippings from contaminated pastures (Figure 17-1). Cattle may become infected similarly if they are grazed on the same pastures as sheep. Since Q fever organisms replicate in mammary gland tissue, milk may become infected, but pasteurization of cow's milk effectively prevents human infection by the milk-borne route. Tick vectors have been implicated in natural cycles of infection in Montana, USA where wild rodents *(Citellus sp)* are reservoirs, and in Queensland, Australia where bandicoots (rat-like marsupials) are reservoirs.

Laboratory diagnosis is established by demonstration of rising antibody titers during convalescence, using as antigen Q fever organisms in phase 2 (egg passaged) in CF or immunofluorescence tests. In cases of Q fever endocarditis, antibodies may be detected against phase 1 organisms (guinea pig passage) at higher titers than against phase 2 organisms. Treatment is by tetracycline or chloramphenicol.

SYMPTOMATOLOGY: CHLAMYDIAE

CHLAMYDIA PSITTACI

Psittacosis is characterized by fever, chills and sweating, accompanied by headache and myalgia, with photophobia, cough, conjunctivitis and epistaxis occurring less frequently. Patches of bronchopneumonic consolidation may be seen in chest x-rays of more than 50% of patients. The incubation period is 6–15 days and symptoms usually persist 4–14 days. Tetracycline or chloramphenicol are highly effective in treatment of psittacosis.[6]

Birds are natural reservoirs which become infected by inhalation of dust contaminated by chlamydia-laden feces of infected birds. Chlamydiae replicate in the tracheobronchial tree and they may be expectorated in sputum, but they also become blood-borne and undergo further replication in the spleen. Chlamydiae are excreted in high concentrations in feces of caged birds which become ill.

Psittacosis may afflict humans, either (i) in epidemics such as employees in the kill-and-pick, evisceration and packaging departments of turkey processing plants; or (ii) as sporadic cases, for example a vivarium technician or a pet shop operator who works consistently with birds especially parrots and pigeons (psittacine birds).

Laboratory diagnosis is established by demonstration of rising antibody titers by CF against the chlamydia group antigen or by microimmunofluorescence in paired sera from patients. Chlamydiae may be isolated from sputum by centrifugation on cycloheximide-treated tissue culture monolayers of McCoy cells, using immunofluorescence (not iodine staining) to detect inclusion body formation.

CHLAMYDIA TRACHOMATIS

Several clinical entities are associated with infection by a variety of serotypes.

TRACHOMA arises from infection with serotypes A, B, Ba, C. Characteristic signs are keratoconjunctivitis with follicles, papillary hyperplasia, pannus and cicatrization i.e., the conjunctiva shows vascularization and cellular infiltration extending on to the cornea which eventually may develop scar tissue, and the heavily vascularized conjunctiva of the upper eyelids causes droopiness. The follicles comprise accumulations of epithelial cells of the conjunctiva which contain basophilic cytoplasmic inclusions (Halberstaedter-Prowazek bodies) in which the chlamydial elementary bodies are enmeshed in a carbohydrate matrix which stains with iodine. Trachoma is spread by direct finger-to-eye contact or by fomites, so that infections involving entire families or clusters of children are common. Trachoma is widely prevalent throughout the Middle East, Africa and the Pacific Rim of the Orient, but pockets of infection have also been found in North and South America and Australia. Tetracycline administered both topically and orally is currently recommended for treatment,[7] which should be administered to all members of the affected family or group simultaneously. Sulfonamides administered similarly have also provided effective therapy.

INCLUSION CONJUNCTIVITIS is attributed to infections with some serotypes D through K. Mucopurulent conjunctival discharge appears within 5–14 days after birth and persists for several weeks without treatment. The newborn baby becomes infected by passing through the infected birth canal of the mother. Erythromycin induces a prompt therapeutic response, but tetracycline or sulfonamides provide adequate therapeutic alternatives.

Neonatal chlamydial infections other than conjunctivitis include radiologically-confirmed pneumonia during the first two weeks of life.

Laboratory diagnosis of trachoma and inclusion conjunctivitis is achieved by centrifugation of suspensions of conjunctival swabs or scrapings on monolayer tissue cultures of McCoy cells (continuous synovial cells) with maintenance medium containing 1 ug/ml cycloheximide. Staining by iodine or Giemsa or immunofluorescence using polyclonal or monoclonal antichlamydial antibodies will reveal chlamydial inclusions after incubation for 1–2 days at 37° C. Direct examination of conjunctival scrapings after staining by iodine or immunofluorescence may reveal chlamydial inclusions within 1–2 hours of collection, but microscopy-negative specimens should always be inoculated on McCoy cells to detect chlamydial concentrations below those revealed by direct microscopy.

NON-GONOCOCCAL URETHRITIS due to infection with some serotypes D through K induces urethral discharge and dysuria in men from whom *Neisseria gonorrhoeae* cannot be cultivated, yet regularly Gram-stained smears of urine contain more than 4 polymorphonuclear leukocytes per high power field. A group of Seattle men with non-gonococcal urethritis showed a 42% chlamydial infection rate, compared to 7% without urethritis and 19% with gonorrhea, and postgonococcal urethritis developed in 11 of 11 (100%) men infected with chlamydiae. Chlamydiae were also recovered from the endocervix of a female consort of 68% non-gonococcal urethritis men who yielded chlamydiae, but in only 8% consorts of patients without chlamydial infections, thus demonstrating sexual transmission of chlamydiae. Erythromycin or tetracycline have provided effective therapy for non-gonococcal urethritis induced by chlamydiae,[7] but also by *Ureaplasma urealyticum* which may induce concomitant infections.

Laboratory diagnosis is achieved similarly to trachoma and inclusion conjunctivitis by detection of chlamydia inclusions in McCoy cells after incubation following centrifugal inoculation of suspensions of urethral discharge or urine, using iodine staining or immunofluorescence.

LYMPHOGRANULOMA VENEREUM due to infection with serotypes L1, L2, L3 presents with inguinal lymphadenopathy (buboes), often accompanied by chills and fever in men, or disorders of the gastrointestinal tract including fistula or anogenital disease in women. The disease is prevalent in Central America, South America and Southeast Asia. It is sexually transmitted. It affects men about 20 times more commonly than women. Diagnosis is achieved serologically by complement fixation or microimmunofluorescence tests on paired sera or by isolation of chlamydiae from aspirates of buboes by inoculation of mice intracerebrally (encephalitis is induced), or development of plaques after inoculation of tissue cultures of L cells. Treatment is achieved optimally by administration of tetracycline or erythromycin.[7]

REFERENCES

[1]Bell EJ, Stoenner HG: Immunological relationships among the spotted fever group of rickettsias determined by toxin neutralization tests in mice with convalescent animal serums. J Immunol 84:171, 1960.

[2]Bergey's Manual of Systematic Bacteriology, ed. NR Krieg and JG Holt, Williams and Wilkins, Baltimore, 1984.

[3]Center for Disease Control: Imported scrub typhus - Connecticut. MMWR 23:105, 1974.

[4]Center for Disease Control: Laboratory-acquired endemic typhus - Maryland. MMWR 27:215, 1978.

[5]Center for Disease Control: Q fever - United Kingdom. MMWR 28:230, 1979.

[6]Center for Disease Control: Epidemic typhus - Georgia. MMWR 33:618, 1984.

[7]Medical Letter Handbook of Antimicrobial Therapy: The Medical Letter Inc., New Rochelle, New York, 1984.

PART III

CHAPTER 18

RESPIRATORY INFECTIONS

Virus infections of the respiratory tract are classified clinically according to the location of the greatest extent of inflammatory response within the air-containing passages (Table 18-1). For convenience, virus infections involving mainly the pleura and pericardium are grouped with respiratory infections. (Figure 18-1).

CORYZA

CLINICAL

The common cold (coryza) is a virus infection restricted to the mucous membrane of the nose and nasal turbinates. Intense watery nasal discharge (rhinorrhea) accompanied by sneezing and mild fever comprise the principal signs of infection, necessitating the use of at least 15 disposable tissue handkerchiefs (Kleenex® or similar) per day. The causative agent is one of more than 110 numbered serotypes of Rhinovirus.[1,18]

The incubation period of coryza due to rhinovirus infection is 1 day. Symptoms persist usually 2–3 days. Rhinovirus infections are communicable for 2–3 days after onset of sneezing. Although rhinovirus infections are transmitted by inhalation of infected droplets, they are also transmitted efficiently by contamination of hands with virus-laden nasal secretions.[17]

LABORATORY DIAGNOSIS

Laboratory diagnosis of rhinovirus infections is usually undertaken only during epidemiological investigations. Nasal secretions or throat garglings are collected in 5–10ml saline or tissue culture maintenance medium containing 10% fetal bovine serum, centrifuged for 10 minutes at 2000xg to deposit bacteria and cell debris, and 0.5ml portions of supernatant are diluted 1:10 by addition to 4.5ml maintenance medium containing 10% fetal bovine serum. A pair of drained tissue culture plates or tubes containing monolayers of primary monkey kidney (rhesus or cynomolgus) cells and another pair of diploid human fibroblasts (prepared locally from human foreskins or derived from MRC-5 or WI-38 diploid human cell lines) are each inoculated with

TABLE 18-1
TIME CHARACTERISTICS OF VIRAL RESPIRATORY INFECTIONS

Syndrome	Virus species (family)	Incu-bation period	duration of		Virus identification			Antibodies (paired sera) (paired sera)		
			comm.	illness	same day EM	IF	virus isolation	test	initial detection	persis-tence
Coryza (common cold)	Rhinovirus 1-111 (Picornaviridae)	1–2d	0 to +3d	2–3d	n/a	n/a	MK33° C DH	NT (type)	2w	3 mo
Pharyngo-conjunctival fever	Adenovirus, 3, 4, 7. (Adenoviridae)	5–8d	0 to +3d	4–5d	+	+	PH DH	HI (type) CF (group)	2w 2–3w	1+ yr 6 mo
Influenza	Influenza A, B (Orthomyxoviridae)	1–2d	0 to +4d	3–7d	+	+	MK33, 37° C DH	HI (curr) S-CF	7–10d 1w	2+ yr 6 mo
Croup, tracheo-bronchitis	Parainfluenza 1,3 (Paramyxoviridae)	1–3d	0 to +3d	2–3d	+	+	MK33, 37° C DH	HI (type)	1–2w	5+ yr
Bronchiolitis broncho-pneumonia	RS (Paramyxoviridae)	1–3d	0 to +3d	2–7d	+	+	PH DH	NT CF	1–2w 2–3w	5+ yr 1 yr
Pleurodynia, pericarditis	Coxsackie B1-B6 (Picornaviridae)	4–8d	0 to +4d	3–7d	n/a	n/a	MK37° C	NT	4–7d	10 yr

Day 0:	day of onset of illness	DH:	continuous diploid human fibroblasts	NT: neutralization
comm:	communicability	MK:	primary monkey kidney cultures	curr: current year's serotype
+4:	four days after onset	PH:	continuous polyploid human cells	group: serogroup
EM:	electron microscopy (negative stain technique)	CF:	complement fixation	type: serotype
IF:	indirect immunofluorescence	S-CF:	soluble antigen in CF test	
n/a:	not applicable	HI:	hemagglutination inhibition	

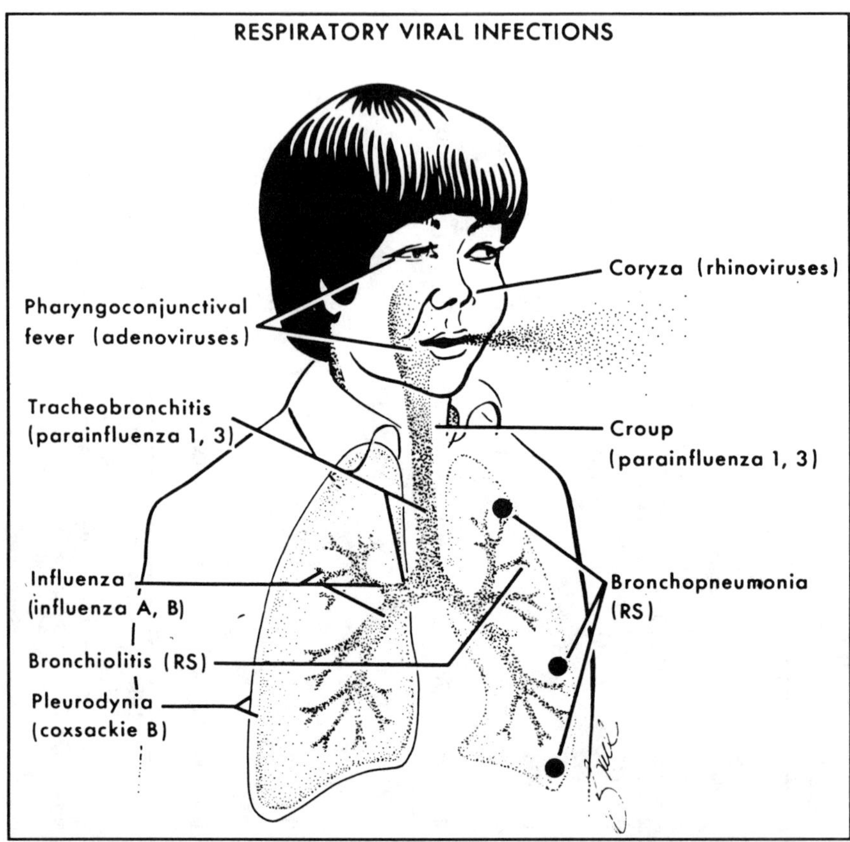

Figure 18-1: Sites of virus proliferation which induce symptoms of acute respiratory infection.

1.0ml aliquots of the diluted supernatant, and incubated in 5% CO_2 for 7–10 days at 33° C. Polyploid human cells (HeLa, HEp-2) may be used as well as diploid cells. Cytopathic effects comprising shrinkage of cells followed by pyknosis are observed after 3 or more days of incubation; these indicate the isolation of a rhinovirus. Serotyping of the fresh isolate is achieved by neutralization tests in tissue culture using appropriate typing antisera. On account of the brief duration and mildness of symptoms of the common cold, serological investigation of individual cases is not clinically indicated, but in epidemiological surveys for the prevalence of a particular serotype, antibodies are measured by neutralization tests in tissue culture.

EPIDEMIOLOGY

Common colds are transmitted naturally either by: (i) inhalation of virus-laden droplets within a radius of 2 meters of an infected subject who expels virus by sneezing or coughing; (ii) contact of nose or mouth with hands contaminated by infected nasal or oropharyngeal secretions of an infected person. Recent epidemiological investigations[17] have emphasized the importance of spread of coryza by hands. Colds spread more frequently during the cooler months of autumn and winter than during the warm summer months, probably due to greater crowding in meeting rooms or public transit where exchange of air is reduced during cool weather. Several rhinovirus serotypes may circulate simultaneously; since there is no cross-immunity between different serotypes, more than one rhinovirus infection may affect a subject during the winter season. When no outside visitors arrive into a closed community, such as an Antarctic research station during 6 months of winter isolation, virtually no respiratory virus infections afflict the staff.[31] However both rhinovirus and parainfluenza virus infections are associated with a high incidence of respiratory tract illness shortly after the arrival of new personnel during spring. Thus a continuous re-introduction of rhinoviruses is required in order to maintain high prevalence of respiratory illness.

PHARYNGOCONJUNCTIVAL FEVER

CLINICAL

Pharyngoconjunctival fever is an infection involving the pharynx and the conjunctiva, induced by one of several serotypes of adenovirus. Symptoms include acute redness and injection of the conjunctivae with gritty sensation in the eyes, together with an acutely reddened and sore pharynx, cough and nasal discharge, and patients are usually febrile.

The incubation period is 5 to 8 days. Symptoms usually persist no longer than 4–5 days. Adenovirus infections are communicable by droplets or expectoration or in tears for about 3 days after onset.

LABORATORY DIAGNOSIS

Laboratory diagnosis of adenovirus infections causing pharyngoconjunctival fever is established by inoculation of nasopharyngeal secretions or throat garglings or conjunctival swabs into primary and continuous tissue culture monolayers as described above for rhinoviruses.[25] After incubation for 4–7 days, cytopathic effects comprising shrinkage of cells which develop intranuclear inclusions, accompanied by pronounced acidity of the supernatant fluid, are observed mainly in continuous diploid or polyploid cells. Tissue culture supernatant fluid is removed, and typed in polyploid cell cultures by neutralization tests. This procedure is serotype-specific. However the tissue culture supernatant fluid may be used as antigen in a complement fixation test using antiserum to any adenovirus serotype, which confirms that the new isolate is within the adenovirus group.

EPIDEMIOLOGY

Adenovirus types 3, 4, 7 are commonly encountered in pharyngoconjunctival fever. Swimming pools provide a particularly effective means of transmission amongst bathers, especially during summers.[2,5,10] Adenoviruses spread particularly effectively among populations of military recruits during winter[19,36] most likely by the airborne route, inducing acute respiratory disease usually without conjunctivitis. Adenoviruses are also transmitted readily by fomites such as a common roller towel in a washroom during winter[16] where type 8 or type 19 viruses induced keratoconjunctivitis, or face cloths used to mop sweaty brows at a refugee camp during summer where the disease induced by adenovirus 8 was keratoconjunctivitis.[37] Among 18,000 Washington D.C. children[3] who were surveyed between 1957 and 1967 for viral respiratory illnesses, the peak 15.7% rate of adenovirus infection occurred in May. The peak 10.6% monthly rate of adenovirus-associated illnesses was noted during July among inpatients, but in outpatients both the peak virus isolation rate of 19.7% and the peak 9.7% rate of adenovirus-associated illnesses occurred during the spring month of April.

Other syndromes attributed to adenovirus infection include pertussis-like illness among children,[35] particularly during the warmer months; cystitis associated with adenovirus-11 where patients developed dysuria, frequency and hematuria;[29] a rash clinically resembling rubella due to adenovirus types 4 and 7;[15] meningo-encephalitis due to types 6, 7A and 12;[20] gastroenteritis due to non-cultivatable enteric adenoviruses affects about 6% of all children with acute gastroenteritis in Vancouver[26] and other Temperature Zone communities; gastroenteritis due to adenovirus-3 has affected an entire family.[12] Occasionally, fatal cases of pneumonia with necrotizing patchy alveolar fibropurulent exudate plus necrotizing bronchiolitis due to adenovirus types 3 and 7[4,30] have affected native children during winter.

PREVENTION BY VACCINE

Epidemics of acute respiratory disease due to adenovirus types 4 and 7 among military recruits have been effectively controlled through the administration by mouth of enteric coated capsules containing living vaccine strains of adenovirus-4 and adenovirus-7.[11]

INFLUENZA

CLINICAL

Influenza is an infection involving the mucous membranes of the nose pharynx, trachea, bronchi and bronchioles, which is induced by serotypes of influenza virus within two principal species termed type A and type B. Symptoms include high fever, glazed reddened mucous membranes of the nose and pharynx, dry cough, severe generalized malaise and aches and pains throughout the musculature of the back and limbs (myalgia). Although fever and myalgia usually abate after 2–3 days, malaise accompanied by cough may persist for one week longer. Secondary bacterial infection frequently follows 2 or 3 days after onset of influenza, inducing bronchitis with increased cough, copious sputum and coarse rhonchi through the lung fields. Bronchopneumonia may complicate influenza, both in infants and particularly in elderly patients. They exhibit severe constitutional upsets accompanied by rales and crepitations throughout the lung fields plus radiological evidence of patches of pulmonary consolidation, and death may occur despite administration of antibiotics.

The incubation period of influenza is 1–2 days. Influenza is communicable by droplets expelled by coughing or sneezing for 3–4 days after onset.

LABORATORY DIAGNOSIS

Laboratory diagnosis of influenza is conducted effectively in clinical settings by a combination of the same-day procedures of electron microscopy and immunofluorescence.[26] Nasopharyngeal secretions collected by suction are preferred as specimens from children under 5 years of age (Figure 18-2); throat garglings in water are preferred to throat swabs from older children and adults.

SPECIMENS

Throat garglings, or suspensions in 1 ml water of nasopharyngeal suctions or throat swabs, are mixed promptly with equal quantities of transport medium (tissue culture maintenance medium containing 10% inactivated fetal bovine serum or 0.75% bovalbumin fraction V). If feasible, drops of the aqueous suspension should be applied to electron microscope grids at the patient's bedside; otherwise the transport medium should be added immediately to the specimen before its transmittal to the laboratory. Upon arrival in the virus laboratory, the specimen is centrifuged for 10 minutes at 2000xg in order to deposit epithelial cells and bacteria. The supernatant is pipetted off for attempts at virus isolation; smears of the deposit are placed in each of 12 wells of teflon-coated slides for immunofluorescence testing.

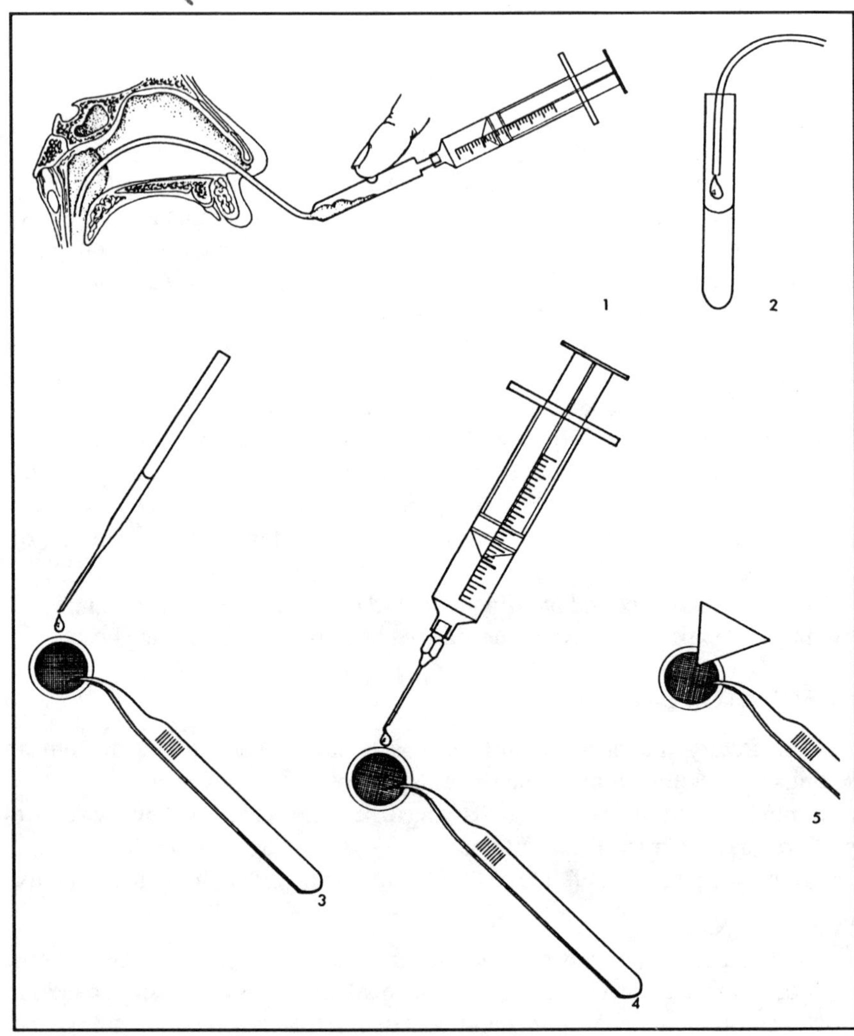

Figure 18-2: Collection of nasopharyngeal secretions by Auger suction. Preparation of grid for electron microscopic examination.

1. Pass catheter through nose into nasopharynx, aspirate secretions.
2. Place secretions into sterile saline.
   If patient is able to cooperate, gargle 10 ml sterile saline and expectorate garglings into sterile container.
3. Place drop of saline suspension on EM grid.
4. Add drop of phosphotungstic acid.

Reproduced with permission from McLean DM and Wong KK, 1984. Same-day Diagnosis of Human Virus Infections. CRC Press, Boca Raton, FL, p. 9.

ELECTRON MICROSCOPY

Drops of garglings, or nasopharyngeal secretions dispersed in 1 ml water, are applied to formvar coated 300-mesh electron microscope grids, air dried, then drops of 2% phosphotungstic acid pH 6.2–6.5 are applied for 30 sec, excess fluid is removed by blotting with filter paper and the grid is allowed to dry in air for 5 minutes. Grids are examined in an electron microscope, scanning initially at 2000x magnification, but proceeding by steps up to 200,000x magnification. Virus particles appear as lighter objects against a darkly stained background. Influenza virions are enveloped with total diameters 80–120nm and they show spikes of hemagglutinin and of neuraminidase 12–15nm protruding outward from a helical nucleocapsid containing strands 9nm diameter which exhibit a typical herringbone appearance due to cross striations each 4nm (Figure 18-3).

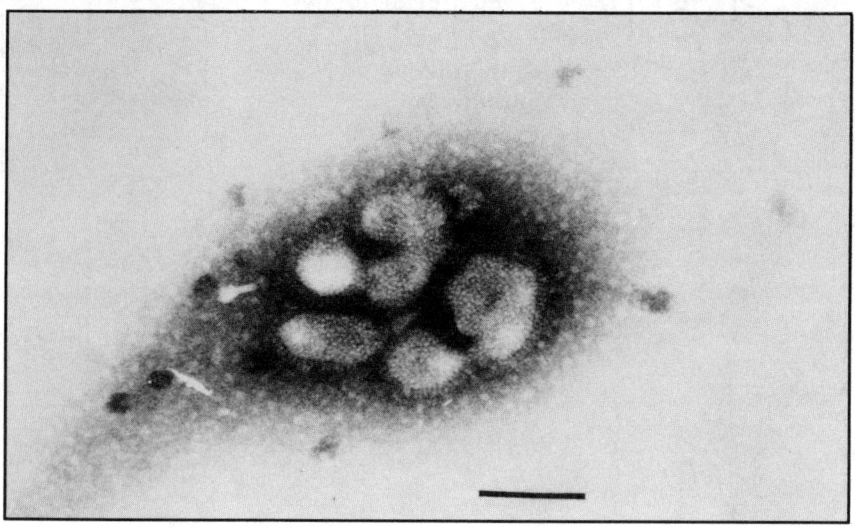

Figure 18-3: Influenza virus particles in nasopharyngeal secretions of a boy aged 4 months with influenza (X 157,420). Reproduced with permission from McLean DM and Wong KK, 1984. Same-day Diagnosis of Human Virus Infections. CRC Press, Boca Raton, FL, 57.

IMMUNOFLUORESCENCE

Slides for immunofluorescence are dried on a warming plate at 40° C, then fixed in chilled acetone for 10 minutes. The indirect immunofluorescence procedure is conducted as follows (Figure 18-4). Place drops of antiserum, prepared in rabbits against serotypes of influenza A (H3N2) and (H1N1) and influenza B, at 1:10 dilution in phosphate-buffered saline (PBS)

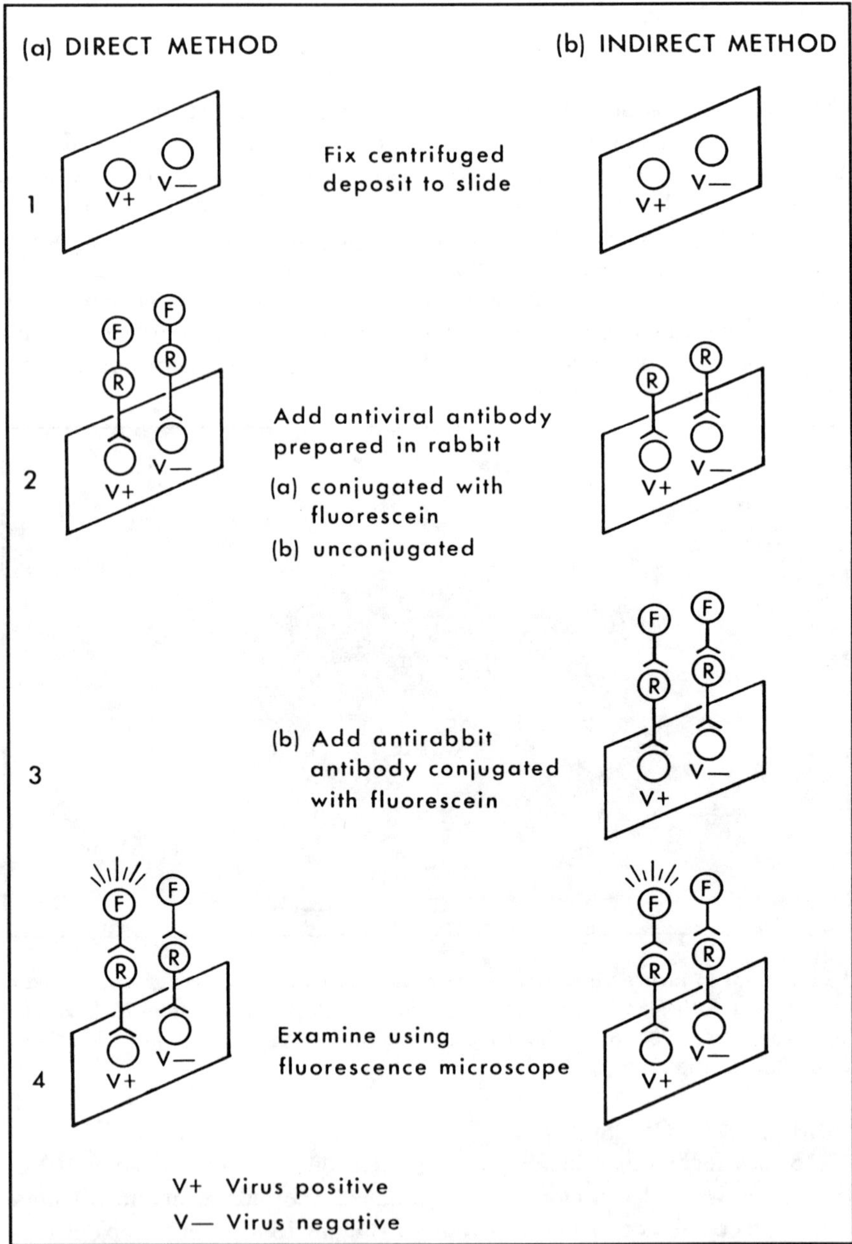

Figure 18-4: Immunofluorescence for detection of virus in throat secretions. Reproduced with permission from McLean DM, 1980. Virology in Health Care, Williams and Wilkins, Baltimore, p. 38.

pH 7.0 on pairs of wells, then incubate in a humidified chamber or incubator for 30 minutes at 37° C, wash 3 times with PBS. Add drops of fluorescein-labelled antiserum prepared in goats (usually) against rabbit immunoglobulin diluted 1:20 and incubate a further 30 minutes, wash with PBS, counterstain for 1/2 minute with 0.1% naphthalene black in PBS and wash thoroughly in PBS for 5 minutes. Examine each well using incident ultraviolet light in a microscope fitted with a dichroic prism and a x 50 water-immersion microscope objective. Bright apple-green fluorescent dots throughout the cytoplasm of cells treated with H3N2 antiserum, but not in wells treated with other antisera, denotes that the patient was infected with influenza A (H3N2) virus. This procedure is completed within 2–3 hours. Combination of electron microscopy with immunofluorescence therefore provides both a presumptive and a serotypic identification of influenza virus infection on the same working day of collection of the specimen.

VIRUS ISOLATION

Supernatant fluids from throat specimens are diluted 1:10 in tissue culture maintenance medium and inoculated on monolayer tissue cultures of primary monkey kidney and continuous diploid human fibroblasts. Duplicate cultures are incubated at 33° C and 37° C as long as 1 week. After 3 days, and again at 7 days, tissue culture fluid is pipetted aseptically into sterile tubes, and a 0.1% sterile suspension of guinea pig erythrocytes is placed in each tissue culture well or tube. Each culture is examined using an inverted microscope for evidence of hemadsorption. Supernatant fluids from culture showing hemadsorption are titrated in hemagglutination tests using 0.5% suspensions of guinea pig and goose erythrocytes. Serotyping of these fresh isolates is performed in hemagglutination inhibition tests using 4 agglutination doses and antisera pretreated with heat and periodate against the current serotypes of influenza A (H3N2) and (H1N1) and influenza B. Virus isolation usually requires 3 days incubation, commonly at 33° C, but incubation for 7 days may be required for some strains. Serotyping is a same-day procedure. Virus isolation provides the best evidence that a patient was actually infected by a particular influenza virus serotype.

SEROLOGIC TESTS

Hemagglutination inhibition is the best test for detection of influenza virus infection by serological techniques. In common with all serological procedures it suffers the drawbacks that two serum specimens are required; the first specimen (acute phase) is collected shortly after onset of illness and the second specimen (convalescent phase) is collected 1–3 weeks after defervescence. Antibodies are first detected by HI about 7–10 days after onset and they persist for several years. Detection of fourfold or greater increases of HI titer against a current influenza serotype indicates a recent infection with that agent. Complement fixation tests using the soluble or nucleocapsid (S-CF) antigen may reveal rising antibody titers within one week after onset of illness, but results merely indicate that the infection was due to influenza type A or type B.

EPIDEMIOLOGY

Influenza epidemics typically involve substantial members of the population of many communities almost simultaneously during a 4–6 week period of winter. Influenza may affect Temperate Zone communities within the Northern Hemisphere between November and March, and in the Southern Hemisphere between May and August, but the influenza "season" is less distinct in the Tropics. Influenza A may reach epidemic proportions about 2 years in 3, particularly in the United States between 1968 and 1977,[6] whilst substantial clusters of influenza B infections occur about 1 year in 4. Influenza A and influenza B may each cause peaks of epidemic prevalence during a particular winter.[27]

Quantitative manifestations of influenza epidemics[33] include: (i) more than twice the usual daily number of visits to family physicians or emergency departments of downtown hospitals with acute respiratory illnesses; (ii) daily school absentee rates more than 2 standard deviations above the average daily expected rate for the period, rates often increase beyond 15%; (iii) weekly reportings of deaths attributed to pneumonia and influenza above the expected average rate for the period, which in mid-winter is 4.5% in the United States[8] (Figure 18-5). Threshold was adjusted to 6.5% for winter 1989–90.

Excess mortality rates due to pneumonia and influenza provide the best documentary evidence of influenza epidemics. Deaths principally affect elderly persons above 60 years of age and infants aged less than 1 year, when rapidly progressing pneumonia complicates the influenza virus infection, but deaths may sometimes occur in young persons aged 20–40 years through a fulminant course of influenza virus infection alone. Chronic bronchitis with or without emphysema in elderly patients, or chronic cardiopulmonary disease in children resulting from cystic fibrosis, bronchiectasis or congenital heart disorders, comprise important predisposing factors to development of pneumonia causing death following influenza virus infection.

Influenza A virus of a particular serotype spreads extensively throughout the world for 1–3 seasons, until it is superseded by a different serotype which rapidly becomes dominant. Since the first isolation of influenza A virus from a human in 1933, there have been two major *antigenic shifts* in the characteristics of the hemagglutinin (H), from H1 to H2 in 1957 and H2 to H3 in 1968. During 1957, the neuraminidase (N) antigen also shifted from N1 to N2 (Table 18-2). Antigenic shift from, for example H2 to H3, operates thus:

antibodies induced by infection with H3 strains inhibit hemagglutination by both H3 and H2 strains, but antibodies to H2 strains inhibit hemagglutination by H2 strains only, not H3 strains. Within a particular antigenic category e.g., H3, successive minor *antigenic drifts* within the hemagglutinin have been noted after every one or two influenza seasons. Antibody to the most recent strain, e.g., A/Philippines/2/82(H3N2) inhibits hemagglutination by strains from all previous years, but antibody to earlier strains such as A/Texas/1/77(H3N2) inhibits hemagglutination by the 1982 isolate at titers substantially lower than the 1977 strains. Apart from one antigenic shift of neuraminidase from N1 to N2 in 1957, virtually no antigenic drift has been found with N2 isolates from succeeding years. Only one antigenic shift of hemagglutinin within the influenza type B was recorded in 1954, and an antigenic drift from B/Singapore/222/79 occurred in 1983 to B/USSR/100/83.

An attack of influenza confers immunity for at least 2 years against further infections with the virus of the same antigenic constitution. Attack rates exceeding 30% are common in communities, following which a high proportion of the population within a community acquires antibodies which inhibit growth of virus, thus halting further epidemic spread of the particular serotype. However, mutations of antigenic composition of influenza viruses occur intermittently, so that a new mutant will survive in the presence of antibodies to pre-existing strains and thus supersede them as the serotype causing a fresh epidemic.

The doctrine of "original antigenic sin"[13] is frequently encountered during serological investigations of influenza prevalence. Antibody response to the first serotype which infected the patient during childhood occurs regularly at higher titers than antibodies against more recent serotypes which caused infections during subsequent years.

PREVENTION BY VACCINE

Preventive measures against clinical attacks of influenza have been implemented for many years through the subcutaneous administration of influenza vaccine containing killed preparations of the most recent serotypes of influenza A and influenza B. Since two antigenic categories of influenza A, H3N2 and H1N1, have circulated simultaneously in many communities since 1978, in addition to type B strains, current vaccines are trivalent, e.g., the formulation for the 1984–84 influenza "season" contained 15 micrograms of hemagglutinin for each of the most recently emerged serotypes: A/Philippines/2/82 (H3N2), A/Chile/1/83 (H1N1) and B/USSR/100/83.[7]

Influenza vaccines which are marketed currently comprise: (a) *whole* virus vaccines in which the influenza virus infectivity has been inactivated

TABLE 18-2
ANTIGENIC DRIFT AND SHIFT OF INFLUENZA A VIRUS INFECTING HUMANS FROM 1931 TO 1985[a,b]

H subtype	Reference strains	Year of prevalence	N subtype	Reference strain	Year of prevalence
H1	A/Swine/1976/31(H1N1)	1931–1978	N1	A/PR/8/34(H1N1)	1933–1946
	A/WS/1/33(H1N1)	1933–1946		A/FM/1/47(H1N1)	1947–1957
	A/PR/8/34(H1N1)			A/Chile/1/83(H1N1)	1977–1985
	A/FM/1/47(H1N1)	1947–1957			
	A/FW/1/50(H1N1)				
	A/USSR/90/77(H1N1)	1977–1985			
	A/Brazil/11/78(H1N1)				1967
	A/Chile/1/83(H1N1)				
H2	A/Singapore/1/57(H2N2)	1957–1967	N2	A/Singapore/1/57(H2N2)	1957–1967
	A/England/12/64(H2N2)				
	A/Tokyo/3/67(H2N2)				
H3	A/Hong Kong/1/68(H3N2)	1968–1985		A/Philippines/2/82(H3N2)	1968–1985
	A/England/42/72(H3N2)				
	A/Port Chalmers/1/73(H3N2)				
	A/Victoria/3/75(H3N2)				
	A/Texas/1/77(H3N2)				
	A/Bangkok/1/79(H3N2)				
	A/Philippines/2/82(H3N2)				

Adapted from: a Bulletin of the World Health Organization 1971, 45:119-124.
 b Morbidity and Mortality Weekly Report 1980, 29:514-515.

TABLE 18-3
VIRUS ISOLATION RATES FROM PATIENTS WITH CROUP

	Toronto[a,b]		Newcastle[c]	Washington[d]	Melbourne[e]	Seattle[f]	Chapel Hill[g]
	Percentage virus isolations from patients						
Serotype	1960–63	1964–67	1969–70	1957–61	1981–82	1966–71	1966–75
Parainfluenza-1	30.3	43.9	19.1	20.0	12.7	12.9	67.3*
Parainfluenza-2	0.5	–	10.6	4.4	18.2	1.4	*
Parainfluenza-3	3.5	5.5	5.3	4.4	6.3	2.9	*
Influenza A	0.4	0.3	3.2	–	0.9	1.0	4.6
Influenza B	1.1	1.3	–	–	0.9	1.0	2.8
Respiratory syncytial	–	–	10.6	–	7.3	1.0	9.6
Other viruses	–	–	6.4	–	0.9	7.2	5.5
Total positive %	35.9	51.0	55.3	28.6	47.2	29.8	35.4
Total cases tested	794	380	94	206	110	210	793

* Represents 189 strains of parainfluenza types 1, 2 and 3; proportions of each were not stated.

a McLean et al. Can Med Ass J 89:1257, 1963.

b McLean et al. Can Med Ass J 96:1449, 1967.

c Gardner et al. Brit Med J 2:7, 1971.

d Parrott et al. Am J Pub Health 52:907, 1962.

e Fairfield Hospital, Melbourne, Australia, Annual Report, 1982.

f Foy et al. Am J Epidemiol 97:80, 1973.

g Chapman et al. Am J Epidemiol 114:768, 1981.

by formalin, but the virus particles are morphologically intact; (b) *split product* vaccines in which the outer coat of influenza virion is disrupted by ether to yield a preparation containing hemagglutinin. Adverse reactions (reactogenicity) to influenza vaccine are usually minimal after administration of the split product, but adverse reactions to the whole virus are usually negligible following vaccine purification by rate zonal centrifugation. Adverse reactions may comprise pain, redness and swelling at the site of injection, together with fever and malaise appearing 1–2 days after injection. Split product vaccine is usually advocated for administration to children aged less than 5 years who also may require two doses one month apart.

Influenza vaccines should be administered to susceptible recipients within 2 weeks to 3 months before an outbreak of influenza e.g., during October immediately preceding the North American influenza "season" November through March. In most recipients HI antibody titers increase within 2–4 weeks after one dose of vaccine, particularly in those with pre-existing antibodies following past influenza virus infections or vaccine injections, but in elderly subjects the antibody response may be delayed. In several epidemics, the overall protective efficacy of influenza vaccine was about 50–60%.[27,28] Vaccine-induced antibodies usually decline to minimal titers after 6–12 months, so that subjects require fresh doses of vaccine immediately before each influenza "season" in order to achieve protective antibody levels.

ANTIVIRALS

Oral administration of Amantadine 200 mg once daily for 10 days during an influenza A (H2N2) epidemic in 1964 has reduced the clinical attack rate by 73% as compared with untreated controls.[34] However it is ineffective against influenza B. This approach to influenza prophylaxis is unsuitable in most clinical settings[7] due to inability to maintain amantadine dosage throughout the 6 weeks of the influenza season, together with some intolerance of amantadine by some patients. Recently, significantly shorter duration of fever and systemic illness due to influenza A (H1N1) was observed following inhalation for 1 day or more of aerosols containing Ribavirin as compared with untreated controls.[21] Somewhat higher mean HI antibody titers were found in treated subjects than in controls.

CROUP AND TRACHEOBRONCHITIS

CLINICAL

Croup is an infection involving the mucous membranes of the vocal cords, trachea and bronchi, characterized by croupy cough, loud inspiratory stridor, diminished air entry into the lungs and indrawing of the chest wall around the rib cage, sternum and supraclavicular areas. About 80% of patients exhibit a cough and runny nose 1–3 days before onset of croup. Patients are usually afebrile. Chest x-ray examination may reveal diminished inflation of the lungs. Occasionally the epiglottis is grossly swollen and reddened (epiglottitis), but more commonly this arises from infection with *Haemophilus influenza* type b than virus infection.

Parainfluenza 1 virus is the commonest cause of croup (Table 18-3), but other paramyxoviridae such as parainfluenza types 2 and 3 and respiratory syncytial (RS) viruses may induce croup, and occasionally influenza A or B, measles or chickenpox viruses may cause croup.

Tracheobronchitis in children who present clinically with deep cough and rhonchi but without croupy cough or inspiratory stridor may also be caused by infection with parainfluenza viruses type 1 and 3.

The incubation period of these two conditions is about 1–3 days, but it is often difficult to determine this time exactly due to the variable duration of the runny nose before onset of croup. Patients with croup and respiratory distress (rapid pulse, indrawing) are nursed in plastic tends supplied with cooled humidified oxygen ("croupettes") and they are given a sedative to allay restlessness. Usually within 1–2 days, respiratory distress has abated, indrawing has ceased and the croupy cough has diminished greatly. Croup due to parainfluenza viruses is communicable by droplets expelled by coughing or sneezing for 2–3 days after onset.

LABORATORY DIAGNOSIS

Laboratory diagnosis of parainfluenza virus infections is achieved on the same day of collection of nasopharyngeal secretions from patients by the Auger suction technique (Figure 18-2), using a combination of electron microscopic and immunofluorescence techniques identical with those described for influenza virus (page 241). Attempts should always be made to isolate parainfluenza viruses by inoculation of centrifugally clarified nasopharyngeal suspensions into primary tissue cultures of monkey kidney cells; hemadsorption is observed in virus-positive specimens after incubation for 3–7 days at 37° C and the fresh virus isolate is serotyped by HI, as for influenza virus.

Although HI antibodies to parainfluenza viruses may develop in older children after one virus infection, antibody response in infants may not occur until the patient has sustained several infections with the same serotype. Antibody determinations are not usually helpful in diagnosis.

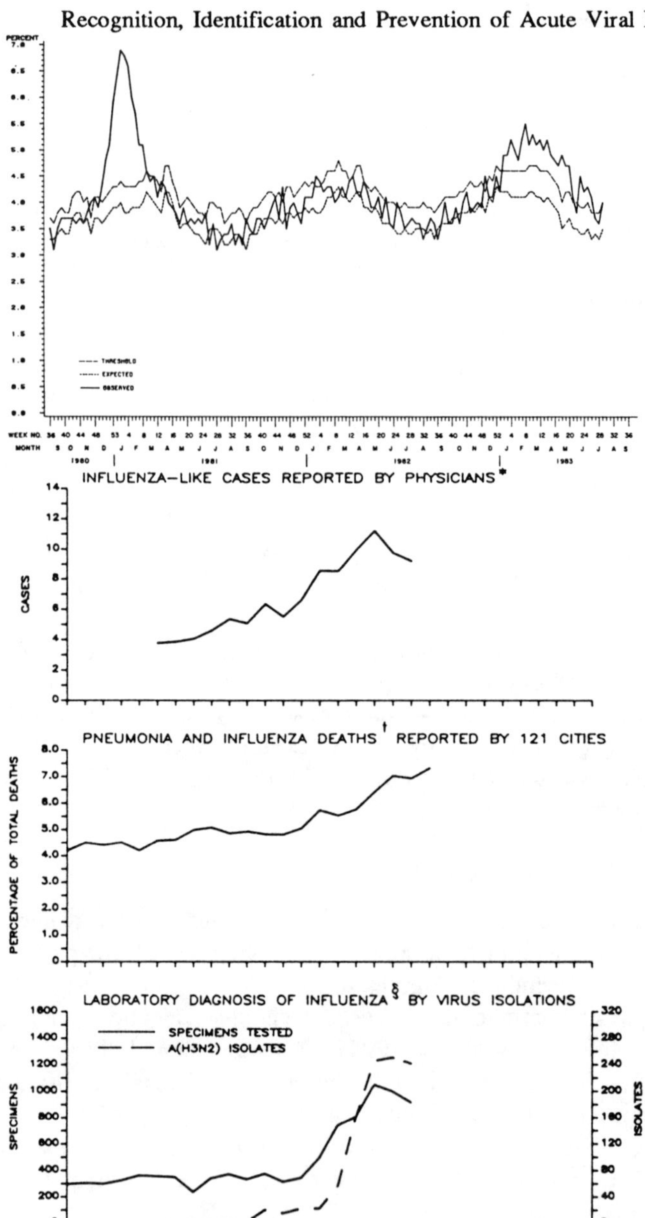

Figure 18-5: Observed and expected ratio of deaths attributed to pneumonia and influenza in 121 cities - United States: (a) 1980–1983 (MMWR 32:377, 1983); (b) 1984–85 (MMWR 34:115, 1985). Reproduced with permission from Centers for Disease Control.

EPIDEMIOLOGY

Croup due principally to parainfluenza virus infection occurs commonly during the cooler months of each year in most temperate zone communities, usually between October and March in North America, and virus isolation rates are highest during this period. For example in Toronto, Canada when parainfluenza 1 virus was isolated from 30.3% and parainfluenza 3 from 3.5% of 794 children who were hospitalized with croup between November 1960 and March 1963, the peak monthly incidence rate of 72% for isolation for parainfluenza 1 virus was achieved during November 1962[22] (Table 18-3). During winters 1965–65 and 1966–67, 43.9% of 380 patients were infected with parainfluenza 1 and 5.5% with parainfluenza 3 virus, with a peak virus isolation rate of 60% for parainfluenza 1 during January 1967.[24] Influenza A and influenza B viruses were isolated infrequently from croupy patients, despite their epidemic prevalence during successive winters when they caused numerous cases of clinically typical influenza among adults. Similarly in 5 other centers in North America, England and Australia, parainfluenza viruses, especially type 1 were commonly isolated from croupy children, but RS and influenza viruses were isolated less frequently.

Croup attacks children aged less than 3 years more frequently than older children or adults. For example in Toronto between November 1962 and March 1963 when parainfluenza viruses were isolated from 41% of 224 croupy children, virus excreters comprised 46% of 166 aged less than 3 years and 33% of 58 older children.[22]

BRONCHIOLITIS AND BRONCHOPNEUMONIA

CLINICAL

Bronchiolitis is a catarrhal inflammation of the bronchioles, caused typically by infection with RS virus. Symptoms include excessive production of mucous secretions accompanied by wheezing, increased coughing and difficulty with respirations resulting in rib-cage retraction plus a barrel-shaped chest indicating obstruction to the outflow of air. A runny nose and cough usually appear 1–2 days before the copious secretions and wheeze. Fever is minimal. Radiological examination reveals over-inflated lungs. Patients require nursing in croupettes, with frequent nasopharyngeal suction to remove the mucous secretions; bronchoscopic suction may be required to provide an adequate airway. Symptoms usually abate after 2–3 days.

The incubation period is about 1–3 days, but due to the runny nose which occurs early in the course of illness, it is difficult to determine the time of onset of symptoms of bronchiolitis. Patients may transmit virus in droplets expelled during the initial 3 days after onset.

Bronchopneumonia is recognized principally by auscultation of rales over portions of both lung fields, together with severe cough, difficulty with respiration, and fever. Patchy consolidation is detected throughout the lung fields on radiological examination. Clinical improvement usually occurs within 4–7 days. Although RS virus alone may induce bronchopneumonia, often there is overgrowth of resident bacterial flora such as *Haemophilus influenzae* which may aggravate the illness, and antibiotics such as Ampicillin are frequently prescribed as adjunct therapy.

Acute upper respiratory illness comprising cough, increased nasopharyngeal secretions, runny nose, mild fever, irritability and crankiness, but without wheeze or respiratory distress may be induced in young children by RS virus, but these symptoms are indistinguishable from those associated with other virus infections. On the contrary, RS virus has occasionally been implicated as the cause of death in infants with bronchiolitis and bronchopneumonia.[14] In Great Britain, RS virus has comprised the major cause for hospitalization of infants and children with acute respiratory infections.[9]

LABORATORY DIAGNOSIS

Laboratory diagnosis is performed effectively using the same-day procedures of electron microscopy in combination with immunofluorescence on nasopharyngeal suctions or throat swabs, comparable to influenza virus (page 241). Detection of enveloped virions about 200 nm or greater diameter with helical nucleocapsids 18 nm diameter by electron microscopy provides presumptive evidence of RS virus (Figure 18-6), and serotyping as RS virus by indirect immunofluorescence is accomplished within 2–3 hours. Isolation of RS virus is achieved by inoculation of continuous diploid and polyploid human tissue cultures, when syncytia formation is observed after 3–7 days incubation at 37° C. Serotypic identification of the new isolate as RS virus is achieved by complement fixation or neutralization tests.

EPIDEMIOLOGY

Respiratory syncytial virus is clearly the dominant paramyxovirus serotype isolated from children with bronchiolitis and bronchopneumonia in three North American centers and Newcastle-upon-Tyne, England (Table 18-4). Typically bronchiolitis occurs in short sharp peaks towards the end of winter and it is largely confined to children aged less than 2 years. However RS virus has been isolated from several elderly patients within small clusters who developed influenza - like illness during winter of 1976 and 1980.[32]

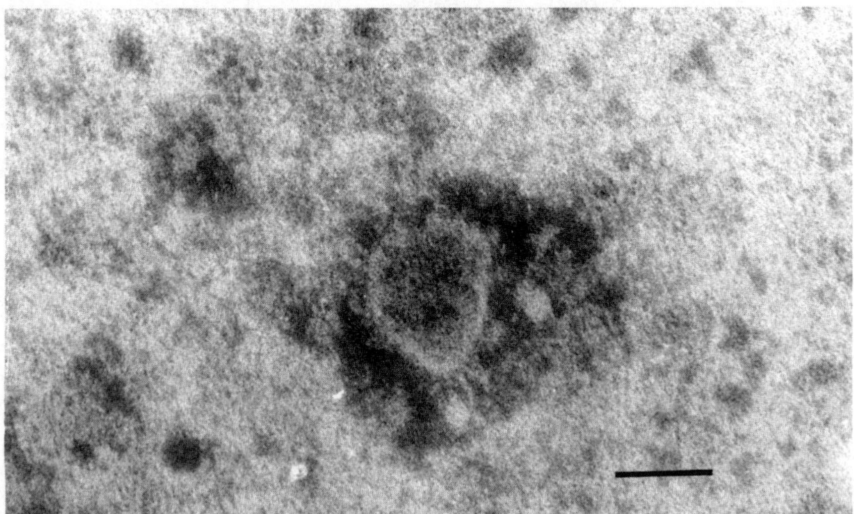

Figure 18-6: Respiratory syncytial virion in nasopharyngeal secretions from a boy aged 5 months with bronchiolitis (X150,150). Reproduced with permission from McLean DM and Wong KK, 1984. Same-day Diagnosis of Human Virus Infections. CRC Press, Boca Raton, FL, p. 82.

PLEURODYNIA AND PERICARDITIS

CLINICAL

Although pleurodynia and pericarditis arise from viral infections of the serous membranes surrounding the lungs and the heart respectively, and therefore they are not strictly infections of the respiratory tract, for convenience they are considered along with respiratory infections. They are caused by any of the 6 serotypes of group B coxsackievirus.

Pleurodynia is manifested by the sudden onset of sharp pains on one side of the chest which are aggravated by deep breathing or coughing. A pleural friction rub is heard over the painful site, accompanied by mild fever. Usually there is no effusion. Additionally patients may develop sharp severe pains in skeletal muscles of the trunk and limbs (myositis). Usually the painful respirations, friction rub and fever disappear after 2–4 days, but recurrences may sometimes affect the same or different location in the chest during the succeeding week.

Pericarditis is characterized by severe pain over the heart accompanied by a pericardial friction rub and moderate fever. Although pericardial effusions

TABLE 18-4
PARAINFLUENZA VIRUS ISOLATES FROM CHILDREN WITH ACUTE LOWER RESPIRATORY INFECTIONS

Serotype	Location		Percentage virus isolation in each clinical category		
		Croup	Tracheobronchitis	Bronchiolitis	Pneumonia
Parainfluenza-1	Newcastle 1969–70[a]	19.1	1.5	2.1	1.1
	Washington 1957–61[b]	20.0	1.0	1.0	0.6
	Seattle 1966–71[c]	12.9	–	2.6	0.2
	Chapel Hill 1966–75[d]	23.8*	5.9	5.5	20.0
Parainfluenza-2	Newcastle	10.6	0	0	0
	Washington	4.4	0.4	0.3	0.1
	Seattle	1.4	–	1.3	0
	Chapel Hill	*	*	*	*
Parainfluenza-3	Newcastle	5.3	2.7	6.4	3.2
	Washington	4.4	2.0	4.0	1.6
	Seattle	1.4	–	1.3	1.1
	Chapel Hill	*	*	*	*
Respiratory syncytial	Newcastle	10.6	+	40.8+	+
	Washington 1959–61[e]	3.0	2.0	25.0	10.0
	Seattle	1.0	–	9.8	2.3
	Chapel Hill	3.4	4.7	7.5	26.1

a Gardner et al. Brit Med J 2:7, 1971.
b Parrott et al. Am J Pub Health 52:907, 1962.
c Foy et al. Am J Epidemiol 97:80, 1973.
d Chapman et al. Am J Epidemiol 114:786, 1981.
e Chanock et al. Am J Pub Health 52:918, 1962.
* serotypes were not stated in the publication.
+ overall RS isolation rate from respiratory infections other than croup.

develop rarely, sufficient fluid may accumulate to impede the pumping action of the heart i.e., cardiac tamponade. This necessitates removal of fluid by paracentesis. Electrocardiograms typically show flattening and inversion of the T waves in the precordial leads V3 through V5. Occasionally pleurodynia and pericarditis may affect the same patient simultaneously. Symptoms persist usually for 3–5 days after which complete recovery occurs. Occasionally patients may develop progressive fibrous thickening of the pericardium, leading eventually to constrictive pericarditis, for which surgical removal of sclerotic pericardium may be required to improve cardiac function.

Serous peritonitis may be induced occasionally by group B coxsackievirus infections, in addition to pleurodynia or pericarditis, or apart from those conditions. Patients develop severe generalized abdominal pain and tenderness with fever, but the leukocyte count remains normal. If a laparotomy is performed upon suspicion of acute appendicitis, there is generalized hyperemia beneath the peritoneum, with or without free fluid in the peritoneal cavity, and ileocecal lymph nodes may be enlarged. Serous peritonitis resolves within 3–5 days.

The incubation period of pleurodynia and pericarditis is about 4–8 days. Serous membrane infections due to coxsackieviruses are communicable by fecal contamination of fomites for as long as one week after onset.

LABORATORY DIAGNOSIS

Laboratory diagnosis of pleurodynia and other serous membrane infections requires isolation of coxsackievirus from feces or a rectal swab collected within 3 days after onset. Feces or rectal swabs are extracted with 2 ml tissue culture maintenance medium, centrifuged at 2000 xg for 10 minutes to deposit bacteria and gross particles and 0.1 ml quantities of supernatant are inoculated into primary tissue cultures of monkey kidney cells which are incubated at 37° C. Cytopathic effects typical of enteroviruses (Chapter 7) are observed after 2–7 days incubation and the new isolate is serotyped by neutralization in tissue culture. Same-day methods for identification of enteroviruses have not yet been developed reliably, due to their small particle size. Serological evidence that the new enterovirus isolate (group B coxsackievirus) actually caused the infection at the time of illness is obtained by performance of neutralization tests on paired sera (2 ml clotted blood specimens) collected initially on the day of onset of pleurodynia and 2–5 days subsequently, after disappearance of fever and other symptoms. Detection of antibodies in the second blood sample but not the first, or at least a four fold increase of antibody titer between the two sera indicate current infection.

EPIDEMIOLOGY

Pleurodynia arises from infection with any of the 6 coxsackievirus serotypes B1 through B6. For example, in Toronto, Canada between 1958 and 1965, enteroviruses were isolated from feces of 46 of 62 cases of pleurodynia, including 9 isolates of coxsackievirus B1 and 22 of coxsackievirus B5, whilst smaller numbers of cases were attributed to infection with types B2, B3, B4 coxsackievirus.[23] In 1958, coxsackievirus B5 only was isolated from pleurodynia patients and it was the dominant strain among aseptic meningitis patients, but throughout subsequent years when pleurodynia was associated with any of 5 group B coxsackievirus serotypes, most cases of aseptic meningitis were associated with echoviruses. Comparable experience has been summarized from many Temperate Zones communities.[23] In all outbreaks, pleurodynia occurred during summer months, simultaneously with aseptic meningitis, pericarditis, myositis or other enterovirus-induced illnesses.

REFERENCES

[1]A collaborative report: Rhinoviruses - extension of the numbering system. Virology 43:524, 1971.

[2]Bell JA, Rowe WP, Engler JI, Parrott RH, Huebner RJ: Pharyngo-conjunctival fever. Epidemiological studies of a recently recognized disease entity. JAMA 157:1083, 1955.

[3]Brandt CD, Kim HW, Jeffries BC, Pyles G, Christmas EE, Reid JL, Chanock RM, Parrott RH: Infections in 18,000 infants and children in a controlled study of respiratory tract disease II. Variation in adenovirus infections by year and season. Am J Epidemiol 95:218, 1972.

[4]Brown RS, Nogrady MB, Spence L, Wiglesworth FW: An outbreak of adenovirus type 7 infection in children in Montreal. Can Med Ass J 108:434, 1973.

[5]Caldwell GG, Lindsey NJ, Wulff H, Donnelly DD, Bohl FN: Epidemic of adenovirus 7 acute conjunctivitis in swimmers. Am J Epidemiol 99:230, 1974.

[6]Centers for Disease Control. MMWR Annual Summary 1977, issued Sept. 1978.

[7]Centers for Disease Control. Prevention and control of influenza. MMWR 33:253, 1984.

[8]Choi KW, Thacker SB: An evaluation of influenza mortality surveillance 1962–1979. II. Percentage of pneumonia and influenza deaths as an indicator of influenza activity. Am J Epidemiol 113:227, 1981.

[9]Clarke SKR, Gardner PS, Poole PM, Simpson H, Tobin JO'H: Respiratory syncytial virus infection: admission to hospital in industrial, urban and rural areas. Brit Med J 2:796, 1978.

[10]D'Angelo LJ, Heirholzer JC, Keenlyside RA: Anderson LJ, Martone WJ: Pharyngoconjunctival fever caused by adenovirus type 4: report of a swimming pool-related outbreak with recovery of virus from pool water. J Infect Dis 140:42, 1979.

[11]Dudding BA, Top FH Jr, Winter PE, Buescher EL, Lamson TH, Leibovitz A: Acute respiratory disease in military trainees. The adenovirus surveillance program 1966–1971. Am J Epidemiol 97:187, 1973.

[12]Duncan IBR, Hutchinson JGP: Type-3 adenovirus infection with gastrointestinal symptoms. Lancet 1:530, 1961.

[13]Francis T Jr: On the doctrine of original antigenic sin. Proc Am Philos Soc 104:572, 1960.

[14]Gardner PS, McQuillan J, Court SDM: Speculation on pathogenesis in death from respiratory syncytial virus infection. Brit Med J 1:327, 1970.

[15]Gutekunst RR, Heggie AD: Viremia and viruria in adenovirus infections. Detection in patients with rubella or rubelliform illness. New Eng J Med 264:374, 1961.

[16]Guyer B, O'Day DM, Hierholzer JC, Schaffner W: Epidemic keratoconjunctivitis. A community outbreak of mixed adenovirus type 8 and type 19 infection. J Infect Dis 132:142, 1975.

[17]Gwaltney JM Jr: Understanding and controlling rhinovirus colds. IV International Symposium on Medical Virology, Anaheim CA, 9 Nov. 1984.

[18]Hamparian VV: Rhinoviruses. In Diagnostic procedures for Viral, Rickettsial and Chlamydial Infections, 5th ed. EH Lennette and N Schmidt editors, American Public Health Association, Washington, DC, 1979, p. 535.

[19]Hilleman MR: Epidemiology of adenovirus respiratory infection in military recruit populations. Ann NY Acad Sci 67:262, 1957.

[20]Kelsey DS: Adenovirus meningoencephalitis. Pediatrics 61:291, 1978.

[21]Knight V, McClung HW, Wilson SZ, Waters BK, Quarles JM, Cameron RW, Greggs SE, Zerwas JM, Couch RB: Ribavirin small-particle aerosol treatment of influenza. Lancet 2:945, 1981.

[22]McLean DM, Bach RD, Larke RPB, McNaughton GA: Myxoviruses associated with acute laryngotracheobronchitis in Toronto 1962–63. Can Med Ass J 89:1257, 1963.

[23]McLean DM: Coxsackieviruses and echoviruses. Am J Med Sci 251:351, 1966.

[24]McLean DM, Bannatyne RM, Givan KF: Myxovirus dissemination by air. Can Med Ass J 96:1449, 1967.

[25]McLean DM: Immunological Investigation of Human Virus Diseases. Vol. 5, Practical Methods in Clinical Immunology, Series Editor RC Nairn. Churchill Livingstone, Edinburgh, 1982.

[26]McLean DM, Wong KK: Same-day Diagnosis of Human Virus Infections. CRC Press, Boca Raton, FL, 1984.

[27]Maynard JE, Dull HB, Hanson ML, Feltz ET, Berger R, Hommes L: Evaluation of monovalent and polyvalent influenza virus vaccines during an epidemic of type A2 and B influenza. Am J Epidemiol 87:148, 1968.

[28]Meiklejohn G, Eickhoff TC, Graves P, Josephine I: Antigenic drift and efficacy of influenza virus vaccines 1976–1977. J Infect Dis 138:618, 1978.

[29]Numazaki Y, Kumasaka T, Jano N, Yamanaka M, Miyazawa T, Takai S, Ishida N: Further study on acute hemorrhagic cystitis due to adenovirus type 11. New Eng J Med 289:344, 1973.

[30]Parker WL, Wilt JC, Stackiw W: Adenovirus infections. Can J Public Health 52:246, 1961.

[31]Parkinson AJ, Muchmore HG, Scott LV, Kalmakoff J, Miles JAR: Parainfluenza virus upper respiratory tract illnesses in partially immune adult human subjects: a study at an antarctic station. Am J Epidemiol 110:753, 1979.

[32]Public Health Laboratory Service Communicable Disease Surveillance Centre: Respiratory syncytial virus infection in the elderly 1976–82. Brit Med J 287, 1619, 1983.

[33]Rubin RJ, Gregg MB: Influenza surveillance in the United States, 1972–74. Am J Epidemiol 102:225, 1975.

[34]Stanley ED, Muldoon RE, Akers LW, Jackson GG: Evaluation of antiviral drugs. The effect of amantadine on influenza in volunteers. Ann NY Acad Sci 130:44, 1965.

[35]Sturdy PM, Court SDM, Gardner PS: Viruses and whooping cough. Lancet 2:978, 1981.

[36]Van der Veen J, Dykman JH: Association of type 21 adenovirus with acute respiratory disease in military recruits. Am J Hyg 76:149, 1962.

[37]Zweighaft RM, Hierholzer JC, Bryan JA: Epidemic keratoconjunctivitis at a Vietnamese refugee camp in Florida. Am J Epidemiol 96:399, 1977.

CHAPTER 19

EXANTHEMATA

RASHES, CONJUNCTIVITIS, MUMPS

Virus infections causing skin rashes or inflammation of mucous membranes and their accessory organs (Table 19-1) include: (i) maculopapular rashes induced by measles, rubella and some enteroviruses; (ii) conjunctivitis induced by enterovirus 70 and some adenoviruses; (iii) vesicular rashes caused by herpes simplex and varicella-zoster which are classified within the Herpesviridae family whilst mononucleosis and cytomegalovirus disease are febrile affections caused by additional Herpesviridae members; (iv) mumps induces inflammation of the parotid and submandibular salivary glands, without rash.

Maculopapular rashes appear as red blushes with irregular margins 2–5 mm diameter (macules) in the centers of which are raised white "pin-heads" 1 mm diameter (papules), so that the skin resembles red stucco cement. Vesicular rashes show clusters or individual lesions 1–3 mm diameter which contain serous fluid and they are surrounded by reddened areolae 1–2 mm diameter.

Vaccinia virus induces vesicular eruptions at the site of inoculation with antismallpox vaccine, and occasionally the virus may be spread to eczematous areas or mucocutaneous junctions by mechanical transfer, inducing numerous vesicles. Since the last naturally occurring case of smallpox was documented in October 1977 and because antismallpox vaccine (vaccinia virus) is no longer manufactured or distributed, vaccinia complications are unlikely to be encountered in 1985 or subsequent years. Therefore vaccinia virus will not be discussed in this book.

MEASLES

CLINICAL

Measles (red measles, rubeola) presents with acute onset of fever, maculopapular rash and Koplik's spots, due to infection with measles virus. The temperature usually increases to 39° C. The maculopapular rash comprising

TABLE 19-1
TIME COURSE AND LABORATORY DIAGNOSIS OF VIRAL EXANTHEMATA

| Syndrome | Virus species (family) | Incubation period | Duration of | | Virus identification | | | | Antibodies (paired sera) | | |
			comm.	illness	specimen	EM	IF	virus isolation	test	initial detection	persistence
Measles	Measles (Paramyxoviridae)	12–14d	–2 to +4d	2–3d	throat	+	+	GMK	HI IF ELISA CF	2–4d 14–21d	20+ yr 6 mo
Rubella	Rubella (Togaviridae)	16–18d	–2 to +7d	1–3d	throat	n/a	n/a	GMK RK-13	HI IF ELISA RIA CF	2–4d 14–21d	20+ yr 6 mo
Enteroviral rash	Echovirus-9	4–8d	0 to +4d	3–5d	feces, throat	n/a	n/a	MK	NT	2–5d	10+ yr
conjunctivitis	Enterovirus-70 (Picornaviridae)	1–2d	0 to 3+d	3–5d	eye swab	n/a	n/a	DH	NT	2–5d	10+ yr
Herpes simplex	Herpes 1, 2	2–3d	0 to +4d	2–4d	scraping	+	+	DH	IF	7–14d	10+ yr
Varicella-Zoster	Varicella-Zoster	14–18d	–2 to +4d	2–4d	scraping	+	+*	(DH)	IF CF	4–7d 14–21d	10+ yr 6 mo
Mononucleosis	EBV	2–7w	0 to +8d	1–3w	n/a				IF	1–3w	1+ yr
Cytomegalovirus	CMV (Herpesviridae)	congenital	2+ yr	chronic	urine	+	+*	(DH)	IF CF	1–3w 1–3w	1+ yr 1+ yr
Mumps	Mumps (Paramyxoviridae)	16–18d	–2 to +4d	2–4d	throat	+	+	MK	HI S-CF	2–4d 2–4d	20+ yr 6 mo

Day 0: day of onset of illness	DH: continuous diploid human fibroblasts	HI: hemagglutination inhibition
–2: two days before onset	MK: primary monkey kidney cultures (rhesus)	NT: neutralization
+4: four days after onset	GMK: primary monkey kidney cultures (grivet)	ELISA: enzyme-linked immunosorbent assay
EM: electron microscopy (negative stain)	RK-13: continuous polyploid rabbit kidney	RIA: radioimmunoassay
IF: indirect immunofluorescence	CF: complement fixation (virus particle)	
*: anticomplement immunofluorescence	S-CF: soluble antigen in CF test	

red blotches, reminiscent of stucco walls, involves mainly the face and trunk, extending over the upper arms and legs (Figure 19-1), but the palms of the

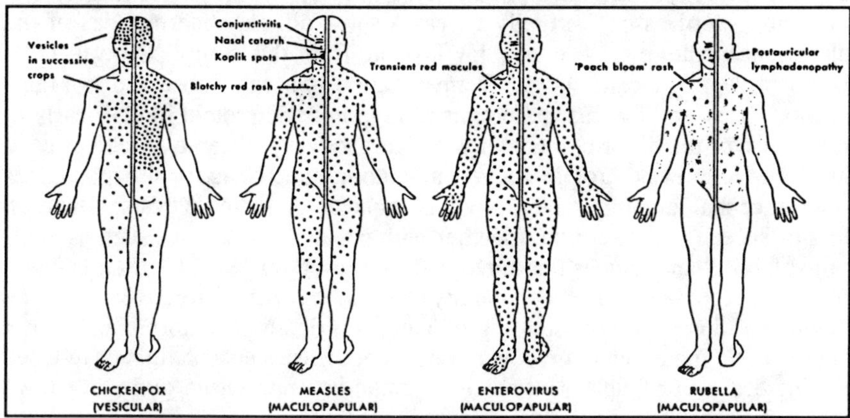

Figure 19-1: Distribution over the body surface of maculopapular rashes due to measles, enteroviruses, rubella, and vesicular rash due to chickenpox (varicella).

hands and soles of the feet are usually devoid of rash. Koplik spots are pathognomonic of measles; they comprise raised white 'grains of sand' on bluish red spots 2–3 mm diameter over the buccal mucosa inside the cheeks and lips, and they disappear 1–2 days after onset of the skin rash (exanthem). Characteristically the rash of measles is preceded by a runny nose, harsh cough and mild fever, reddened watery eyes with drooping eyelids 1–2 days earlier, so that the typical measles patient exhibits a dejected appearance ("measly look").

The incubation period of measles is about 14 days to the onset of rash and fever, or about 12 days to the onset of the catarrhal stage preceding the rash. The period of communicability, by droplets expelled by coughing or in nasal discharges, extends from 2 days before to 4 days after onset of the rash. Fever persists for 2–3 days after onset of rash, the maculopapular eruption undergoes brownish discoloration after 4 days and the rash disappears after 7 days. Recovery is usually complete, and performance of children at school remains unchanged.[19,33]

COMPLICATIONS

Complications frequently involve the respiratory tract, giving rise to croup (occasionally) or bronchopneumonia affecting as many as 1 in 15 cases of measles in a British series.[43] Encephalitis may affect 0.22 to 1.39 per 1000 reported cases of measles in USA from 1963 to 1979.[6] Febrile convulsions without encephalitis may occur in another 1 in 700 reported cases.[43]

Encephalitis usually begins 2–7 days after onset of the measles rash[1,30,31,36] with a temperature exceeding 39° C, drowsiness deepening into stupor or coma, irritability, neck stiffness and lymphocytes in CSF exceeding 10 per mm^3 in 75% of cases. Virtually all cases show diffuse abnormalities of the electroencephalogram. The case fatality rate from this complication in USA is 5.3 to 29.4%, mean 14.0%.[6] Demyelination is usually observed in brains of fatal cases, and increased amounts of myelin basic protein in CSF early in the course of the disease, together with lymphocyte proliferative responses to human myelin basic protein suggest an autoimmune basis for this postinfectious encephalomyelitis.[30] Neurological sequelae including paresis, athetosis, loss of speech and dementia, together with personality changes such as emotional lability and temper tantrums, may be present in 18–23% of cases upon discharge from hospital.[1,25] Personality changes may persist for 1 year or more. Administration of corticosteroids or adrenocorticotrophic hormone has not significantly increased the recovery rate from measles encephalitis or reduced the incidence of sequelae,[31,63] nor has human immune serum globulin shown any therapeutic benefit.[25]

Subacute sclerosing panencephalitis (SSPE) is a slowly progressing encephalopathy which complicates 6–22 per million cases of reported measles,[6] and symptoms appear after a mean interval of 7 years following measles. If there is any risk of contracting SSPE after measles vaccine, this risk is 1:5 to 1:40 lower than the risk of SSPE after natural measles.[6] The syndrome comprises progressive dementia, myoclonic jerks, pyramidal and extrapyramidal signs, an electroencephalogram with regular periodic complexes, and a paretic type of colloidal gold reaction in CSF.[16] Measles antigen has been detected in brains of these patients[16] and measles antibody has been found both in IgM and IgG of both CSF and serum from SSPE patients[17] several months after onset, but not in CSF of measles patients without SSPE.

Atypical measles has been encountered on repeated occasions[39] since its initial description in 1967.[23] Petechial and sometimes vesicular eruptions may cover the trunk, accompanied by unusually severe constitutional upsets and bronchopneumonia is demonstrated radiologically. Atypical measles affects children who contract natural measles several years after administration of killed measles virus vaccine. Since killed measles vaccine was withdrawn from the commercial market after 1967, future occurrence of atypical measles is unlikely.

Immunosuppressed states which occur naturally as in leukemia, or during therapy as in prolonged corticosteroid therapy, may predispose to unusually severe attacks of measles, resulting in bronchopneumonia[44] with typical radiological findings of extensive bilateral nodular infiltration of the lung fields. Frequently this leads to death with 2 weeks, and multinucleate giant cells, which show specific immunofluorescence reactions for measles antigen, are found within smears or sections of lung tissue. This is termed giant cell pneumonia.

The measles case-fatality rate in USA has declined substantially from 0.086% reported cases in 1960, before measles immunization to virtually zero from 1979 through 1981[6] some 18 years after licensure of measles vaccine. However the case-fatality rate among hospitalized measles patients in Sydney, Australia was 1.2%,[1] and it attained 5.7–21% in underdeveloped rural areas of tropical Africa.[46] The principal cause of death from measles in developed countries comprised respiratory and encephalitic complications; malnutrition contributed to the high death rate in underdeveloped countries.

LABORATORY DIAGNOSIS

Laboratory diagnosis of measles is accomplished rapidly in clinical settings using same-day techniques of electron microscopy in combination with immunofluorescence[42] as described for influenza virus (Chapter 18, page 240). Briefly, nasopharyngeal secretions or throat garglings are collected preferably within one day after onset of rash. Electron microscopic examination of grids moistened with throat specimens and stained negatively with phosphotungstic acid reveal paramyxovirus virions with total diameters about 200 nm and they contain herringbone strands of helical nucleocapsid 18 nm diameter (Figure 8-10). Smears of cellular deposit from throat specimens reveal immunofluorescent staining in the presence of anti-measles serum by the indirect technique.

Isolation of measles virus from throat secretions or from leukocytes within the buffy coat of plasma collected with 1 day after onset of rash, may be achieved, with considerable difficulty by inoculation of primary tissue cultures of grivet monkey which may exhibit syncytia formation after 7–10 days incubation. Measles virus is liberated into the supernatant fluid and it agglutinates grivet monkey erythrocytes in buffered diluents at pH 7.0 and 37° C. Addition of anti-measles serum to an appropriate dilution of supernatant fluid inhibits hemagglutination, thus confirming the serological identification of the fresh isolate as measles virus. Some batches of primary human amnion or continuous polypoid human (HeLa) tissue cultures have been employed successfully for isolation of measles virus from throat specimens or blood leukocytes.

Detection of fourfold or greater increases of measles antibody titers, in sera collected within 2 days after onset and subsequently after a further 2 or more days[41] (one day or more after defervescence), is achieved readily on the same day of collection of the second serum by hemagglutination inhibition or indirect immunofluorescence, or on the next day by enzyme immunoassay (ELISA). Peak antibody titers are attained 1 month to 1 year after onset, and after about a fourfold decline within 5 years after onset, titers remain stationary lifelong. Complement fixing antibody titers are first detected 14–21 days after onset and they persist about 6 months.

EPIDEMIOLOGY

Before the licensure of measles vaccine in 1963, the annual incidence rate of measles was between 200 and 400 cases per 100,000 population in the United States (Figure 19-2). Following widespread use of vaccine during the succeeding 5 years, measles incidence had fallen to 10 cases per 100,000 but

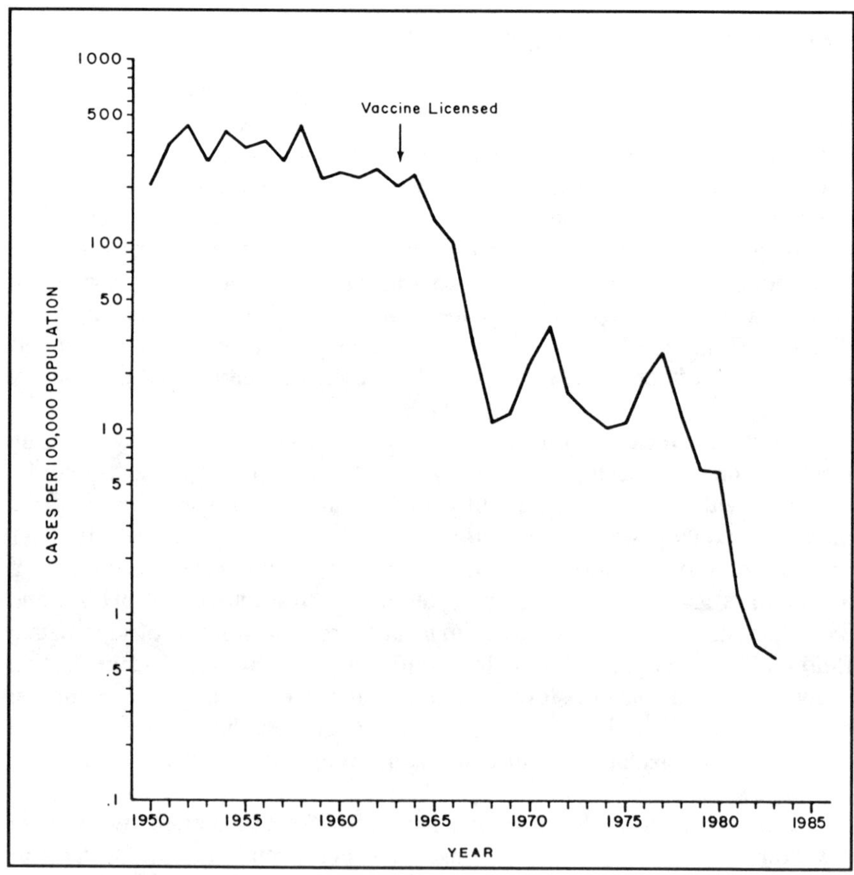

Figure 19-2: Reported measles incidence (cases per 100,000 per annum), United States 1950–1983. Reproduced with permission from Centers for Disease Control. MMWR 33:106, 1984.

with less comprehensive measles vaccination programs in the early 1970's the measles incidence increased to 30 cases per 100,000 representing 57,345 reported cases in 1977.[6] Following commencement of the Measles Elimination Program in October 1978, a steady decline in the incidence of measles was noted from 1979 onwards (Figure 19-3), so that during the first 39 weeks of

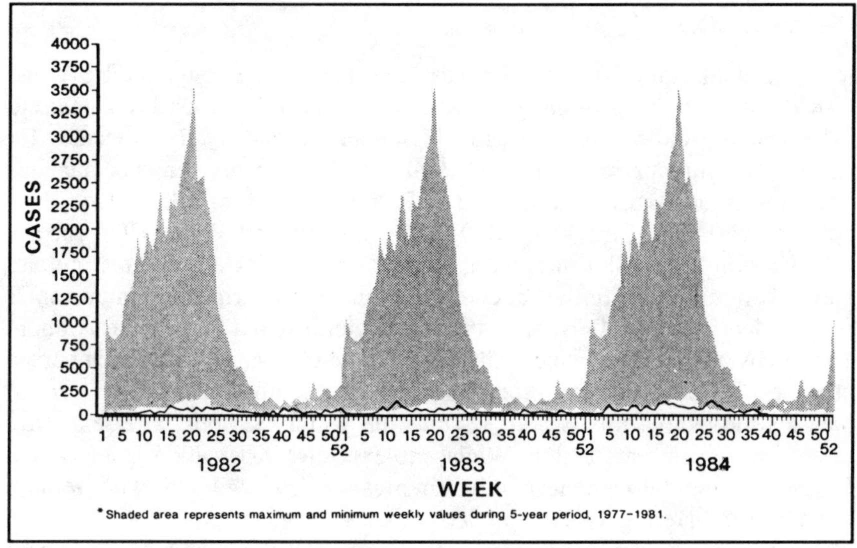

Figure 19-3: Reported measles cases - United States 1982–1984. Reproduced with permission from MMWR 33:673, 1984.

1984, a total of only 2322 measles cases (incidence rate 1.0 per 100,000) was reported throughout USA,[15] despite intensive measles surveillance. During 1984, 11.3% measles cases were associated with international or out-of-state importations. Most cases of measles in USA occur each year within the first 26 weeks (winter and spring). Incidence rates are highest in preschool and school-age children aged less than 10 years. In the pre-vaccine era 1960–1964, this age group comprised 90% of all reported cases of measles. After some 15 years of routine vaccination, in 1976–80, this age group comprised 54% of reported cases, when the incidence of measles had declined by about 95% from the pre-vaccine era.[6]

Measles is endemic in many countries where measles vaccination programs are not provided universally. Unvaccinated travelers who become infected with measles whilst in these countries develop clinically obvious measles after arrival in USA and transmit infection to unvaccinated contacts by the airborne route. For example an infant who contracted measles infection whilst in Korea developed a measles rash during November 1982, for which she was taken to a pediatricians' office 2 days later.[10] Measles occurred 14 days later in 4 unvaccinated pediatric patients who attended the office within 60–75 minutes after the departure of the index case, and 2 of these subsequently transmitted measles to family contacts.

PREVENTION

Excellent control of measles has been achieved throughout USA and Canada through virtually universal administration of live measles vaccine to infants and/or children before entry to school. Frequently live vaccines for rubella and mumps are combined with measles vaccine for subcutaneous injection as one does of trivalent MMR live vaccine, of which each does contain 1000 TCD_{50} measles, 5000 TCD_{50} mumps and 1000 TCD_{50} rubella vaccine strains. Measles vaccine is propagated in chick embryo cell culture and it comprises the further attenuated strain of the original Edmonston B strain. Measles or MMR vaccines are best administered to children at about 15 months of age,[7] after which 95% develop measles antibodies which persist at least 16 years, and they protect against disease after natural exposure to measles throughout this period. Vaccination within 72 hours after exposure may provide some protection. Whilst pre-exposure vaccination is advocated for all infants throughout North America, a few children who remain unimmunized are highly susceptible following exposure to an imported case of measles.[10] In this instance intramuscular injection of pooled human immune globulin 0.25 ml/kg within 6 days of exposure will prevent or modify measles,[7] but passive immunity wanes after 3 months. Measles vaccine induces relatively few adverse reactions such as mild fever about 6 days after vaccination in 5–15% recipients and transient rashes in 5% vaccines. Encephalitis or encephalopathy have been reported in 1 per million recipients, but this is lower than the rate of encephalitis of undetermined etiology. Contraindications to live measles vaccine include pregnancy, febrile illness, administration of immune globulin within the preceding 3 months, tuberculosis and immunosuppressed states.

RUBELLA

CLINICAL

Rubella (German Measles) presents with acute onset of mild fever, maculopapular rash and postauricular lymphadenopathy, due to infection with rubella virus. The temperature does not usually increase beyond 38° C. The maculopapular rash is bright red and resembles peach bloom; it extends principally over the face and trunk (Figure 19-1), but it does not involve the palms and soles. Enlarged lymph nodes behind the ears are pathognomonic of rubella infection, and they are always present at onset of fever and rash.

The incubation period of rubella is 16–18 days (Table 19-1). The period of communicability by infected droplets extends from 2 days before onset of rash regularly until 7 days after onset, but some patients have shed virus as long as 21 days. Fever persists 1–2 days and patients usually feel well by 3 days. The rash usually persists 2–4 days, and no longer than 5 days, but no skin staining is observed after disappearance of the rash. The eyes may appear suffused, with a gritty sensation and occasionally photophobia may be experienced, but in contrast to measles there is no running of the eyes. The buccal mucous membrane appears normal.

COMPLICATIONS

Arthritis characteristically affects the fingers, wrists, elbows, knees or ankles of 1% or less of subjects who contract rubella naturally or who received earlier formulations of rubella vaccine which are no longer marketed. Swelling and pain in one or more joints commences within 6 days before to 4 days after onset of rubella rash, and persists for a few days to 3 weeks. The incidence is highest in women aged more than 20 years.

Encephalitis may complicate about 1:5000 cases of rubella. In an outbreak involving about 30,000 cases of rubella among Pittsburgh, PA school children during 1964, 6 cases of encephalitis, including 3 deaths, were encountered within 2–4 days after onset of rubella.[59]

CONGENITAL RUBELLA SYNDROME denotes the anomalies which are observed in newborn infants which result from intrauterine infections of their mothers during the first trimester of pregnancy. Anomalies affected 70 infants at 4 North American Medical Centers after the last major rubella epidemic of 1964–65 in the following proportions:[40] cataracts or other ocular anomalies 71%, cardiac anomalies, usually patent ductus arteriosus 81%, thrombocytopenic purpura with platelet counts as low as 10,000–30,000/mm³, giving the baby the appearance of a blueberry muffin 55%, birth weight below 2500 g despite normal gestational age 70%, hepatomegaly with or without splenomegaly 42%, radiological changes in the metaphysis of the humerus or femur, giving the appearance of a frayed celery stalk 38%. Clinical history of rubella during the first trimester was obtained in mothers of 77% infants, and exposure to rubella but without development of rash was noted in 11% mothers, one of whom received human immune globulin 24 hours after her husband contracted rubella.[40] Although deafness was not detected in the above North American series, due to technical difficulties with its assessment in newborn infants, it was encountered among 37% children aged 4–8 years in Australia[56] and significant loss of hearing was detected in 19% school children aged 8–11 years in Britain,[58] following clinical evidence of rubella in their mothers during the first trimester. Mental retardation was noted in 14% cases in USA,[45] delay development of motor activity was detected in 4% cases in Australia,[56] but the distribution of intelligence quotients among children who contracted intrauterine rubella infections in Britain paralleled that observed in offspring of mothers without clinical evidence of rubella during pregnancy.[58]

The risk of development of congenital rubella syndrome was found, in a large prospective study before the advent of laboratory confirmation of rubella, to be 50% when rubella affected mothers from the 1st to the 4th week of gestation, 25% at 5–8 weeks, 17% at 9–12 weeks, 11% at 13–16 weeks, 6% at 17–24 weeks and none at later stages of pregnancy. The category of congenital anomaly was related to the gestational age at which rubella affected the mother clinically.[56,58] Cataracts and cardiac anomalies occurred following maternal rubella during the initial 8 weeks of pregnancy, deafness usually followed rubella at 5–15 weeks gestation, and multiple anomalies were encountered only with rubella before the 9th gestational week.

Rubella virus is excreted in the throat of infants with the congenital rubella syndrome regularly during the initial 20 weeks of life and infrequently up to 12 months of age, thus providing a source of infection for susceptible health care professionals who attend these infants.[40] Virus is excreted in urine during the initial 8 weeks and in feces up to 2 weeks of life. In infants with congenital cataracts, rubella virus is found in conjunctival swabs or eyes during the initial few weeks of life, or from the eye lens up to 18 months of age. Virus has also been found in CSF up to 1 year of age and in peripheral blood leukocytes to 6 months of age.

LABORATORY DIAGNOSIS

Rubella is diagnosed optimally by isolation of rubella virus from throat garglings or swabs collected within the initial 3 days after onset of rash. After centrifugation of suspensions of these samples in maintenance medium to deposit bacteria and cell debris, the supernatant is inoculated into primary tissue cultures of grivet monkey kidney and continuous polyploid cultures of rabbit kidney RK-13 cells. Evidence of isolation of rubella virus from a patient is achieved: (i) in grivet monkey cultures after 7 days incubation, by demonstration of interference with the growth of echovirus 11 (ii) observation of cytopathic effects 2–4 days after inoculation of RK-13 cultures, when the isolate is serotyped by neutralization tests. Due to a small particle size (40 nm) of rubella virions and their relatively low concentration (10,000 TCD_{50} per ml) in throat samples, same-day methods of identification by electron microscopy and immunofluorescence have proved unsatisfactory as diagnostic procedures.

Serological methods have provided the most convenient and precise approach to diagnosis of rubella in clinical settings, despite their inherent delay to await collection of the second of a pair of sera 2 or more days after defervescence. For routine purposes detection of a fourfold or greater increase of HI titer to rubella virus during convalescence[41] provides good evidence of current rubella virus infection. Parallel results are obtained using ELISA tests. In doubtful cases, or where a single serum only is available early in convalescence, ELISA or radioimmunoassay is employed to detect rubella-specific IgM,[54] since antibody titers within this immunoglobulin fraction are high during the initial 6 weeks after natural or vaccine-induced rubella. Surveys for prevalence of rubella infection in communities are performed conveniently by radial hemolysis tests.

EPIDEMIOLOGY

Before licensing of live rubella vaccine in USA during 1969, rubella was an endemic childhood disease which spread principally during winter and spring every year, and epidemic peaks occurred approximately every 3 years. The last, and greatest epidemic peak for any year, occurred during winter-spring 1964 with an annual incidence rate per 100,000 approaching 600,[3] in contrast to previous peaks of about 450 in 1935 and 1943, and rates as low as 25 to 30 per 100,000 during intervening years (Figure 19-4). Follow-

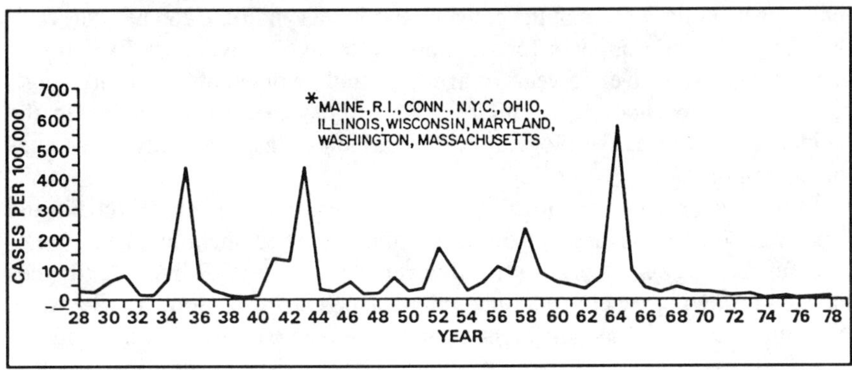

Figure 19-4: Rubella incidence in 10 States within U.S.A. 1928–1978. Reproduced with permission from Centers for Disease Control Rubella Surveillance Jan 1976–Dec 1978, issued May 1980, p 3.

ing intensification of rubella vaccination programs during the late 1970's the annual incidence rate has fallen below 2 per 100,000 since 1980[13] (Figure 19-5). This represents a total of 745 reported cases throughout USA during 1984, which is substantially lower than the previous five year median of 2308 cases annually between 1979 and 1983. Although age-specific attack rates were highest among infants and children below 10 years of age before 1969, adolescents and young adults aged 15-24 years experienced the highest attack rates during the mid 1970's. Since 1981, attack rates among all age categories have decreased substantially, with rates in those over 15 years following the overall trend to a total all-time low of 0.3 per 100,000 representing 745 cases during 1984, and low rates persisted through 1989.

In contrast to the rapid and profound decline in reported clinical cases of rubella shortly after initiation of widespread rubella vaccination in USA during 1969, the annual incidence rate of congenital rubella syndrome of 102 per 100,000 live births remained relatively unchanged between 1969 and 1979 (Figure 19-5), when 27 to 93 affected infants were born each year.[13] Since 1979 when 62 new cases were reported, there has been a steady decline each year in the number of infants born with congenital rubella syndrome, with an all-time low of 3 infants during 1984, which was maintained through 1989.

PREVENTION

The objective of any program to control and eventually eliminate rubella infections nationwide is to eliminate occurrence of the congenital rubella syndrome. Epidemiological evidence available in USA during mid 1984 indicates that elimination of the congenital rubella syndrome can be achieved[12] through concentration of efforts towards effective delivery of live rubella vaccine to persons over 15 years of age, especially women of childbearing age, and also to preschool-aged children. With the vast overall decline in the incidence of rubella, serological confirmation of suspected cases becomes vitally important.

Protection rates exceeding 90% against both clinical attacks of rubella and subclinical infections (asymptomatic viremia) have been demonstrated repeatedly for as long as 15 years after live rubella vaccine.[12] Rubella antibodies induced following vaccine administration have persisted as long as 18 years.[53] Administration of four different rubella vaccine strains to adult human volunteers evoked development of peak rubella-specific IgG antibodies within 6 months after vaccination,[54] in radioimmunoassay tests which are more highly sensitive than HI tests. Fourfold decline of titer was noted during the next 2–5 years, after which antibodies remained relatively stationary, and 98% vaccinees retained antibodies 8–12 years after vaccination. Rubella-specific serum IgA antibody responses were found, at titers lower than IgG, in virtually all subjects between 3 weeks and 6 months after vaccination by each strain, and persisted as long as 8–12 years. Rubella-specific serum IgM titers which peaked 3–6 weeks after vaccination declined to low or undetectable amounts by 6–12 months. Rubella-specific IgA and IgG titers in nasopharyngeal

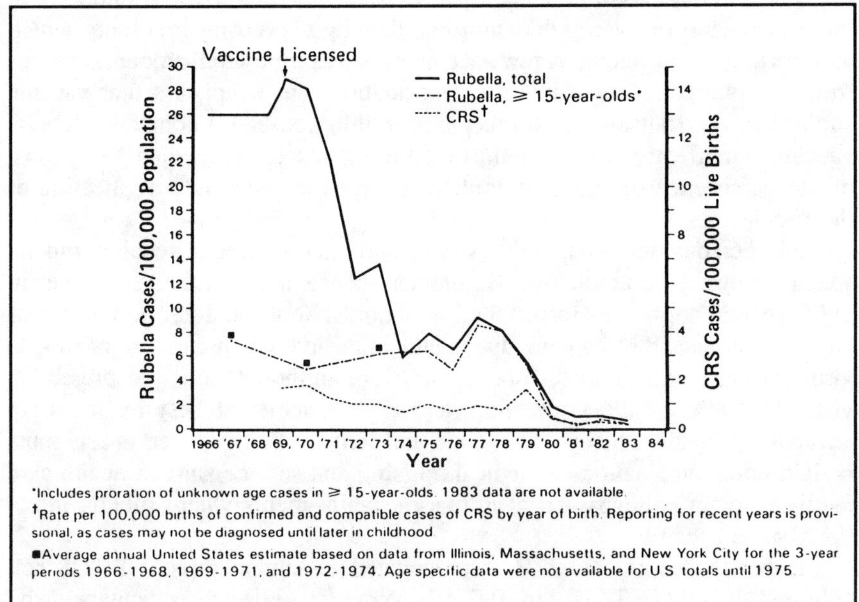

Figure 19-5: Incidence rate (per 100,000 per annum) of reported rubella and congenital rubella syndrome (CRS) cases - United States 1966–1983. Reproduced with permission from Centers for Disease Control. MMWR 33:529, 1984.

secretions were detected as long as 3 years after vaccination with the currently marketed RA 27/3 vaccine strain, but for shorter durations after administration of 3 previously marketed vaccine strains. Although natural reinfections were detected in some recipients of the 3 previously marketed vaccines by detection of abrupt increases to RIA antibody titer several years after initial vaccination, reinfections were not encountered in this group of RA 27/3 recipients, although reinfections have been detected in recipients of RA 27/3 vaccine elsewhere. It seems likely that long persistence of both IgA and IgG rubella antibodies in both serum and nasopharyngeal secretions after RA 27/3 vaccine mediates the enhanced degree of immunity against natural reinfection. Results of the above RIA assays published in January 1985 confirm earlier results obtained by the less sensitive HI assays, which led to the replacement of earlier vaccine by RA 27/3 vaccine in January 1979.

Rubella vaccine RA 27/3 strain should be administered to all persons aged more than 12 months,[12] unless they are immune. Documentary evidence of immunity comprises either serological evidence of previous rubella infection or an immunization certificate showing administration of rubella vaccine after the first birthday. A single dose of rubella vaccine has induced antibody in more than 95% of susceptible subjects, thereby conferring immunity which appears to persist lifelong. A few vaccinees may excrete small amounts of virus from the pharynx 7–28 days after vaccination, but it appears that vaccine strains are not transmitted to other susceptible household contacts. Rubella vaccine is ineffective when administered to infants aged less than 12 months, due to persistence of maternal antibodies which interfere with replication of the vaccine.

All persons including adolescents and adults should receive rubella vaccine unless contraindicated. Before commencement of rubella vaccines in 1969, rubella antibodies were found in about 85% of the adult population of North America and elsewhere, due to endemic and epidemic spread of rubella virus. In order to eliminate rubella infection, antibodies must be present in virtually 100% of the population, and this is achieved best by intensive vaccination of all subjects, both male and female. Particular emphasis must be laid upon vaccination of medical, nursing and service staff in health care facilities[9] or in colleges and at military establishments where rubella infections spread readily.

Rubella vaccine RA 27/3 is propagated in human diploid WI-38 cell cultures and 1000 TCD_{50} in 0.5 ml volume is injected subcutaneously, preferably in combination with 1000 TCD_{50} live measles vaccine and 5000 TCD_{50} live mumps vaccine.

Contraindications to rubella vaccination include: (i) infants aged less than 12 months where maternal immunity may interfere with the vaccine "take"; (ii) children who have received immune globulin for measles or hepatitis prophylaxis within the preceding 3 months; (iii) pregnant women; (iv) severe febrile illness, when vaccination should be postponed until recovery; (v) persons who developed anaphylactic reactions (not contact dermatitis) following neomycin injections because the vaccine contains trace amounts of neomycin; (vi) persons with immune deficiency diseases such as leukemia and generalized malignancy, or those on long-term immunosuppressive chemotherapy and corticosteroids.

Adverse reactions to rubella vaccine are relatively infrequent; they may comprise mild fever, rash, lymphadenopathy and pain in the small joints, but frank arthritis affects less than 2%. No evidence of congenital malformations was detected in 216 offspring born to 214 mothers who inadvertently received rubella vaccine during the first trimester of pregnancy.[12] Thus the vaccine does not appear to place the unborn child at risk; this is substantiated by isolates of rubella virus from aborted material from 1 of 32 (3%) mothers who received RA 27/3 vaccine inadvertently during pregnancy in contrast to 17 of 85 (20%) mothers who received previously licensed vaccine strains.

Striking effectiveness of rubella vaccination strategies in USA which were initiated in 1969 and intensified from 1978 onwards, concentrating on infants after their first birthdays, children at school entry and before leaving school, and susceptible adult workers in high-risk occupations has been demonstrated by reports of merely 745 rubella cases and an all-time low of 3 infants with congenital rubella syndrome during 1984,[13] thus approaching the goal of elimination.

ENTEROVIRUS RASHES AND CONJUNCTIVITIS

CLINICAL

ENTEROVIRAL RASHES appear commonly during seasons of high prevalence of some enteroviruses, especially echovirus 9.[40] Other causative echoviruses include types 4, 6, 16 and 30. Transient maculopapular eruptions resembling measles[35] involve largely the trunk and limbs, including the palms and soles (Figure 19-1), accompanied by mild fever. Unlike measles there is no runny nose or conjunctivitis. About one-third of cases with a rash also develop aseptic meningitis (Chapter 23).

The incubation period is 4–8 days. The period of communicability, principally by the feces, extends about 4 days after onset. Fever and rash persist usually for 3 days, or a maximum of 5 days, but there is no residual skin staining as in measles.

Enteroviral rashes are distinguished readily from measles by the lack of nasal and conjunctival catarrh and the presence of rash on the palms, which usually does not occur in measles. Enteroviral rashes are differentiated from rubella by the peripheral distribution of the rash which involves mainly the face and trunk in rubella, and the absence of enlarged postauricular nodes which are always found in rubella. Furthermore enteroviral rashes occur in summer and autumn, measles and rubella occur mainly during winter and spring.

ENTEROVIRAL CONJUNCTIVITIS first affected large numbers of residents of tropical Africa and Asia between 1969 and 1971[34] and it was caused by enterovirus 70. Patients suddenly develop severe inflammation of the conjunctivae bilaterally, accompanied by subconjunctival hemorrhages and photophobia.[64] Although patients are unable to work for a few days, complete recovery normally ensues, but rarely it is complicated by neurological syndromes such as radiculomyelitis and cranial nerve involvement. Coxsackievirus A24 has been implicated in some recent outbreaks.

The incubation period is 1–2 days. Symptoms usually persist for 3–5 days. The period of communicability, principally by direct contact and by fomites, extends from the onset of symptoms for 3 or more days until clinical recovery.[64]

LABORATORY   DIAGNOSIS

Laboratory diagnosis of enteroviral infections is accomplished best by isolation of the causative virus from the feces or throat of patients with rash, or from eye swabs or feces of patients with conjunctivitis. Feces, rectal swabs or throat swabs are collected in vials containing 2 ml tissue culture maintenance medium, centrifuged at 2500 x g for 10 minutes to deposit bacteria, and supernatant fluids are inoculated into primary monkey kidney tissue cultures which are incubated at 37° C until cytopathic effects are observed 2–7 days later. Enterovirus 70 is best isolated in human diploid fibroblast cultures.[29] The fresh virus isolate is serotyped by neutralization tests in tissue culture. This entire isolation and serotyping procedure frequently requires 10 days or longer to achieve a definitive result. Same-day methods of morphological and immunofluorescent identification are not applicable to enteroviruses, due to their small particle size which is confused easily with subcellular debris.

Serological identification of enterovirus infections is accomplished conveniently by neutralization tests in tissue culture against the same serotype which infected the patient. Antibodies are first detected about 2 days after onset, and fourfold increases in titer are frequently demonstrated 2–3 days subsequently.

EPIDEMIOLOGY

Enterovirial rashes in North America, Europe and Australia occur principally during summer and autumn, which in USA comprises June through October[5] (Figure 23-1). Rash comprised the major clinical feature in 192 of 16,978 patients (1.1%) who yielded an enteroviral isolate throughout the USA between 1970 and 1979. Echoviruses infected 85 of these 192 subjects (44%), and the commonest serotype was echovirus 9, which was isolated from 36 rash patients (19%). Rash was observed in as many as one-third of patients during outbreaks of echovirus 9 infection in Great Britain[35] and North America between 1955 and 1965, and rash was encountered less frequently during epidemic spread of echovirus type 4 and 6 during the same era.[37] Enteroviral rashes affect mainly children under 5 years of age, who comprised 69% of virus positive patients between 1970 and 1979;[5] males and females were affected equally frequently.

Acute hemorrhagic conjunctivitis due to enterovirus 70 usually affects densely populated coastal communities in Tropical countries.[64] Although Asian epidemics affected mostly young adult males, a recent outbreak in Florida involved mainly school-age children and adult females. The disease spreads readily through households by direct contact and by fomites. Epidemic activity was first recognized in both Ghana and in Java during early 1969. From Ghana the disease spread along the West African coast to reach Morocco and other North African countries by 1971; it also spread southwards into Zaire by 1972. Meanwhile the disease spread from Java through Malaysia, easterly into Thailand and India, and northwards as far as Japan through 1971. Acute hemorrhagic conjunctivitis first appeared in southern Florida,[29] Puerto Rico[64] and several Central American republics during 1981.

HERPES SIMPLEX

CLINICAL

Herpes simplex (herpes) is a crop of vesicles 1 mm diameter frequently involving portions of the face and lips which is caused usually by human herpesvirus 1, or the external genitalia where it is usually due to infections by herpesvirus 2.

Primary herpesvirus infections in infants aged less than 1 year usually induce gingivostomatitis with vesicular eruptions, becoming confluent over the mucous membrane of the mouth and gums, plus the anterior two-thirds of the tongue. This is accompanied by fever, irritability and refusal to drink fluids on account of the painful mouth, so that dehydration may become sufficiently severe to require administration of fluids intravenously. The raw, extremely tender surface beneath the burst herpetic vesicles may become infected with opportunistic organisms such as *Candida albicans* which induces yellowish plaques, or fusospirochaetes (Vincent's organisms) which induce a smelly blackened appearance to the mucosa. Vesicles may also appear on the lips, and after bursting they present a scabby appearance.

In older children and adults, vesicles 1 mm diameter are usually confined to the lips and immediately adjacent facial skin. Initially they appear watery, but rupture within 2 days, after which a scab persists about 1 week. Recurrences appear in the same location after abnormal external stimuli such as extreme heat or cold, or internal stimuli such as severe infections, or emotional trauma such as death of a close relative. Virus cannot be detected on the lips when lesions are absent i.e. the virus becomes latent, but it can be isolated readily from vesicle fluid during recurrences of eruptions, despite the presence of neutralizing antibodies in patients' sera.

Herpesvirus vesicles may erupt on the skin anywhere over the body in addition to the face and lips. Denuded areas of skin following abrasions, burns or atopic eczema are at high risk of herpesvirus implantation by direct contact with exuding vesicles either on the same patient or other subjects. Fomites such as toys in daycare centers, which are contaminated by infected saliva or vesicular exudate, provide an effective means of virus transmission between patients. When the eczema extends over a major proportion of an infants' skin surface, herpesvirus infection (eczema herpeticum or Kaposi's varicelliform eruption) may be disseminated by the blood to the liver and other organs, with fatal outcome. Characteristically vesicles are 1 mm or more in diameter and show raised edges after the vesicles burst.

Herpetic whitlows may develop on the fingers of health care personnel who care for tracheotomy stomas infected by herpesvirus. These comprise herpetic infection of the pulp space; the finger becomes extremely painful, reddened and swollen.

Herpesvirus infections of the conjunctiva are uncommon, but the infection may spread to the cornea (keratitis) either superficially or including the stroma. This may result in corneal scarring and opacity formation. Cataracts, iridocyclitis and panuveitis are also attributed to herpesvirus infections.

Herpetic encephalitis is rare, affecting 77 patients, of whom 31 died during 1978.[4] Several days after the appearance of an herpetic vesicle, on the lip or elsewhere, the patient develops high fever, clouding of consciousness, disorientation and may convulse or show spastic weakness of limbs. Herpesvirus 2 may involve newborns, which contract infection during transit of the birth canal, and herpesvirus 1 usually involves older subjects, except in immuno-compromised patients where either serotype may cause encephalitis.

Genital herpes is usually due to type 2 infections,[66] but occasionally type 1 infections may be implicated. In the male, painful 1 mm vesicles appear over penile shaft and the glans penis. In the female, extremely painful vesicles appear at the vaginal introitus on the labial folds, and sometimes on the cervix.

Herpetic infections of the newborn are acquired during passage of the infant through a birth canal infected usually with type 2 virus. Extensive vesicular eruptions appear over the scalp and face, accompanied by high fever, refusal to feed and irritability or extreme lassitude. Infants frequently die several days later, with extensive vesicular lesions in the liver and other viscera, meningitis and destruction of cerebral neurones.

LABORATORY DIAGNOSIS

Herpes simplex infections of the skin and mucous membranes are diagnosed readily by the same-day procedures[42] of electron microscopy combined with immunofluorescence (Figure 19-6). Electron microscope grids and teflon-coated immunofluorescence slides are applied directly to vesicle fluid immediately after puncturing the vesicle, or scrapings of the base of vesicles are smeared immediately on grids and slides. Grids are air-dried, treated with phosphotungstic acid and examined by electron microscopy;

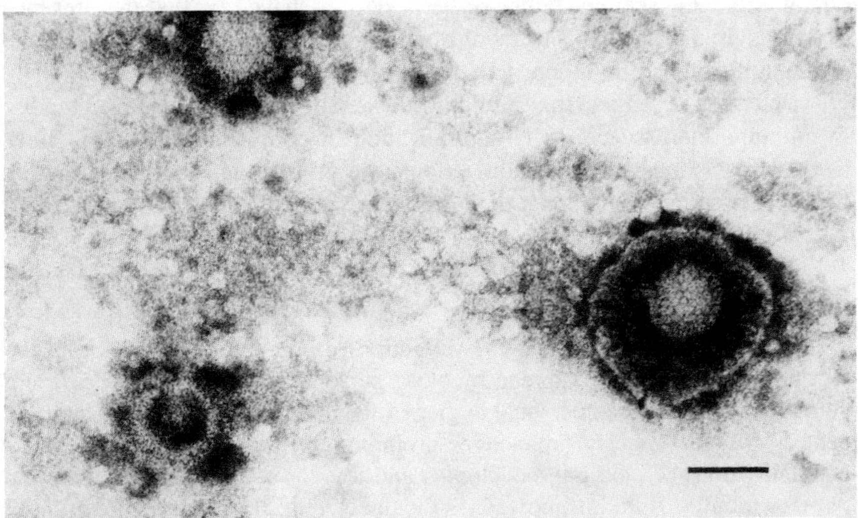

Figure 19-6: Herpesvirus-1 virions in facial vesicles (x120,120). Reproduced with permission from McLean DM and Wong KK 1984. Same-day Diagnosis of Human Virus Infections. CRC Press, Boca Raton FL, p 46.

herpesvirus virions are visualized within 1–10 minutes of examining grids from virus-positive patients. Thus a presumptive diagnosis of herpesvirus infection is given to the patient whilst he or she waits in the adjacent examination room. Effective antiviral therapy is prescribed, if appropriate, before the patient departs. Serotyping of the herpesvirus is accomplished with 1 hour by direct immunofluorescence tests, using fluorescein-labelled antisera, preferably with monoclonal antibodies[24] to type 1 and type 2 viruses.

Virus isolation is attempted by inoculation of diploid human fibroblast tissue cultures with suspensions of vesicle fluid or scrapings. Cytopathic effects consisting of grape-like clusters of cells, some of which are multinu-cleated and contain intranuclear inclusions, are observed after 1–4 days incubation at 37° C, and an increased acidity is imparted to the tissue culture medium. Fresh virus isolates are typed by immunofluorescence, as for direct smears, or by kinetic neutralization tests in tissue cultures. In herpes encephalitis, if a brain biopsy is undertaken, this material should be cut into fine pieces using two scalpels, and these fragments should be co-cultivated with a receptor monolayer culture of human diploid fibroblasts. Cytopathic effects are observed in the monolayer and the new virus isolate is serotyped by immunofluorescence or neutralization. Recent investigations using a tritium-labeled probe containing 300–400 nucleotides of herpesvirus 1 have revealed the presence of herpesvirus genome in smears of brain from one patient with acute herpetic encephalitis and in brain smears from 3 elderly psychiatric patients.[57]

Detection of herpesvirus antibodies in sera of patients is achieved readily by immunofluorescence or by neutralization or complement fixation. Since herpesvirus induces persistent infections, the presence of antibodies merely indicates an infection at some time during the patient's lifetime, and is of no use in clinical diagnosis.

EPIDEMIOLOGY

Herpes simplex is an endemic infection of communities throughout the world. Herpesviruses are spread by close personal contact, so that crowding combined with laxity in personal hygiene favours virus transmission. In urban centers, where formerly orphanages promoted spread of herpes by salivary contaminations of clothing, bedclothes and toys or other articles that can be put into mouths of infants, nowadays the daycare offers the same opportunity for virus transmission. Initial infections usually occur in infants between their first and third birthdays, which coincides with, (a) loss of maternally acquired immunity, (b) increased play activity with indiscriminate use of toys. After initial infections, patients develop neutralizing antibodies in their sera. Although recurrences of herpetic eruptions may occur at the site of initial infection on many occasions during subsequent years, antibody titers increase promptly (the secondary or booster response), and the vesicular eruptions abate within 2–3 days. During recurrences of vesicles however, patients serve as important spreaders of infections.

Heightened public awareness of herpesvirus infections, particularly those transmitted venereally, has stimulated nationwide interest in virus isolations from patients. In Canada during 1984, about 11,000 herpesvirus isolations were reported through laboratories collaborating with the World Health Organization, an increase from about 6000 in 1982, 2000 in 1980 and 1000 in 1975. Improved serotyping procedures during the 1980's have shown a type 1:type 2 ratio of about 2:3.

ANTIVIRAL THERAPY

Successful treatment of herpetic keratitis with idoxuridine suspensions in 1961 and the subsequent demonstration of therapeutic effectiveness of idoxuridine in cream applied topically to herpetic skin vesicles, stimulated the development of newer and improved antiviral agents against herpesvirus infections. Acyclovir has come into general use for topical therapy of herpesvirus infections of the lips[21] and the genitals[18] during the 1980's. Application of 5% acyclovir in a polyethylene glycol ointment 5 times daily for 5 days, shortly after eruption of herpes vesicles on the lips significantly shortened the times to formation of ulcer or crust and to complete healing, and although the duration of symptoms in treated patients was shorter than that of controls, the difference was not significant.[21] Topical application of acyclovir cream in polyethylene glycol ointment reduced the mean duration of virus shedding and shortened the healing time in primary genital herpes, and recurrent genital herpes in men but not women.[18] Oral ingestion of 200 mg acyclovir tablets 5 times daily for 5 days reduced the duration of viral excretion and shortened the healing time in primary and recurrent genital herpes.[49] Despite these encouraging early reports however, practical experience has shown less therapeutic effectiveness of acyclovir in recurrent genital herpes than in primary infections, and it should be reserved for treatment of patients with frequent recurrences.[50]

Herpetic encephalitis, although rare, has a high mortality rate, and severe neurological impairment often adversely affects the quality of life of survivors. A recent Swedish investigation,[60] involving 53 virologically confirmed cases, showed that intravenous administration of acyclovir 10 mg/kg every 8 hours significantly reduced the mortality rate to 10%, from 56% in those who received the previously licensed antiviral vidarabine; 56% of acyclovir-treated patients had returned to normal life 6 months subsequently, in contrast to 13% vidarabine-treated patients.

CHICKENPOX AND HERPES ZOSTER

CLINICAL

Chickenpox (varicella) presents with acute onset of fever and vesicles 2–3 mm diameter surrounded by red areolas 1–2 mm thick appearing over the face, scalp, trunk and proximal parts of the limbs, but rarely involving the palms of the hands or soles of the feet (Figure 19-1). Successive crops of vesicles appear over a period of 4 days. Fever usually abates after the initial 2 days. Vesicles burst after 1–2 days and become covered with scabs which separate within 7 days.

The incubation period is 14–18 days. Patients may transmit virus by droplets expelled during coughing from about 2 days before to 4 days after onset of vesicles. Apart from scabbed-over vesicles, the generalized illness resolves with 2—4 days.

Complications are rare in children. Occasionally they present with croup, due to catarrhal inflammation of the trachea and larynx. Encephalitis, which may develop 1–3 weeks after chickenpox, affected 26 per 100,000 cases in

USA during 1978,[4] with an average case fatality rate of 23%. Chickenpox may infect adults occasionally; primary varicella pneumonia is particularly likely to involve adults aged more than 50 years.

Immunosuppressed patients, especially those with leukemia or other malignancies of the reticuloendothelial system who are receiving antineoplastic chemotherapy, are at high risk for development of disseminated chickenpox. Vesicles develop in the liver and other parenchymatous organs, frequently with a fatal outcome.

Herpes zoster (shingles) comprises clusters of chickenpox-like vesicles over certain dermatomes i.e. cutaneous distribution of sensory nerves associated with a dorsal root ganglion in the spinal cord, or the trigeminal ganglion. Characteristically the vesicles affect one side only, and they do not cross the midline. For example a cluster of vesicles may extend over the 7th thoracic nerve distribution on the left side of the chest, or over the right forehead which is the cutaneous distribution of the ophthalmic division of the trigeminal nerve. In the latter instance, there is a high risk of development of corneal ulcers. Onset of vesicular formation is usually sudden, and accompanied by moderate fever; it is usually precipitated by severe emotional trauma such as sudden death of a spouse, or by severe illness, especially where immune function is suppressed as in leukemia.

The incubation period of herpes zoster is prolonged, because usually it arises from reactivation of chickenpox infection which has remained latent in posterior root or trigeminal ganglia for many years. Rarely herpes zoster may be the presenting feature of an initial chickenpox infection in an immunologically normal child, appearing 14–18 days after contact with a case of chickenpox. Usually the degree of communicability of herpes zoster is low, because transmission regularly occurs by fomites contaminated by exudates from ruptured vesicles. An immunosuppressed patient who develops pneumonia, and subsequently herpes zoster, may transmit VZ virus to relatives and health care workers.[20] Thus it is important to nurse hospitalized VZ patients in respiratory isolation facilities in order to prevent spread of infection within hospitals.

LABORATORY DIAGNOSIS

Since the causative viruses in chickenpox and herpes zoster are antigenically, culturally and morphologically identical, they are frequently termed varicella-zoster (VZ) virus and the same laboratory procedures are applied to both conditions.

Diagnosis by same-day techniques is eminently suitable in VZ infections.[42] Electron microscopic examination of negatively stained vesicle fluid or scrapings reveals typical herpesvirus virions (Figure 19-7). Antigen within

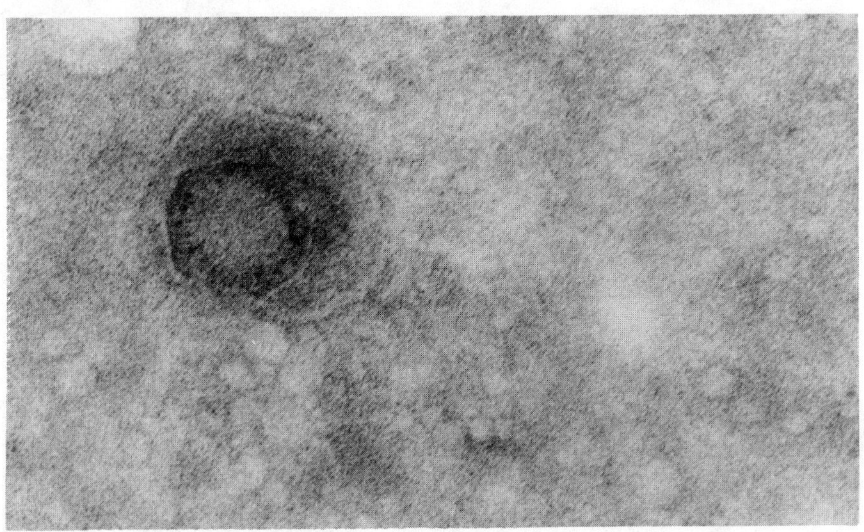

Figure 19-7: Chickenpox virions in neck vesicles of a schoolgirl with chickenpox (x120,120). Reproduced with permission from McLean DM and Wong KK 1984. Same-day Diagnosis of Human Virus Infections, CRC Press, Boca Raton FL, 108.

infected cells of vesicle fluid is serotyped as VZ using the anticomplement immunofluorescent technique.[41]

Isolation of VZ virus has been achieved with considerable difficulty by inoculation of vesicle scrapings (containing infected epithelial cells) into primary monolayer cultures of human amnion or continuous diploid human fibroblasts. Cytopathic effects consisting of grape-like clusters of swollen multinucleate cells with acidophilic intranuclear inclusions appear after 2–6 weeks incubation. Virus is passaged to additional tissue cultures by transfer of infected cells within the supernatant. The fresh virus isolate is serotyped by anticomplement immunofluorescence. A human VZ isolate, after many passages in diploid human cultures and subsequently adapted to fetal guinea-pig cells, has infected strain-2 guineapigs in a manner comparable to VZ infections in humans.[47]

Serological evidence of recent VZ infection is obtained conveniently by demonstration of rising VZ antibody titers in paired sera collected 2–4 weeks apart, using complement fixation, immune adherence hemagglutination, or indirect immunofluorescence to the VZ membrane antigen.

EPIDEMIOLOGY

Chickenpox reporting throughout USA between 1972, when nationwide reporting began, and 1982, has remained remarkably steady between 141,495 and 188,396 cases per annum, with peaks of incidence during spring between March and May of every year.[11] Highest attack rates occurred among children aged 5 to 9 years, comprising 60% of the total reported cases, whilst less than 15% of reported cases affected persons aged more than 15 years.

PREVENTION

Isolation of hospitalized varicella or herpes zoster patients, in rooms with air pressure lower than the corridor in order to prevent spread of infected droplets, is the only effective means of prevention of spread of VZ virus to date.

Currently there is no licensed varicella vaccine. In a recent clinical trial in northeastern USA with a live attenuated varicella vaccine (Oka/Merck) containing 8700 plaque forming units in 1 ml doses injected subcutaneously into 461 healthy children without antibodies, 94% showed seroconversions.[65] No cases of varicella occurred in this group during the subsequent 9 months of observation, in contrast to 39 cases among 446 placebo recipients, giving a protective efficacy of 100%.

Prophylaxis against varicella in high risk patients, especially those who are immunocompromised, is recommended using intramuscular injection of zoster-immune globulin.[51]

Treatment of immunocompromised patients who develop varicella or herpes zoster may show some clinically beneficial effects after intravenous administration of acyclovir or vidarabine, or intramuscular courses of interferon-alpha, when these antiviral substances are given less than 3 days after onset of vesicles.[51] Since each antiviral shows similar therapeutic effectiveness, acyclovir is recommended due to substantially lower costs and fewer adverse reactions.

MONONUCLEOSIS

CLINICAL

Mononucleosis presents with mild fever and malaise increasing in intensity over 3–4 days, when yellow exudate appears on the fauces accompanied by generalized non-tender enlargement of the lymph nodes in the neck, axillae and groin. Transient enlargement of the spleen and/or liver may also be noted, and traces of jaundice may appear for short intervals in a few patients. Characteristically, the peripheral blood smear shows 10% or more atypical monocytes. Mononucleosis is regularly caused by Epstein-Barr (EB) virus. Some infants may develop mild fever and pharyngitis without accompanying lymphadenopathy and atypical monocytosis following primary infection with EB virus, but these symptoms have occurred with comparable frequency among infants without EB virus infection.

The incubation period is 2–7 weeks. Symptoms persist 4–20 days after which convalescence may be slow. The duration of communicability by close personal contact between mucous membranes, as in kissing, extends for 8 days after onset. Mononucleosis may also be spread by blood transfusions, particularly when the recipient is immunosuppressed.

LABORATORY DIAGNOSIS

Isolation of EB virus from throat specimens and the buffy coat of plasma is extremely difficult and it is not undertaken routinely. Inoculation of primary cultures of human leucocytes is required; these are derived either from peripheral blood of adults after phytohemagglutinin stimulation and placing on feeder layers of human placental cells, or from umbilical cord blood. The cells undergo lymphoblastoid transformation after 3–5 weeks of incubation at 37° C, when they exhibit rounding, heaping up, and they impart increased acidity to the maintenance medium.

Serological tests provide several routine procedures for laboratory diagnosis of mononucleosis due to EB virus infection.

(a) The Paul Bunnell (heterophil agglutinin) reaction becomes positive 1 week or more after onset. Sheep erythrocytes are agglutinated regularly by sera from mononucleosis patients at titers of 32 or higher, after absorption with guineapig kidney and beef cell antigens to remove non-specific reactants. This is a technically simple procedure. However it will not detect cytomegalovirus infection which accounts for about 15% of cases with clinically typical mononucleosis.[32]

(b) Immunofluorescence tests are employed routinely to detect antibodies to several components of EB virus following infection.[22] (i) After primary infection in infants, antibodies to the viral capsid antigen (VCA), initially within the IgM component, are first detected at 2–4 weeks. Although the IgM antibody becomes undetectable within 2 months, the IgG antibody persists many years. Antibodies to the restricted component of the early antigen (EA) are first detected at 6–8 weeks, and persist 6–12 months. Antibodies to the diffuse component of EA appear in older patients with infectious mononucleosis 3–4 weeks after onset and persist about 6 months, but they do not appear in infants. Antibodies to the Epstein-Barr nuclear antigen (EBNA) are first detected 3–4 months after infection and persist many years. The single most valuable serological test for detection of EB virus infection is demonstration of VCA antibodies, particularly in the IgM component of serum.

EPIDEMIOLOGY

Clusters of mononucleosis cases usually occur among teenagers or young adults 2–7 weeks after periods of close personal contact including kissing, which presumably promotes direct transfer of infected saliva. Typically, students in residential colleges develop mononucleosis several weeks after their return to North American campuses following the Christmas vacation. Clinically inapparent primary EB infections have occurred among 17.5% infants in Philadelphia.[22]

In tropical East Africa, the clinical manifestation of EB virus infection among the native population is Burkitt's lymphoma.[2]

CYTOMEGALOVIRUS

CLINICAL

Cytomegalovirus (CMV) infection in immunologically normal youths and adults is usually asymptomatic, and it is detected, for example in pregnant women during antenatal surveillance, by seroconversions or IgM antibody determination.[55,62] Immunologically compromised children and adults, however, are at high risk of developing clinically manifested CMV infections which resemble mononucleosis with high fever, often accompanied by lymphocytosis with more than 10% abnormal leukocytes, but the Paul Bunnell and EB-VCA-IgM tests remain negative. Cytomegalovirus pneumonia is an important and severe opportunistic infection in recipients of transplants of bone marrow where it affects 15% of subjects and carries a 90% mortality rate.[27] Other immunosuppressed patients who frequently develop CMV opportunistic infections are recipients of organ transplants, especially kidneys[52] and those with the acquired immunodeficiency syndrome (AIDS).

Cytomegalovirus infection, which is acquired antenatally, is manifested clinically in newborn babies as one or more of microcephaly, mental retardation, chorioretinitis, optic atrophy, hepatosplenomegaly, jaundice and thrombocytopenic purpura. Infants may die within a few weeks or months, or they may survive at least 2 years and show microcephaly, spastic quadriplegia, optic atrophy, severe psychomotor retardation, bilateral hearing loss and pneumonitis, especially in those with birth weight light for gestational age.[55]

Congenital CMV infection may be transmitted transplacentally to the fetus at any stage during pregnancy that the mother contracts a primary or recurrent CMV infection. In London, England, the rate of congenital CMV infections in infants was 3 per 1000[55] and in Birmingham, Alabama it was 5 per 1000[62] but only 50% of maternal infections were transmitted to infants. About 60% of infected newborns showed no anomalies and remained asymptomatic 2 years later, 7% continued to show severe neurological damage and 33% had minor or transient abnormalities in the English series[55] whilst in the Alabama series about 75% of infected infants were asymptomatic, 9% has severe neurological damage and 16% had hepatosplenomegaly and jaundice.[62] Urinary excretion of CMV persisted at least 12 months in asymptomatically infected infants, at mean titers of 3000 TCD_{50}/ml, which was about tenfold lower than the mean at birth.[62] Infants with congenital anomalies also excrete CMV in urine for more than one year. Experience in many hospitals has shown that when allied health and medical personnel vigorously follow "isolation procedures" i.e. wearing of gloves and gowns and wash the hands thoroughly between attending each patient, there is no addition risk of contraction of CMV infection above the normal risk of the entire community.

LABORATORY DIAGNOSIS

Urine is the best specimen for attempts at isolation of CMV by inoculation of diploid human fibroblast cultures, which develop grape-like clusters of rounded cells and multinucleate cells after 1–4 weeks of incubation. Passage of the new isolate to other fibroblast cultures requires transfer of cells as well as supernatant fluid, because the virus is strongly cell-bound. Immediate inoculation of tissue cultures with freshly passed urine is highly desirable, but the specimen may be held overnight at 4° C (not frozen), if fibroblast cultures are not available immediately. However the virus in patients' urine is inactivated rapidly by freezing. Fresh virus isolates are serotyped in tissue culture neutralization tests or by the anticomplement immunofluorescence technique. The same procedures are used for attempts at isolation of CMV from various organs of fatal cases.

Rapid detection of CMV antigen in exfoliated cells in urine, saliva, blood and bronchoalveolar lavage specimens, has been achieved by detection of early antigen fluorescent foci in diploid human fibroblast cultures after 24 hours incubation, using monoclonal antibodies in mouse ascitic fluid.[26] Frozen sections of lung biopsies from CMV-infected patients with hematological malignancies revealed CMV antigen readily in immunofluorescence tests employing mouse monoclonal antibodies.[27] In situ hybridization with a biotinylated CMV probe has also detected CMV infection in formalin-fixed paraffin-embedded sections of lung biopsies within one day.[48]

Serological methods are important for detection of past and present CMV infections. Whilst good results are obtained using the relatively insensitive complement fixation test, enzyme immunoassay (ELISA) and indirect immunofluorescence provide convenient and more sensitive contemporary techniques.

EPIDEMIOLOGY

Serological evidence of past CMV infection was found among 56% pregnant women attending antenatal clinics in London, England[55] and 65% antenatal patients in Birmingham, Alabama.[62] In the latter center, 45% were susceptible to CMV infection among members of the upper socioeconomic group and 1.4% developed primary CMV infection during pregnancy, in contrast to 18% susceptibles among the lower socioeconomic category, of whom 2.2% developed primary CMV infections during pregnancy. Recurrences of CMV infection during pregnancy involved 0.5% and 3.5% women in the two groups respectively. However only 1 of 21 primary infections exhibited symptoms resembling mononucleosis. Transplacental attack rates among offspring of infected mothers were 3 per 1000 in England and 5 per 1000 in Alabama.

Heterosexual contact appears to be an important mechanism of transfer of CMV among some young adult couples. Antibody to CMV by ELISA tests was found in 74% of 42 men whose female consorts were seropositive, in contrast to 31% of 16 men whose partners were seronegative.[28] Semen or urine from 22% of 18 men yielded CMV isolates when their female partners excreted CMV from the cervix or urine, in contrast to none of 42 men whose partners did not yield CMV isolates. Common strains were found to infect two couples, using DNA restriction enzyme typing of the CMV isolates.

Among renal transplant patients, CMV infection may involve 60% seronegative recipients, and 90% seropositive patients who are immunosuppressed and therefore highly susceptible to an opportunistic CMV infection. Reactivation of CMV infection probably occurs in seropositive recipients. Recipients of blood transfusions may also acquire primary CMV infections. In most cases the infections are asymptomatic.

In an intensive care unit where 8 infants excreting CMV were nursed during a period of 4 months, CMV strains from 3 babies were identical in restriction-endonuclease-digestion analyses.[61] It seemed likely that one baby transmitted CMV to the other 2 infants through contaminated unidentified fomites. Provided that adequate "isolation nursing" procedures are carried out rigorously, the health care personnel in intensive care units are not at increased risk of contracting CMV infection.

Present evidence indicates that acyclovir, interferon-alpha and other antiviral substances have little or no effectiveness in the prophylaxis and treatment of CMV infections.[51] Ganciclovir [9-(1,3 dihydroxy-2-propoxymethyl)] guanine has shown promising therapeutic effectiveness.

MUMPS

CLINICAL

Mumps presents with swelling of one or both parotid glands, along with redness and pouting of the orifices of the parotid (Stensen's) duct, dryness of the mouth and moderate fever with temperature 38–39° C; it is caused by infection with mumps virus. Bilateral parotitis occurs in about 70% of cases. Parotitis characteristically causes painful bulging of the skin around and under the angle of the mandible anterior to the sternomastoid muscle, thus distinguishing it from cervical lymphadenopathy which causes painful swelling deep and posterior to the sternomastoid. Submandibular salivary glands may be enlarged and tender in 5–10% of cases.

The incubation period of mumps is 14–18 days. The period of communicability by droplets or saliva usually ranges from 2 days before to 4 days after onset of parotitis and fever. Fever and malaise usually persist 2–3 days, swelling of the parotid and/or submandibular glands may persist 4–7 days.

Complications of mumps commonly include: (i) orchitis affecting overall about 5% of males, but attaining 18% in adult men; (ii) oophoritis affecting about 5% of postpubertal females; (iii) pancreatitis affecting about 7% cases; (iv) meningitis (meningoencephalitis) affecting 0.5–2% of cases. Less frequent complications include: (v) presternal edema or thyroiditis; (vi) arthritis; (vii) polyneuritis plus central hypertension; (viii) encephalitis with perivascular demyelination in 154 per 100,000 cases of mumps in USA during 1978[4] with an average case fatality rate of 1.3%; (ix) deafness which although rare, is usually permanent.

Mumps meningitis begins 6 days before to 14 days after onset of parotitis. Meningitis without swelling of parotid or submandibular glands may occur in about one third of laboratory confirmed cases of mumps meningitis.[38] Mumps meningitis affects males 2–3 times more commonly than females. Clinical features include high fever, neck stiffness, positive Kernig's or Brudzinski's signs, vomiting, headache, irritability and a high count of lymphocytes in CSF without significant alteration of the glucose, protein or chloride contents. Febrile convulsions may herald the onset of mumps meningitis in 5–10% children. Meningeal signs usually resolve within 2–3 days, especially after lumbar puncture, but neck stiffness, irritability and fever may persist as long as 1 week in 1:6 subjects.

LABORATORY DIAGNOSIS

Mumps virus is isolated from patients with parotitis by inoculation of primary monkey kidney tissue cultures with saliva suspended in maintenance medium. Infected cultures show syncytia after 3–7 days' incubation at 35–

37° C. The isolate is typed by HI or immunofluorescence as for influenza virus.

In mumps meningitis, CSF is collected by lumbar puncture as a regular clinical diagnostic procedure. Same-day identification of mumps virus in CSF[42] is achieved readily by observation of paramyxovirus particles (Figure 8-8) in negatively stained preparations examined by electron microscopy which are serotyped as mumps by immunofluorescence. Mumps virus is isolated readily from CSF by inoculation of monkey kidney tissue cultures.

Serological techniques of HI and S-CF reveal the presence of mumps antibodies in patient's sera 1–2 days after defervescence which occurs usually 2–4 days after onset.[41] Neutralizing and HI antibodies persist 20 years or more, S-CF antibodies become undetectable after about 6 months.

EPIDEMIOLOGY

During 1967, when live attenuated mumps vaccine was first licensed in USA, 185,691 cases were reported. During the preceding 50 years, the annual incidence rates per 100,000 ranged from about 90 to 220, with peaks of incidence approximately every third year (Figure 19-8).[14] The incidence has

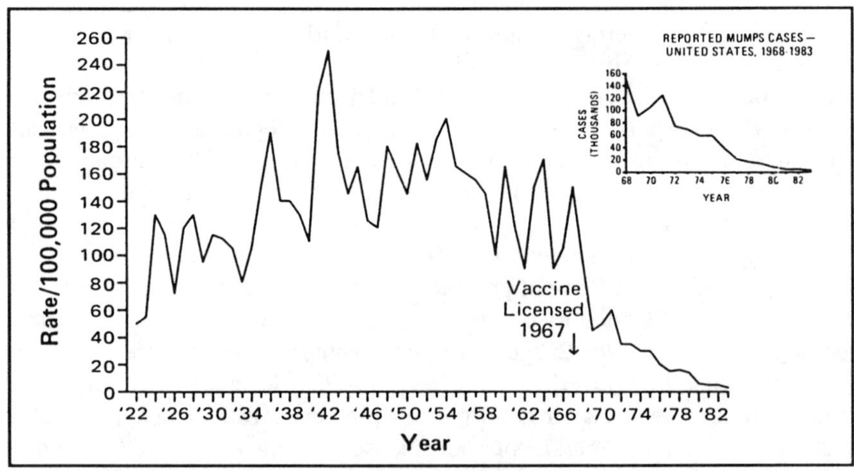

Figure 19-8: Mumps incidence rates (per 100,000 per annum) United States 1922–1983. Reproduced with permission from Centers for Disease Control MMWR 33:533, 1984.

declined steadily from 1972 with 74,215 cases (38 per 100,000), to 1983 with 3355 cases (1.4 per 100,000). Currently the incidence rates, as in the prevaccine era, are highest among school-age children 5–14 years old. In common with measles and rubella, mumps attack rates are usually highest during winter and spring. Mumps meningitis also occurs largely during the cooler months, in contradistinction to enteroviral meningitis which occurs mainly during summer and autumn (Chapter 23).

PREVENTION

Live attenuated mumps vaccine containing 5000 TCD_{50} per dose is administered subcutaneously to all infants at 12–15 months, usually in combination with live measles and rubella vaccines as a trivalent product. This induces mumps antibodies in more than 90% susceptible recipients; both antibodies and protection against natural infection persist at least 15 years.[8] The protective efficacy is about 75–90%. Adverse effects are minimal. Rigorous implementation of a nationwide policy of vaccination of all infants immediately after their first birthdays, combined with vaccination upon school entry of children who did not receive mumps vaccine during infancy, has resulted in the virtual elimination of indigenous mumps from United States residents since 1983. In 1989, meningoencephalitis was reported in less than 1 per million vaccine recipients.

REFERENCES

[1]Broughton CR: Morbilli in Sydney: a review of 3601 cases with consideration of morbidity, mortality and measles encephalomyelitis. Med J Austral 2:859, 1964.

[2]Burkitt DP: Determining the climatic limitations of a children's cancer common in Africa. Brit Med J 2:1019, 1962.

[3]Centers for Disease Control: Rubella Surveillance, Jan 1976–Dec 1978, issued May 1980.

[4]Centers for Disease Control: Encephalitis Surveillance Annual Summary 1978, Issued May 1981.

[5]Centers for Disease Control: Enterovirus Surveillance Report, 1970–1979, Issued Nov. 1981.

[6]Centers for Disease Control: Measles Surveillance Report No. 11, 1977–1981, issued September 1982.

[7]Centers for Disease Control: Measles Prevention. MMWR 31:217, 1982.

[8]Centers for Disease Control: Mumps Vaccine MMWR 31:617, 1982.

[9]Centers for Disease Control: Rubella in Hospitals - California. MMWR 32:37, 1983.

[10]Centers for Disease Control: Imported measles with subsequent airborne transmission in a pediatrician's office - Michigan. MMWR 32:401, 1983.

[11]Centers for Disease Control: Annual Summary 1982. MMWR 31(54), 1983.

[12]Centers for Disease Control: Rubella prevention. MMWR 33:301, 1984.

[13]Centers for Disease Control: Rubella and congenital rubella syndrome - United States, 1983–1984. MMWR 33:528, 1984.

[14]Centers for Disease Control: Mumps - United States, 1983–1984. MMWR 33:533, 1984.

[15]Centers for Disease Control: Measles - United States, first 39 weeks, 1984. MMWR 33:673, 1984.

[16]Connolly JH, Allen IV, Hurwitz LJ, Miller JHD: Measles virus antibody and antigen in subacute sclerosing panencephalitis. Lancet 1:542, 1967.

[17]Connolly JH, Haire M, Hadden DSM: Measles immunoglobulins in subacute sclerosing panencephalitis. Brit Med J 1:23, 1971.

[18]Corey L, Nahmias AJ, Guinan ME, Benedetti JK, Critchlow CW, Holmes KK: A trial of topical acyclovir in genital herpes simplex virus infection. New Eng J Med 306:1313, 1982.

[19]Douglas JWB: Ability and adjustment of children who have had measles. Brit Med J 2:1301, 1964.

[20]Faizallah R, Green HT, Krasner N, Walker RJ: Outbreak of chickenpox from a patient with immunosuppressed herpes zoster in hospital. Brit Med J 285: 1022, 1982.

[21]Fiddian AP, Yeo JM, Stubbings R, Dean D: Successful treatment of herpes labialis with topical acyclovir. Brit Med J 286:1699, 1983.

[22]Fleischer G, Henle W, Henle G, Lennette ET, Biggar RJ: Primary infection with Epstein-Barr virus in infants in the United States: clinical and serological observations. J Infect Dis 139:553, 1979.

[23]Fulginiti VA, Eller JJ, Downie AW, Kempe CH. Altered reactivity to measles virus. JAMA 202:1075, 1967.

[24]Goldstein LC, Corey L, McDougall JK, Tolentino E, Nowinski RC: Monoclonal antibodies to herpes simplex viruses: use in antigenic typing and rapid diagnosis. J Infect Dis 147:829, 1983.

[25]Greenburg M, Pellitteri O, Eisenstein DT: Measles encephalitis. I. Prophylactic effect of gamma globulin. J Pediat 46:642, 1955.

[26]Griffiths PD, Parjwani DD, Stirk PR, Ball MG, Ganczakowski M, Blacklock HA, Prentice HG: Rapid detection of cytomegalovirus infection in immunocompromised patients by detection of early antigen fluorescent foci. Lancet 2:1242, 1984.

[27]Hackman RC, Myerson D, Myers JD, Shulman HM, Sale GE, Goldstein LC, Rastetter M, Flournoy N, Thomas ED: Rapid diagnosis of cytomegaloviral pneumonia by tissue immunofluorescence with a murine monoclonal antibody. J Infect Dis 151:325, 1985.

[28]Handsfield HH, Chandler SH, Caine VA, Meyers JD, Corey L, Medeiros E, McDougall JK: Cytomegalovirus infection in sex partners: evidence for sexual transmission. J Infect Dis 151:344, 1985.

[29]Hatch MH, Malison MD, Palmer EL: Isolation of enterovirus 70 from patient with acute hemorrhagic conjunctivitis in Key West, Florida. New Eng J Med 305:1648, 1981.

[30]Johnson RT, Griffin DE, Hirsch RL, Wolinsky JS, Roedenbeck S, Lindo de Soriano I, Vaisberg A: Measles encephalomyelitis—clinical and immunological studies. New Eng J Med 310:137, 1984.

[31]Karelitz S, Eisenberg M: Measles encephalitis. Pediatrics 27:811, 1961.

[32]Klemola E, Kaariainen L: Cytomegalovirus as a possible cause of a disease resembling infectious mononucleosis. Brit Med J 2:1099, 1965.

[33]Kogan A, Hall CE, Cooney MK, Fox JP: Measles in readiness for reading and learning. IV. Shoreline School District study. Am J Epidemiol 88:351, 1968.

[34]Kono R: Apollo 11 disease or acute hemorrhagic conjunctivitis: a pandemic of a new enterovirus infection of the eyes. Am J Epidemiol 101:383, 1975.

[35]McLean DM, Melnick JL: Association of mouse pathogenic strain of ECHO virus

type 9 with aseptic meningitis. Proc Soc Exp Biol Med 94:656, 1957.

[36]McLean DM, Best JM, Smith PA, Larke RPB, McNaughton GA: Viral infections of Toronto children during 1965. II. Measles encephalitis and other complications. Can Med Ass J 94:905, 1966.

[37]McLean DM: Aseptic Meningitis, in Recent Advances in Medical Microbiology, ed. AP Waterson, J and A Churchill, London 1967. p. 66.

[38]McLean DM, Larke RPB, Cobb C, Griffis ED, Hackett SMR: Mumps and enteroviral meningitis in Toronto, 1966. Can Med Ass J 96:1355, 1967.

[39]McLean DM, Kettyls GDM, Hingston J, Moore PS, Paris RP, Rigg JM: Atypical measles following immunization with killed measles vaccine. Can Med Ass J 103:743, 1970.

[40]McLean DM: Virology in Health Care. Williams and Wilkins, Baltimore, 1980. pp 60 and 137.

[41]McLean DM: Immunological Investigation of Human Virus Diseases. Churchill Livingstone, Edinburgh, 1982 p 74.

[42]McLean DM, Wong KK: Same-Day Diagnosis of Human Virus Infections. CRC Press, Boca Raton FL, 1984, pp 46–55.

[43]Miller DL: Frequency of complication of measles. Brit Med J 2:75, 1964.

[44]Mitus A, Enders JF, Craig JM, Holloway A: Persistence of measles virus and depression of antibody formation in patients with giant-cell pneumonia after measles. New Eng J Med 261:882, 1959.

[45]Modlin JF, Brandling-Bennett AD, Witte JJ, Campbell CC, Meyers JD: A review of five years' experience with rubella vaccine in the United States. Pediatrics 55:20, 1975.

[46]Morley D: Severe measles in the Tropics. Brit Med J 1:297 and 363, 1969.

[47]Myers MG, Stanberry LR, Edmond BJ: Varicella-zoster virus infection of strain 2 guinea pigs. J Infect Dis 151:106, 1985.

[48]Myerson D, Hackman RC, Myers JD: Diagnosis of cytomegalovirus pneumonia by in situ hybridization. J Infect Dis 150:272, 1984.

[49]Nilsen AE, Aasen T, Halsos AM, Kinge BR, Tjotta EAL, Wikstrom K, Fiddian AP: Efficacy of oral acyclovir in the treatment of initial and recurrent genital herpes. Lancet 2:571, 1982.

[50]Nicholson KG: Antiviral therapy: respiratory infections, genital herpes and herpetic keratitis. Lancet 2:617, 1984.

[51]Nicholson KG: Antiviral therapy: varicella-zoster infections, herpes labialis and mucocutaneous herpes, and cytomegalovirus infections. Lancet 2:677, 1984.

[52]Nunan TO, Banatvala JE: Cytomegalovirus infections in renal transplant recipients. Brit Med J 288:1477, 1984.

[53]O'Shea S, Best JM, Banatvala JE, Marshall WC, Dudgeon JA: Persistence of rubella antibody 8–18 years after vaccination. Brit Med J 288:1043, 1984.

[54]O'Shea S, Best JM, Banatvala JE, Shepherd WM: Development and persistence of class-specific antibodies in the serum and nasopharyngeal washings of rubella vaccinees. J Infect Dis 151:89, 1985.

[55]Peckham CS, Chin KS, Coleman JC, Henderson K, Hurley R, Preece PM: Cytomegalovirus infections in pregnancy: preliminary findings from a prospective study. Lancet 1:1352, 1983.

[56]Pitt D, Keir EH: Results of rubella in pregnancy. Med J Austral 2:647 and 739, 1965.

[57]Sequiera LW, Jennings LC, Carrasco LH, Lord MA, Curry A, Sutton RNP: Detection of herpes-simplex viral genome in brain tissue. Lancet 2:609, 1979.

[58]Sheridan MD: Final report of prospective study of children whose mothers have rubella in early pregnancy. Brit Med J 2:536, 1964.

[59]Sherman FE, Michaels RH, Kenny FM: Acute encephalopathy (encephalitis) complicating rubella. JAMA 192:675, 1965.

[60]Skoldenberg B, Forsgren M, Alestig K, Bergstrom T, Burman L, Dahlquist E, Forkman A, Fryden A, Lovgren K, Norlin K, Norrby R, Olding-Stenkirst E, Stiernstedt G, Uhnoo I, De Vahl K: Acyclovir versus vidarabine in herpes simplex encephalitis. Lancet 2:707, 1984.

[61]Spector SA: Transmission of cytomegalovirus among infants in hospital documented by restriction-endonuclease-digestion analyses. Lancet 1:378, 1983.

[62]Stagno S, Pass RF, Dworsky ME, Henderson RE, Moore EG, Walton PD, Alford CA: Congenital cytomegalovirus infection. The relative importance of primary and recurrent maternal infection. New Eng J Med 306:945, 1982.

[63]Swanson BE: Measles meningoencephalitis. Am J Dis Child 92:273, 1956.

[64]Waterman SH, Casas-Benabe R, Hatch MH, Bailey RE, Munoz-Jimenez R, Ramirez-Ramierez R, Rodriguez-Bigas M: Acute conjunctivitis in Puerto Rico, 1981–1982. Am J Epidemiol 120:395, 1984.

[65]Weibel RE, Neff BJ, Kuter BJ, Guess HA, Rothenberger CA, Fitzgerald AJ, Connor KA, McLean AA, Hilleman MR, Buynak EB, Scolnick EM: Live attenuated varicella virus vaccine. Efficacy trial in healthy children. New Eng J Med 310:1409, 1984.

[66]Wolontis S, Jeansson S: Correlation of herpes simplex virus types 1 and 2 with clinical features of infection. J Infect Dis 135:28, 1977.

CHAPTER 20

GASTROENTERITIS

CLINICAL

Viral gastroenteritis of infants and children presents typically with passage of 4–10 or more loose watery yellow-green stools during the preceding 1–2 days,[9,10] often accompanied by repeated vomiting. This leads to dehydration, the extent of which corresponds to the excessive loss of fluid and electrolyte. Some patients may pass watery green stools explosively, others may pass a series of mushy stools which become more frequent over 2–3 days. Some patients with chronic diarrhea may suddenly or progressively develop acute diarrhea. Signs of dehydration include dry glazed lips and tongue, sunken eyeballs, lack of skin turgor and doughy abdomen. Among pediatric patients hospitalized with gastroenteritis in Vancouver, Canada, correction of dehydration by intravenous infusion of fluids and electrolytes is required in about 25% patients.[9] Occasional deaths have been attributed to rotavirus gastroenteritis.[12] Rotavirus infection has increased the rate of hospitalization of gastroenteritis patients in pediatric practices.[7]

LABORATORY DIAGNOSIS

Causative viruses in gastroenteritis are usually identified by morphological or immunological techniques because most agents are not readily cultivated using routine procedures for virus isolation. Virus species include rotavirus, adenovirus, astrovirus, calicivirus, coronavirus and other small round viruses such as parvovirus and picornavirus-like particles.

Electron microscopy of negatively stained aqueous suspensions of fecal matter collected during the initial 1–5 days after onset of loose stools provides the best single method of detection of all causative viruses in gastroenteritis.[10] Feces is placed in a snap-cap or screw-cap container for transport to the laboratory where it is dispensed in 2 ml water (Figure 20-1), a drop is placed on an electron microscope grid, dried in air, a drop of 2% phosphotungstic acid pH 6.2–6.5 is added, held for 30 seconds, excess fluid is blotted away,

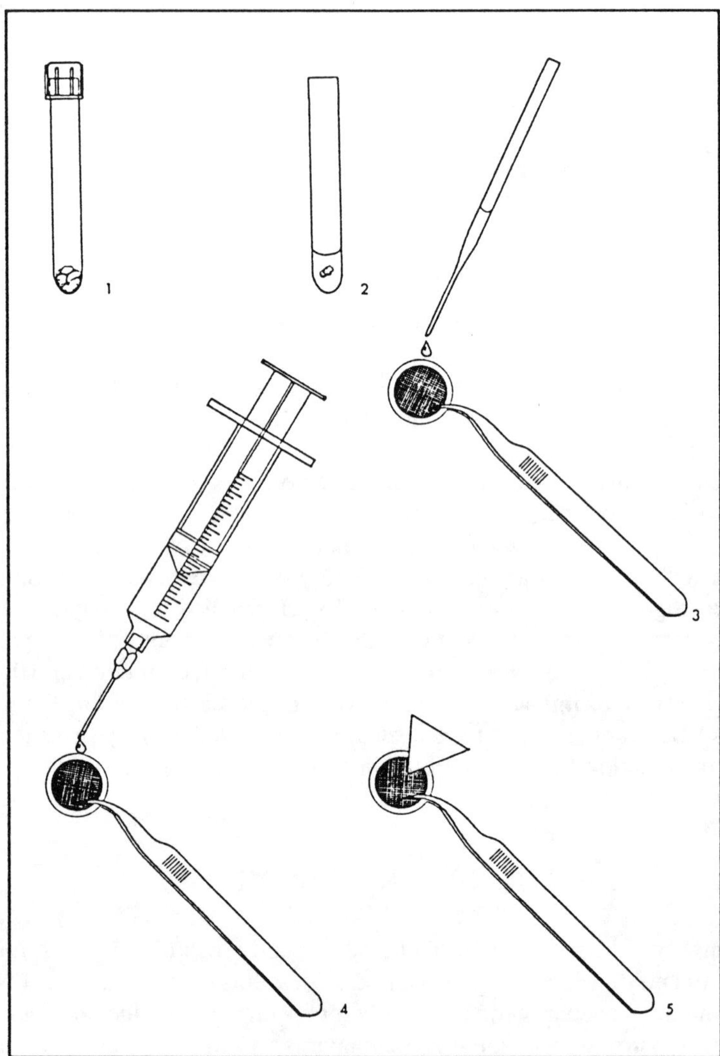

Figure 20-1: Direct electron microscopic examination of feces. Reproduced with permission from McLean DM and Wong KK 1984. Same-day Diagnosis of Human Virus Infections. CRC Press, Boca Raton FL, p 10.

(1) Colelct feces in snap-cap container

(2) Place 1 g (approx.) feces in 2 ml sterile water

(3) Add drop fecal extract to EM grid

(4) Add drop phosphotungstic acid

(5) Blot grid dry, examine in electron microscope

and the grid is dried in air for 5 minutes. The grid is examined in an electron microscope, scanning initially at 2000 x magnification and appropriate areas are examined more closely at magnification up to 200,000 x, where the stain is neither too heavy nor too light. Virions appear as lighter objects against a darkly stained background. Virus particles are regularly observed within the initial 5–10 minutes of examination, thus providing a convenient same-day diagnostic procedure (Figure 20-2). Results are delayed until the next day whenever immunoelectron microscopic techniques are employed.

Enzyme immunoassay (ELISA) offers a convenient alternative same-day test for identification of rotaviruses or other non-cultivable agents in feces of gastroenteritis patients.[16] However it suffers from the substantial disadvantage that only a particular virus species can be detected, in contradistinction to electron microscopy which reveals all of the causative virus species. Briefly 96-well plastic Immulon® plates are coated with goat antiserum to human rotavirus diluted 1:10,000, fecal extracts from patients are added, plates are incubated for 10 minutes at 37° C, then peroxidase-labelled rabbit IgG antibody to rotavirus diluted 1:200 is added without washing, incubated at 37° C for 10 minutes, washed, and substrate (peroxide-O-phenylenediamine) is added. The brown colour which develops within 10 minutes is quantitated in a microplate colorimeter.

EPIDEMIOLOGY

Viral gastroenteritis commonly affects infants and children aged less than 5 years. Although the disease is encountered year-round in most Temperature Zone communities, the highest monthly incidence rates occur during the cooler months of winter and spring which, in Northern Hemisphere communities such as Vancouver, Canada (Table 20-1) is between December and May. For example in Vancouver between 1976 and 1983, virions were identified by electron microscopy in feces from 393 to 1258 (31.2%) consecutive hospital admissions with gastroenteritis.[8] Of the 6 morphological categories of virion visualized, the commonest was rotavirus affecting 20.7% patients with other virions in decreasing frequency: adenovirus 5.6%, coronavirus and picornavirus-like particles each 1.7% and the combined total of astrovirus plus calicivirus 1.5%. The results paralleled those obtained in other centers such as Glasgow, Scotland,[11] Washington D.C.[2] and Michigan.[7] The relative risk of hospitalization of rotavirus gastroenteritis in Michigan practices was 2.8 times greater than non-rotavirus cases.[7] The relative risk increased fourfold between 6 months and 2 years because the absolute risk of hospitalization from non-rotavirus diarrhea decreased more rapidly with age than the absolute risk of rotavirus diarrhea. In pediatric practices, annual

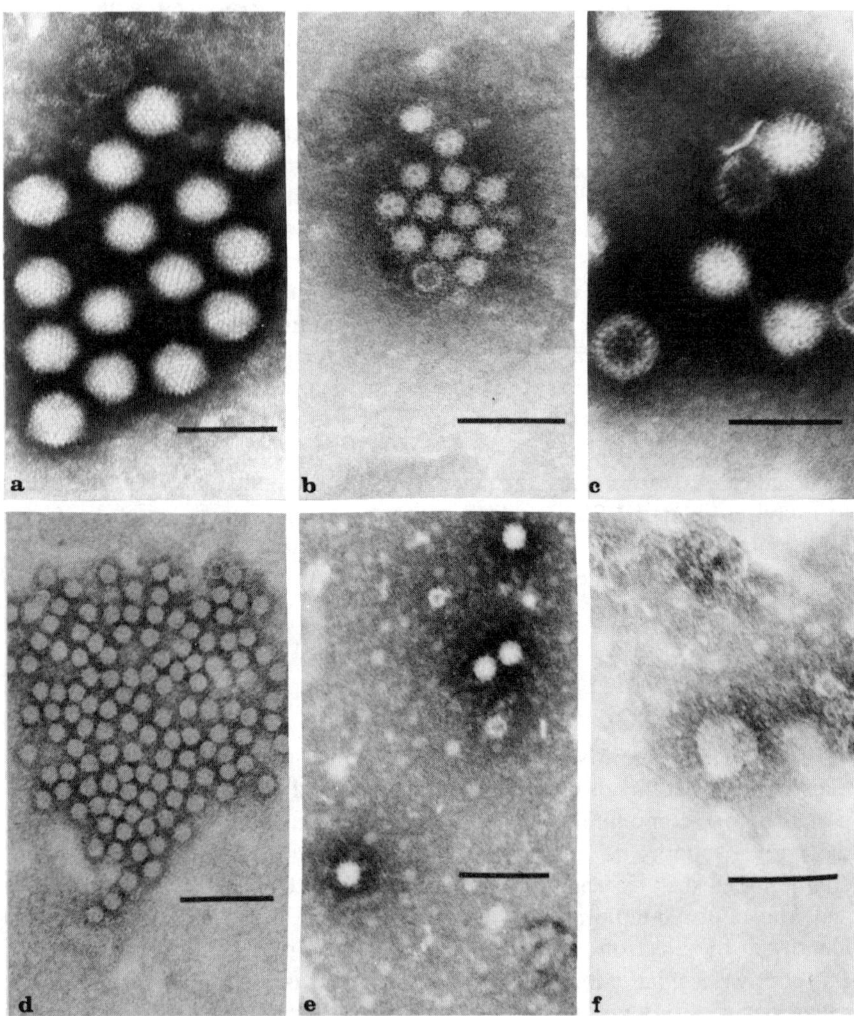

Figure 20-2: Virions in feces of patients with acute gastroenteritis.
a. Adenovirus (x161,700)   b. Calicivirus (x148,500)
c. Rotavirus (x185,625)   d. Picornavirus (x148,500)
e. Astrovirus (x148,500)   f. Coronavirus (x178,200).

rates of diarrhea during the initial 12 months of life were 0.82 per child, falling to 0.42 in the second year and to 0.02 after 5 years of age.

Rotavirus infection of newborn infants in Melbourne, Australia reduced significantly the rate of occurrence of severe and mild gastroenteritis following subsequent reinfection with rotavirus during the initial 3 years of life, although it did not alter the rate of reinfection.[1]

Four serotypes of human rotaviruses are currently recognized through the use of plaque reduction and tube neutralization tests for those strains which can be cultivated serially on MA104 or primary grivet monkey kidney cells.[15] In Birmingham, England a shift was observed in the dominant serotype between 1982 and 1983.[13] A fifth serotype was identified recently.

Episodes of gastroenteritis affecting small communities of adults have been attributed to calciviruses resembling the Norwalk agent at Snow Mountain, Colorado,[4] and also at Rome, Georgia[5] where illness was associated with drinking water from a large municipal water system. An outbreak of gastroenteritis due to the Norwalk-like agent which affected elderly residents in a Baltimore nursing home during December 1980 appeared to be spread by person-to-person contact.[6]

Adenoviruses have comprised a small but persistent proportion (about 5%) of the total cases of pediatric gastroenteritis in several centers,[2,3,10] with a somewhat greater prevalence during winter. Similarly coronaviruses have been associated with a small proportion of gastroenteritis cases in many centers, but in Vancouver they were observed more frequently in patients with anatomical or immunological abnormalities of the alimentary tract more frequently than other virions.[8]

PREVENTION

Prevention of spread of rotavirus and other viruses including gastroenteritis is achieved in hospitals through meticulous attention to adequate handwashing and the use of individual gowns whilst examining each patient, all of whom are nursed in rooms dedicated to enteric isolation.

Recently a live oral rotavirus vaccine of bovine origin has been developed for human administration.[14] Development of antibodies in more than 70% of adult and child recipients of vaccine, in the absence of severe adverse reactions, gives promise of an effective prophylactic against rotavirus gastroenteritis.

REFERENCES

[1]Bishop RF, Barnes GL, Cipriani E, Lund JS: Clinical immunity after neonatal rotavirus infection. A prospective longitudinal study in young children. New Eng J Med 309:72, 1983.

TABLE 20-1
GASTROENTERITIS, VANCOUVER CHILDREN, 1976–1983

Month	Rota				Adeno				Ast Cal			
	76 to 80	81	82	83	76 to 80	81	82	83	76 to 80	81	82	83
Jan.	25	11	20	0	3	0	3	0	1	0	0	0
Feb.	22	7	13	2	6	2	2	0	0	0	0	0
March	21	12	8	3	5	1	0	1	2	0	0	0
April	13	4	5	1	4	0	1	1	0	0	0	1
May	10	10	8	2	5	1	0	0	2	0	0	0
June	8	1	1	1	3	3	0	1	2	0	0	0
July	5	0	0	0	3	0	0	1	0	0	0	0
August	2	1	0	0	3	1	0	0	1	0	0	0
Sept.	2	0	0	1	2	0	1	0	3	0	0	0
Oct.	2	0	0	0	2	1	0	0	0	0	0	0
Nov.	7	0	0	0	7	0	0	0	1	0	0	0
Dec.	19	12	1	1	4	3	0	0	2	0	0	0
TOTAL:	136	58	56	11	47	12	7	4	18	0	0	1
ALL:	261 20.7%				70 5.6%				19 1.5%			

TABLE 20-1 (Continued)
GASTROENTERITIS, VANCOUVER CHILDREN, 1976–1983

Picorna				Corona				Total Annual				Overall	
76 to 80	81	82	83	76 to 80	81	82	83	76 to 80	81	82	83	NO.	%
1	0	1	0	0	0	0	0	30/78	11/26	24/40	0/1	65/145	44.8
2	0	0	0	0	3	1	0	30/92	12/27	16/23	2/4	60/146	41.1
3	3	0	0	0	0	0	1	31/99	16/25	8/16	5/13	60/153	39.2
1	0	0	0	0	1	1	4	18/72	5/19	7/19	7/9	37/119	31.1
5	0	0	0	0	0	0	2	22/85	11/20	8/12	4/10	45/127	35.4
0	0	0	0	0	0	0	2	13/70	4/10	1/1	4/10	22/91	24.2
0	0	0	0	0	0	0	0	8/44	0/6	0/3	1/11	9/64	14.1
1	0	0	0	0	0	0	0	7/43	2/11	0/3	0/5	9/62	14.5
1	1	0	0	0	1	0	1	8/57	2/6	1/9	2/10	13/82	15.9
0	1	0	0	0	0	0	0	4/44	2/8	0/4	0/9	6/65	9.2
0	1	0	0	0	0	0	4	15/61	1/7	0/1	4/21	20/90	22.2
2	1	0	1	0	0	0	1	27/67	16/23	1/3	3/21	47/114	41.2
12	7	1	1	0	5	2	15	213/812	82/188	66/134	32/124	393/1258	31.2
21				22				393/1258				31.2%	
1.7%				1.7%									

[2]Brandt CD, Kim HW, Yolken RH, Kapikian AZ, Arrabio JD, Rodriguez WJ, Wyatt RG, Chanock RM, Parrott RH: Comparative epidemiology of two rotavirus serotypes and other viral agents associated with pediatric gastroenteritis. Am J Epidemiol 110:243, 1979.

[3]Bryden AS, Davies HA, Hadley RE, Flewett TH, Morris CA, Oliver P: Rotavirus enteritis in the West Midlands during 1974. Lancet 2:241, 1975.

[4]Dolin R, Reichman RC, Roessner KD, Tralka TS, Schooley RT, Gary W, Morens D: Detection by immune electron microscopy of the Snow Mountain agent of acute viral gastroenteritis. J Infect Dis 146:184, 1982.

[5]Kaplan JE, Goodman RA, Schonberger LB, Lippy EC, Gary GW: Gastroenteritis due to Norwalk virus: an outbreak associated with a municipal water system. J Infect Dis 146:190, 1982.

[6]Kaplan JE, Schonberger LB, Varano G, Jackman N, Bied J, Gary GW: An outbreak of acute nonbacterial gastroenteritis in a nursing home. Demonstration of person-to-person spread by temporal clustering of cases. Am J Epidemiol 116:940, 1982.

[7]Koopman JS, Turkish VJ, Monto AS, Gouvea V, Srivastava S, Isaacson RE: Patterns and etiology of diarrhea in the three clinical settings. Am J Epidemiol 119:114, 1984.

[8]McLean DM: Viral gastroenteritis in Vancouver children, 1983 - British Columbia. Can Dis Wkly Rep 10:17, 1984.

[9]McLean DM: Wong KSK, Bergman SKA: Virions associated with acute gastroenteritis in Vancouver, 1976. Can Med Ass J 117:1035, 1977.

[10]McLean DM, Wong KK: Same-day Diagnosis of Human Virus Infections. CRC Press, Boca Raton FL 1984, pp 84–98 and p 119.

[11]Madeley CR, Cosgrove BP, Bell EJ, Fallon RJ: Stool viruses in babies in Glasgow. 1. Hospital admissions with diarrhea. J Hyg 78:261, 1977.

[12]Middleton PJ, Szymanski MT, Abbott GD, Bortolussi R, Hamilton JR: Orbivirus acute gastroenteritis of infancy. Lancet 1:1241, 1974.

[13]Sanders RC, Beards GM, Flewett TH: A shift in prevalent human rotavirus strains. Communicable Disease Report 83/14, 1983.

[14]Vesikari T, Isolauri E, Delem A, D'Houdt E, Andre FE, Zissis G: Immunogenicity and safety of live oral attenuated bovine rotavirus vaccine strain RIT 4237 in adults and young children. Lancet 2:807, 1983.

[15]Wyatt RG, James HD, Pittman AL, Hoshino Y, Greenberg HB, Kalica AR, Flores J, Kapikian AZ: Direct isolation in cell culture of human rotaviruses and their characterization into four serotypes. J Clin Microbiol 18:310, 1983.

[16]Yolken RH, Leister F: Rapid multiple-determinant enzyme immunoassay for the detection of human rotavirus. J Infect Dis 146:43, 1982.

CHAPTER 21

HEPATITIS

CLINICAL

Viral hepatitis arises from infection principally by two taxonomically and epidemiologically distinct viruses, hepatitis A (HAV) and hepatitis B (HBV). (Table 15-2). Throughout the world, a variable but small proportion of hepatitis cases is caused by one of several agents which are not readily identifiable—this is termed non-A non-B hepatitis (NANB). In tropical areas, hepatitis may arise from infection by arthropod-borne viruses such as yellow fever which are discussed in Chapter 24.

Clinical features of hepatitis A and hepatitis B are similar, but the onset of hepatitis A is usually sudden, in contrast to an insidious onset of symptoms of hepatitis B. After several days of intense anorexia, together with nausea and vomiting plus elevation of temperature to 38–39° C, jaundice appears, sometimes accompanied by hepatomegaly and/or abdominal pain, following which the temperature returns to normal. Yellow discoloration is observed over the skin and in the conjunctivae, and there may be itching. The urine becomes dark, due to excretion of urobilinogen and bilirubin, and the feces become pale. Characteristic biochemical findings are raised levels of alanine aminotransferase (ALT) (formerly serum glutamic pyruvic transaminase) (normal 6–35 units/ml) and aspartate aminotransferase (AST) (formerly serum glutamic oxalacetic transaminase (normal 15–40 units/ml). Enzyme levels first become elevated 4–7 days before onset of jaundice in hepatitis A and 3 or more weeks beforehand in hepatitis B, and they remain elevated one to several weeks after disappearance of jaundice. Usually patients recover completely, but occasional patients, both children and adults, may develop fulminant hepatitis with abrupt onset of fever, jaundice, drowsiness progressing to stupor and coma followed by death within 2 or 3 days with acute yellow atrophy (massive necrosis) of the liver. Other patients, especially those with hepatitis B, may develop relapsing hepatitis with progression to cirrhosis of the liver and portal hypertension.

Anicteric hepatitis, where subjects develop anorexia and nausea, mild fever and raised ALT and AST blood levels, but not jaundice, may affect about one third cases of hepatitis A infections during outbreaks in institutions, and a comparable proportion of hepatitis B infections may also be anicteric (without jaundice).

The incubation period of hepatitis A ranges from 15 to 40 days, with an average of 30 days (Table 21-1). Fever persists 2–3 days, but anorexia and jaundice persist about 1 week in children and possibly as long as 2–3 weeks in adults who sometimes develop post-hepatitic depression for several weeks thereafter, and serum transminase levels remain elevated about 1 week after disappearance of jaundice (Figure 21-1). Hepatitis A is communicable by fecal contamination of foodstuffs or fomites about 15 days before to 7 days after onset of jaundice.

The incubation period of hepatitis B ranges from 50 to 160 days, with an average somewhat greater than 60 days. Jaundice and constitutional upsets usually persist longer than in hepatitis A patients. Serum transaminase levels usually increase 2 weeks or more before onset of jaundice and remain elevated 2 months or more after onset (Figure 15-1). Regularly there is a history of parenteral transfer of blood from a case or carrier such as by inadvertent needle-stick or by instruments which were not sterilized between their usage on each patient, or there may be sexual contact with a carrier when virus is transferred directly between the mucous membranes of each partner. Hepatitis B is communicable by parenteral inoculation of blood from about 2 weeks before to 1 month or more after onset of jaundice. In subjects whose sera carry HBeAg (Table 15-1) in addition to HBsAg, they may be communicable for many months,[13] or intermittently for several years, as long as HBeAg is detected in their blood.[22]

The incubation period of NANB hepatitis ranges from 14 to 170 days, with an average of 40 days. The insidious onset and clinical course resemble hepatitis B. In the United States, NANB hepatitis most commonly follows transfusion of blood obtained from commercial donors who are known to harbour a variety of human pathogens transmissible by inadequately sterilized injection equipment. Hepatitis C virus is one NANB agent.

LABORATORY DIAGNOSIS

Since no convenient tissue culture system is currently available for routine isolation of hepatitis viruses, immunological methods are employed for detection of various hepatitis antigens and their respective antibodies in patient's sera. Although radioimmunoassay techniques are currently employed widely, they are being superseded by enzyme immunoassay techniques in many laboratories.[29]

TABLE 21-1
TIME COURSE AND LABORATORY DIAGNOSIS OF VIRAL HEPATITIS

| Syndrome | Virus species (family) | Incubation period | Duration of | | Viral antigen | | | | Antibodies | | |
			communi-cability	illness	test	initial detection	persis-tence	test	initial detection	persis-tence
Hepatitis A	Enterovirus 72 (Picornaviridae)	15–40d (av 30)	–15 to +7d	3–7d	EM(HAV) (feces)	–2d	+2d	RIA total RIA IgM	2w 2w	10+yr 6w
Hepatitis B	Hepadnavirus 1 (Hepadnaviridae)	50–160d (av. 60+)	–1/2 to +1 mo	7–21d	RIA(HBsAg) RIA(HBeAg) (serum)	–1 mo –1/2 mo	+3 mo +1 mo	RIA HBc RIA HBs RIA HBe	0 mo 4 mo 4 mo	10+yr 10+yr 1 yr

EM: electron microscopy (negative stain)
RIA: radioimmunoassay (solid phase)*
*similar results with ELISA

HBs: hepatitis B surface antigen
HBc: hepatitis B core antigen
HBe: antigen of DNA polymerase
HAV: hepatitis A virus (27 nm)

HEPATITIS A

Antibodies to HAV appear in the blood 2–4 weeks after onset of jaundice (Figure 21-1). Initially they are contained principally within the serum IgM,

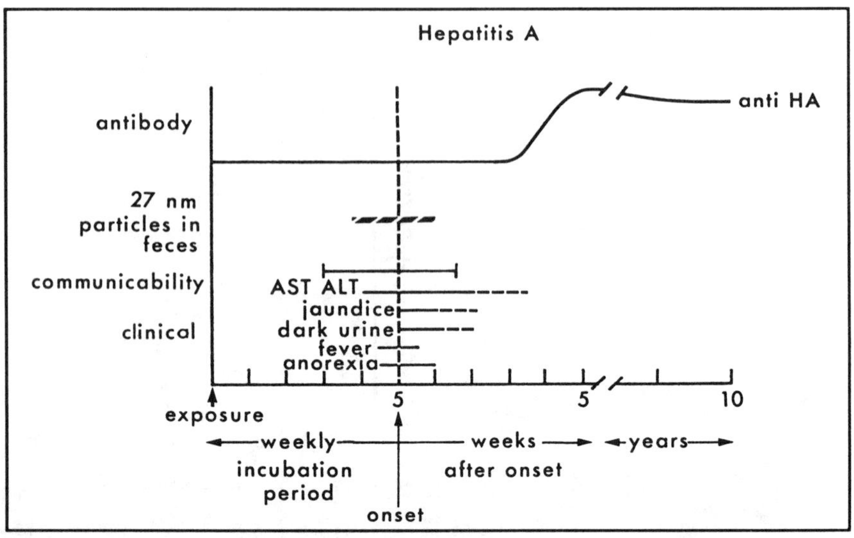

Figure 21-1: Time course of hepatitis A infection. Reproduced with permission from McLean DM 1982. Immunological Investigation of Human Virus Diseases. Churchill Livingstone, Edinburgh p 65.

but after an additional 3–12 weeks the antibodies are contained mainly within the IgG fraction of serum globulins, although IgM antibodies have persisted as long as 164 days after onset.[34] Collect 2–5 ml clotted blood some 2 weeks or more after onset of jaundice, send the serum for determination of anti HAV both in the IgM and IgG components, using appropriate radioimmunoassay[4] techniques which are summarized in a textbook.[25] Detection of anti-HAV in proportionately higher titer in the IgM than the IgG fraction during the first 6 weeks after onset of jaundice provides excellent serological evidence of current HAV infection. This method is recommended for routine diagnostic purposes.

Detection of HAV particles in feces of patients within 1 week before to 1 week after onset of jaundice has been achieved during small outbreaks of hepatitis A by immunoelectron microscopy[16] or by radioimmunoassay.[19] In the latter outbreak which affected a family in Melbourne, Australia during November 1976, the HM175 candidate strain for manufacture of live vaccine was isolated from the feces of a family member on the day of onset of jaundice by inoculation of tissue cultures.[19] Currently however, none of these virus identification methods are employed routinely.

HEPATITIS B

Routine diagnosis of HBV infection is conveniently conducted on one sample of 2–5 ml clotted blood collected during the initial 2–3 weeks after onset of jaundice. Serum is used in the following radioimmunoassay techniques,[22] for detection of anti HBs,[5] anti HBc and HBsAg. Since anti HBc appears in serum at the onset of jaundice or a few days thereafter, at which time HBsAg is circulating, the presence of these two markers denotes current time HBsAg is circulating, the presence of these two markers denotes current HBV infection (Figure 15-1). Often there is an interval of 1–2 months between the disappearance of HBsAg (about 2–4 months after onset of jaundice) and the appearance of anti HBs, but anti HBc is at high titer—the "diagnostic window period." Eventually anti HBs is detected about 6 months after onset of jaundice.

Non-routine tests include radioimmunoassays for HBeAg and anti HBe. Most acute HBV infections show relatively brief circulation of HBeAg for a few weeks around the onset of jaundice. Several weeks to months subsequently anti HBe appears in the circulation, again relatively briefly. However carriers with chronic antigenemia usually show prolonged persistence of HBeAg in serum; these persons pose high risks for transmission of HBV.[13]

Delta antigen, which is associated with HBsAg in chronic antigenemic patients and is replicated with HBV acting as a helper virus, may induce symptoms of acute hepatitis upon superinfection of HBsAg carriers, as in a hemodialysis unit.[15] Both delta antigen and its antibody are detected in sera by radioimmunoassay.

EPIDEMIOLOGY

Annual reported cases of hepatitis A throughout USA have declined each year from 54,074 in 1972 (incidence rate 25.97 per 100,000) to 21,512 in 1984 (9.38 per 100,000).[8] This contrasts with a steady annual increase in the number of reported cases of hepatitis B from 9402 (incidence rate 4.52) in 1972 to 26,102 (incidence rate 11.38) in 1984. During every winter between 1952 and 1977, monthly reporting of hepatitis A increased substantially, but there has been relatively slight variations in monthly attack rates by hepatitis B.[4] For each category of hepatitis, age-specific attack rates were substantially higher in persons aged 15–29 years. Acquisition of hepatitis B with detection of HBsAg in residents of USA was associated significantly with: personal contact, drug abuse, plasmapheresis, percutaneous exposure apart from specified surgical procedures, employment in a health-related field, association with a hemodialysis or renal transplantation team, association with daycare center programs, jaundice and hospitalization for hepatitis.[4] Raw shellfish ingestion was associated significantly with hepatitis A infection. The case fatality rate was less than 1% for persons aged less than 45 years, and about 3% for those over 45 years of age, in conformity with experience over many years.

HEPATITIS A

Acquisition of anti HAV antibodies by residents of metropolitan New York was first noted among children aged 5–9 years in a low socioeconomic group and the rate increased among each ten-year age group thereafter.[12] Rates among middle class New Yorkers were at least 20 percentage points lower than those of comparable age in the former category, and antibody was first acquired at age 20–29 years. In eastern Canada, anti HAV was first acquired by children aged 10–13 years and by 14–16 years 10% had developed antibodies.[11] These observations contrast with an antibody rate of 75–100% among native dwellers on tropical islands in the Southwest Pacific Region[18,36] and a rate of 53% among Inuit children in an isolated community of the Canadian Arctic.[26] In both these native populations, lack of adequate drinking water and sanitation facilities probably promoted extensive spread of hepatitis A virus at an earlier age than in the metropolitan area with good sanitation. The prevalence of anti HAV among healthy blood donors in North America, Europe, Japan and Australia usually ranges from 41 to 62%, but it extends from 12% in Philadelphia and 24% in Bern, Switzerland, to 75% in Dakar, Senegal and 97% in Sarajevo, Yugoslavia.[12]

Hepatitis A is spread naturally by the fecal-oral route. Thus epidemics attributed to virus-infected foodstuffs or drinking water continue to occur since the first documented waterborne epidemic at Sackville, New Brunswick, Canada in 1931.[14] These are reviewed briefly in a textbook.[24] Recent episodes include: (a) consumption of water, derived from a fecally contaminated well, which was supplied to patrons through a water fountain at a rural hardware store;[3] (b) consumption of improperly cooked cockles collected in sewage-polluted estuaries;[27] consumption of green salad, contaminated by the salad-maker who was infected asymptomatically, led to a cluster of cases of hepatitis A among participants at a family reunion;[23] (d) spread of HAV infection occurred asymptomatically among the children at a daycare center. These children transmitted infection to adults in 29% of households with at least one non-toilet trained child, in contrast to 2% of households without such a child.[34]

Following occurrence of hepatitis A among one family member of each of 230 households in Costa Rica, infection was subsequently acquired by

70–83% of household members of all age groups from 1 to 40 years of age,[35] and the rate of asymptomatic infection with seroconversion of anti HAV-IgM status was 1.8 times higher than the attack rate with clinical hepatitis.

Acquisition of hepatitis A infection by homosexual men at a Seattle, Washington clinic for sexually transmitted diseases was correlated with frequent oral-anal sexual contact, but no heterosexual man acquired hepatitis A during the same period of observation.[10] However at a London, England sexually transmitted disease clinic, acquisition of hepatitis A infection was not associated with any particular sexual practice,[9] comparable to experience in New York.[12]

HEPATITIS B

Acquisition of anti HBs antibodies by residents of metropolitan New York increased from less than 5% among lower socioeconomic class minors aged less than 20 years and middle class adults, to about 25% among lower socioeconomic class long-time resident adults, and almost 40% among lower socioeconomic class adults who were born in the Orient.[12] The lower exposure rate among this North American urban population contrasts with the high exposure rate among island residents of the Southest Pacific region where the combined HbsAg plus anti HBs rate of 20–40% among children aged less than 9 years increased to 60% among Fijians aged 20–29 years and 75–90% of residents of Raratonga and other Pacific islands.[18] Further investigation of Fijian residents showed overall HBV infection rates (HBsAg plus anti HBs) of 80–86% among Melanesians and 17–19% among East Indian adults, with rates of HBsAg carriage 10–12% among Melanesians and 0.5–3.2% among East Indians.[37] Taiwanese children aged 1–6 years showed a 15.9% HBV infection rate including 7.8% whose sera carried HBsAg[1] whilst in mainland China, 6.9% of Shanghai residents were HBsAg carriers.[21]

Rate of HBV exposure among North American volunteer blood donors (adults) were 7%[12] in contrast to 5–10 fold higher rates among certain high risk groups including hemodialysis staff (34%), hemodialysis patients (51%), multiply transfused thalassemics (48%), institutionalized mentally retarded persons (68%). All these high risk groups are subject to frequent parenteral exposure to potentially HBV-contaminated blood products or needlestick accidents. Homosexual men in New York City showed a 51% HBV infection rate,[12] comparable to a 56.5% HBV infection rate among homosexual men in London, England.[9] Transmission probably occurs by intimate mucosal contact, since HBsAg has been found in saliva and semen.[20] Frequent exposures to blood or tissues places technicans in biochemistry and hematology laboratories, and morbid anatomists at high risk of HBV infection, but the attack rate was reduced threefold in British laboratories between 1973–1974 and 1975–1976[17] through meticulous practice of techniques designed to avoid blood contamination eg. always use suction bulbs to pipette reagents never aspirate by mouth suction, avoid skin punctures by broken glass, and clean up spilled blood using sodium hypochlorite.

Household spread of HBV infection among Baltimore families was significantly threefold higher,[2] involving 29.9% family members of asymptomatic HBsAg carriers, than 8.8% among families without HBsAg carriers. The HBsAg prevalence rate among female carriers was 4.7 times higher than among contact of male carriers. Children of mothers who were HBsAg carriers had an elevenfold higher HBsAg prevalence than children whose father was the index carrier. Contacts of carriers who had skin lesions during the past year had higher HBV prevalence rates than contact of carriers with intact skin. Within a large Baltimore family of 78 persons,[30] 65% had HBV infection, including 33% who were HBsAg carriers, 4 members had severe chronic liver disease attributed to HBV infection and 72% offspring of HBsAg-positive mothers also circulated HBsAg in blood. Within Taiwan families, the annual asymptomatic HBV infection rate among preschool children was 5%,[1] but of these, 23% became HBsAg carriers; the increased HBV prevalence was associated with the frequency of previous injections. Also in Taiwan, 90–95% children became HBsAg carriers when they were born to mothers who were HBsAg and HBeAg positive, thus illustrating the importance of perinatal transmission.

Persistence of HBeAg for periods as long as 8-1/2 years[22] provides a good indicator of a chronic HBsAg carrier whose serum remains potentially infectious. Among New York residents, the prevalence of HBeAg in persistent HBsAg carriers ranged from 9.1% in carrier blood donors, 23.6% in Chinese-Americans, 35.2% in drug addicts, 61.4% in homosexual men and 71.2% in renal dialysis patients.[32] All patients with acute HBV infections develop transient HBeAg antigenemia but most develop anti HBe subsequently, except those who become chronic antigen carriers.[22,32] An important example of the high communicability of a HBeAg positive HBsAg carrier was the 8% HBV infection rate among gynecological patients who were operated on by a carrier surgeon.[13]

Persistent HBsAg carriers may comprise 200 million persons worldwide.[31] However 0.1–1% residents of North America, western Europe and Australasia are carriers, in contrast to 1–3% in South America, 3–6% in Russia and southern Europe, and 10% or more in Asia and sub-Saharan Africa.

PREVENTION

HEPATITIS A

Emphasis on the necessity to avoid inadvertent fecal contamination of foods by infected food handlers, before they develop jaundice or during anicteric hepatitis through good handwashing techniques, and other procedures which minimize contact of hands with foodstuffs, has reduced substantially the spread of foodborne hepatitis A. Similarly, provision of reticulated water supplies which do not receive fecal discharges and which contain adequate residuals of free chlorine, have minimized water-borne hepatitis A. Water obtained from field sites which are possibly contaminated by sewage should be boiled before use in drinking or washing.

Although no vaccine is licensed currently for use in HAV prevention, two candidate live vaccine strains are currently undergoing development; one after passage through fetal rhesus monkey kidney cells followed by human diploid MRC-5 cells,[28] the other after passage in continuous rhesus kidney (VERO) cells.[19]

Prophylaxis of hepatitis A is achieved by intramuscular injection of 0.05 ml/kg immune globulin (human) as a 16.5% protein suspension prepared by cold ethanol extraction of large pools of human plasma.[4] This should be administered within 1–2 weeks after exposure to the index case. Travelers to Third World countries where hepatitis A is highly endemic, should receive 0.05 ml/kg immune globulin immediately before their departure, and this dose should be repeated every 4–6 months whilst persons are dwelling in those countries.

HEPATITIS B

Avoidance of inadvertent parenteral exposures to blood or secretions of hepatitis B carriers through adequate sterilization of surgical or dental instruments between each patient, careful avoidance of needlestick injuries or laboratory accidents involving jagged glass contaminated by blood. Single use only of disposable syringes and needles for injections or venepuncture, and exclusive use of hemodialysis equipment by individual patients, has minimized substantially the risk of hepatitis B among health care workers.

Inactivated hepatitis B vaccine has been prepared from HBsAg obtained from plasma of chronic carriers and purified by ammonium sulfate concentration, isopycnic banding on sodium bromide, sucrose gradient-rate zonal separation, and enzymatic digestion with pepsin.[31] The purified particles were treated with formalin 1:4000 for 72 hours to kill any possible residual live virus. Preliminary results following intramuscular injection of homosexual men in New York, who were at high risk of HBV infection, with three doses containing 40 micrograms of HBsAg subtype *ad* at zero time, plus 1 and 6 months subsequently showed a protective efficacy of 92.3% against HBV subtype *ad* infection causing hepatitis, and 78.3% against development of any marker of HBV infection.[31] An additional trial of 3 doses of HBV *ad* vaccine among staff of renal dialysis units, who also were at high risk of HBV Infection, showed that 92.6% developed anti HBs after 2 injections and 96% after 3 injections. In renal dialysis units, subtype *ay* is regularly endemic. The protective efficacy rate of HBV *ad* vaccine against cross-type challenge by HBV *ay* was 85.4% for all *ay* infective events and 90.7% for *ay* hepatitis events.[33] This vaccine was first distributed for prophylaxis of persons at high risk of HBV infection in USA during June 1982.[6] These persons include health care workers with frequent exposure to blood or its products, hemodialysis patients, clients and staff of institutions for the mentally retarded, homosexually active males, illicit injectable drug users, recipients of certain blood products such as factor VIII or IX for clotting disorders, household and sexual contacts of HBV carriers, and special high risk populations such as immigrants and refugees from highly endemic regions e.g. eastern Asian and sub-Saharan Africa. By 1989, recombinant HBsAg vaccine has superseded the plasma-derived HBsAg vaccine.

For prophylaxis against hepatitis B following inadvertent exposure such as needlestick accidents or splashing infected blood into eyes or on other mucous membranes, administer 0.06 ml/kg hepatitis B immune globulin intramuscularly within 24 hours, accompanied by 20 microgram doses of HBV vaccine intramuscularly at a separate site, with additional doses 1 month and 6 months subsequently.[7] Babies born to mothers who are HBsAg carriers should receive similar prophylaxis against HBV infection perinatally.

REFERENCES

[1]Beasley RP, Hwang L-Y, Lin C-C, Leu M-L, Stevens CE, Szmuness W, Chen K-P: Incidence of hepatitis B virus infection in preschool children in Taiwan. J Infect Dis 146:198, 1982.

[2]Bernier RH, Sampliner R, Gerety S, Tabor E, Hamilton F, Nathanson N: Hepatitis B infection in household of chronic carriers of hepatitis B surface antigen. Factors associated with prevalence of infection. Am J Epidemiol 116:199, 1982.

[3]Bowen GS, McCarthy MA: Hepatitis A associated with a hardware store water fountain and a contaminated well in Lancaster County, Pennsylvania, 1980. Am J Epidemiol 117:695, 1983.

[4]Center for Disease Control: Hepatitis Surveillance Report No. 42, issued June 1978.

[5]Center for Disease Control: Hepatitis Surveillance Report No 43, issued March 1979.

[6]Centers for Disease Control: Inactivated hepatitis B virus vaccine. MMWR 31:317, 1982.

[7]Centers for Disease Control: Postexposure prophylaxis of hepatitis B MMWR 33:285, 1984.

[8]Centers for Disease Control: Summary—cases of specified notifiable disease, United States, 4 Jan 1985. MMWR 33:720, 1985.

[9]Coleman JC, Evans BA, Thornton A, Zuckerman AJ: Homosexual hepatitis. J. Infection 1:61, 1979.

[10]Corey L, Holmes KK: Sexual transmission of hepatitis A in homosexual men. Incidence and mechanism. New Eng J Med 302:435, 1980.

[11]Crewe MD, Embil JA, Garner JB: Prevalence of antibodies to hepatitis A virus in Nova Scotia children. Can Med Ass J 128:1195, 1983.

[12]Dienstag JL, Szmuness W, Stevens CE, Purcell RH: Hepatitis A virus infection: new insights from seroepidemiologic studies. J Infect Dis 137:328, 1978.

[13]Epidemiological Research Laboratory (Hepatitis), Central Public Health Laboratory: Acute Hepatitis B associated with gynaecological surgery. Lancet 1:1, 1980.

[14]Fraser R: Study of epidemic catarrhal jaundice. Can J Pub Health 22:396, 1931.

[15]Gmelin K, Roggendorf M, Schlipkoter U, Theilmann L, Bommer J, Kommerell B, Deinhardt F: Delta infection in a hemodialyzed patient. J Infect Dis 151, 374, 1985.

[16]Gravelle CR, Hornbeck CL, Maynard JE, Schable CA, Cook EM, Bradley DW: Hepatitis A: report of a common source outbreak with recovery of a possible etiological agent. II. Laboratory studies J Infect Dis 131:167, 1975.

[17]Grist NR: Hepatitis in clinical laboratories 1975–76. J Clin Pathol 31:415, 1978.

[18]Gust ID, Lehmann NI, Dimitrakakis MA: Seroepidemiologic study of infection with HAV and HBV in five Pacific islands. Am J Epidemiol 110:237, 1979.

[19]Gust ID, Lehmann NI, Crowe S, McCrorie M, Locarnini SA, Lucas CR: The origin of the HM 175 strains of hepatitis A virus. J Infect Dis 151:365, 1985.

[20]Heathcote J, Cameron CH, Dane DS: Hepatitis-B antigen in saliva and semen. Lancet 1:71, 1974.

[21]Hu M, Schenzle D, Deinhardt F, Scheid R: Epidemiology of hepatitis A and B in the Shanghai area: prevalence of serum markers. Am J Epidemiol 120:404, 1984.

[22]Krugman S, Overby LR, Mushahwar IK, Ling C-M, Frosner GG, Deinhardt F: Viral hepatitis, type B. Studies on natural history and prevention reexamined. New Eng J Med 300:101, 1979.

[23]Latham RH, Schable CA: Foodborne hepatitis A at a family reunion. Use of IgM-specific hepatitis A serologic testing. Am J Epidemiol 115:640, 1982.

[24]McLean DM: Virology in health Care. Williams and Wilkins, Baltimore, 1980 p 236.

[25]McLean DM: Immunological Investigation of Human Virus Diseases. Churchill Livingstone, Edinburgh 1982 pp 34–35, 64–66.

[26]Minuk GY, Waggoner JG, Jernigan R, Nicolle LE, Postl B, Hoofnagle JH: Prevalence of antibody to hepatitis A virus in a Canadian Inuit Community. Can Med Ass J 127:850, 1982.

[27]O'Mahony MC, Gooch CD, Smyth DA, Thrussell AJ, Bartlett CR, Noah ND: Epidemic hepatitis A from cockles. Lancet 1:518, 1983.

[28]Provost PJ, Banker FS, Giesa PA et al. Progress toward a live attenuated human hepatitis A vaccine. Proc Soc Exp Biol Med 170:8, 1982.

[29]Roggendorf M, Deinhardt F, Frosner GG, Schied R, Bayerl B, Zachoval R: Immunoglobulin M antibodies to hepatitis B core antigen: evaluation of enzyme immunoassay for diagnosis of hepatitis B infection. J Clin Microbiol 13:618, 1981.

[30]Sampliner RE, Loevinger BL, Tabor E, Gerety RJ: Intrafamilial cluster of hepatitis B virus infection: study of a large family in the United States. Am J Epidemiol 113:50, 1981.

[31]Szmuness W, Stevens CE, Harley EJ, Zang EA, Olezyko WR, William DC, Sadovsky R, Morrison JM, Kellner A: Hepatitis B vaccine: demonstration of efficacy in a controlled clinical trial in a high-risk population in the United States. New Eng J Med 303:834, 1980.

[32]Szmuness W, Neurath AR, Stevens CE, Strick N, Harley EJ: Prevalence of hepatitis B "e" antigen and its antibody in various HBsAg carrier populations. Am J Epidemiol 113:113, 1981.

[33]Szmuness W, Stevens CE, Harley EJ, Zang EA, Alter HJ, Taylor PE, De Vera A, Chen GTS, Kellner A and the Dialysis Vaccine Trial Study Group: Hepatitis B vaccine in medical staff at hemodialysis units. Efficacy and subtype cross-protection. New Eng J Med 307, 1481, 1982.

[34]Vernon AA, Schable C, Francis DP: A large outbreak of hepatitis A in a day-care center. Association with non-toilet-trained children and persistence of IgM antibody to hepatitis A virus. Am J Epidemiol 115:325, 1982.

[35]Villarejos VM, Serra J, Anderson-Visona K, Mosley JW: Hepatitis A virus infection in households. Am J Epidemiol 115:577, 1982.

[36]Wong DC, Purcell RH, Rosen L: Prevalence of antibody to hepatitis A and hepatitis B viruses in selected populations of the South Pacific. Am J Epidemiol 110:227, 1979.

[37]Zhuang H, Coupelis AG, Zimmett P. Taylor R, Parshu R, Banure S, Gust ID: Seroepidemiology of infection with hepatitis B virus in Fiji. Am J Epidemiol 116:608, 1982.

CHAPTER 22

ACQUIRED IMMUNODEFICIENCY SYNDROME (AIDS)

CLINICAL

Acquired immunodeficiency syndrome (AIDS) was first defined by the Centers for Disease Control in September 1982[7] as a disease, at least moderately predictive of a defect in cell-mediated immunity, occurring in a person with no known cause for diminished resistance to that disease. Such diseases include Kaposi's sarcoma (KS), *Pneumocystis carinii* pneumonia (PCP) and serious other opportunistic infections (OOI).* Diagnoses are considered to fit the case definition only if based on sufficiently reliable methods, usually histology or culture. Included in this case definition are persons with laboratory evidence of immune deficiency, as revealed by reduction of the OKT4 (helper)/OKT8 (immunosuppressor) T-lymphocyte ratio (<0.9), who show mild to moderate disturbances including fever, weight loss and persistent generalized lymphadenopathy—the lymphadenopathy syndrome (LAS),[5] which may or may not progress eventually into AIDS. Current laboratory evidence clearly demonstrates the human retrovirus, human T-lymphotropic virus type III (HTLV-III), now termed human immunodeficiency virus (HIV), as the usual causative agent of acquired immunodeficiency syndrome and lymphadenopathy syndrome.[3,13] The above case definition was updated by CDC in 1987 and clinical stages I through IV in the evolution of HIV infection were first described.

Following the first published description of AIDS affecting 4 homosexual men in Los Angeles during 1981,[16] 249 cases of AIDS were reported

---

*Other opportunistic infections include pneumonia, meningitis, or encephalitis due to one or more of the following: aspergillosis, candidiasis, cryptococcosis, cytomegalovirus, nocardiosis, strongyloidosis, toxoplasmosis, zygomycosis, or atypical mycobacteriosis (species other than tuberculosis or lepra); esophagitis due to candidiasis, cytomegalovirus, or herpes simplex virus; progressive multifocal leukoencephalopathy; chronic enterocolitis (more than 4 weeks) due to cryptosporidiosis; or unusually extensive mucocutaneous herpes simplex of more than 5 weeks duration.

throughout USA during the first half of 1982[7] to make a total of 593 cases reported since 1979, of whom 41% died. These cases showed 51% with PCP without KS (with or without OOI), 30% had KS without PCP (with or without OOI), 7% had both PCP and KS (with or without OOI) and 12% had OOI with neither PCP nor KS. Of these cases 75% were homosexual men of whom 12.3% used illicit drugs intravenously; 14.2% were bisexual men, 59.8% of whom were illicit drug users; and 5.7% were heterosexual women, 62.5% of whom used intravenous drugs. Haitian residents of USA comprised 6.1% of reported cases, most of whom were neither homosexual nor drug abusers. In Haiti, AIDS was first recognized among members of all strata of Haitian society during 1979,[21] contemporaneously with its first recognition in USA residents. Diarrhea and profound weight loss were the commonest presenting symptoms in Haitian patients[21] and also in patients in the tropical African countries of Rwanda[30] and Zaire.[23]

Homosexual contact appears to be a major factor in transmission of AIDS. Overwhelmingly high incidence of AIDS in male homosexuals in USA[7] and other countries supports this viewpoint. In London, England 17 of 28 homosexual men who had ano-genital intercourse with patients with either AIDS or LAS, developed either of these conditions 1–4 years subsequently, and all 4 patients with AIDS died.[14]

However normal sexual intercourse between married couples may also transmit AIDS. A black Zairian man living in France for more than one year developed fever, weight loss, meningeal syndrome, hepatomegaly, spleno-megaly and lymphadenopathy plus depression of the OKT4/OKT8 ratio in his T-lymphocytes consistent with AIDS in November 1982.[12] His wife developed lymphadenopathy and depression of the OKT4/OKT8 ratio consistent with LAS in February 1984. Peripheral blood T-lymphocytes from these two persons yielded isolates of HIV. Promiscuous out-of-wedlock sexual inter-course may also transmit AIDS.[19]

Blood transfusions are an important non-sexual mechanism for transmis-sion of AIDS. A Frenchman who was transfused with 8 units of Haitian blood following severe trauma in Haiti during 1978 developed AIDS in France during 1982.[1] In USA, 18 of 2157 documented cases of AIDS in August 1983 developed AIDS 15 to 57 months (median 27.5) after receiving blood transfusions[11] and in 7 instances the donors had decreased OKT4/OKT8 ratios consistent with immunodeficiency preceding AIDS.

Hemophiliacs are at high risk for development of AIDS,[6] which strongly suggests transmission by blood products, particularly concentrates of factor VIII or factor IX. Isolation of HIV from peripheral T-lymphocytes of 2 adolescent French boys with hemophilia who were maintained on regular infusions of factor IX concentrate, one of whom developed persistent fever, lymphadenopathy, hepatosplenomegaly, substantial weight loss, severe toxoplasmosis and profound reduction of the OKT4/OKT8 T-lymphocyte ratio consistent with AIDS[31] points strongly towards transmission by plasma factors.

A hemophiliac man aged 26 years received regular infusions of factor VIII concentrate for 9 years preceding the development of splenomegaly and a OKT4/OKT8 ratio reduced to 0.65 in May 1983 followed in January 1984 by lymphadenopathy consistent with LAS.[24] He had monogamous sexual relations with his wife for the 2 years before the birth of their son in March 1984; the wife developed vulvovaginal candidiasis during the second trimester of pregnancy, lymphadenopathy during the third trimester, she became febrile perinatally and subsequently she had a reduced OKT4/OKT8 ratio consistent with LAS. Their son developed persistent oral candidiasis, diffuse bilateral pulmonary infiltrates accompanied by respiratory distress requiring mechanical ventilation, hepatosplenomegaly, lymphadenopathy and reduced OKT4/OKT8 ratio consistent with AIDS. The wife's daughter by a previous marriage, and her former husband had no stigmata of LAS or AIDS. These observations strongly suggest (a) parenteral transmission to the father by factor VIII, (b) monogamous sexual transmission to his wife, (c) transplacental transfer to the son.

Infants have also developed AIDS, particularly those born to Haitian parents in USA.[28] All 9 infants with typical AIDS presented with failure to thrive and reversed OKT4/OKT8 ratio, 77% had persistent *Candida albicans* infection of the oral mucosa, 55% had persistent pulmonary infiltrates, 88% had hepatosplenomegaly and 33% had lymphadenopathy, 44% had PCP, 22% had KS and 55% had OOI apart from PCP. Symptoms first appeared between birth and 6 months of age, and 55% died 2–10 months after onset of symptoms. An additional 5 infants had similar symptoms consistent with AIDS but without opportunistic infections, and 2 died 3–12 months subsequently. Isolation of HIV from T-lymphocytes of a mother who had AIDS and her son age 4 months who also developed AIDS,[32] suggests transplacental transfer to this child, but a twin brother appeared to escape this infection, because he was healthy and devoid of HIV and its antibody at 10 months of age.

The incubation period of AIDS or LAS in 17 men in London, England following homosexual contact was 1–2 years.[14] After development of LAS, some subjects have remained well during the succeeding 2 years, others have progressed to AIDS and died within the next 2–4 years.[14] The incubation period of AIDS after a Frenchman was transfused with Haitian blood was 3-1/2 years, with death occurring 1 year subsequently;[1] in 18 USA patients, AIDS developed 15–57 months (Median 27.5) after blood transfusions.[11] By 1989, the incubation distribution, i.e. time from seroconversion following infection with HIV until onset of AIDS showed a median of 10 years.

LABORATORY DIAGNOSIS

Isolation of HIV virus from T-lymphocytes derived from peripheral blood[12,31,32] or lymph node biopsies[3] of patients with LAS or AIDS provides the best current method for laboratory diagnosis. However, it should be emphasized that this technically sophisticated procedure is performed only in highly specialized laboratories; it is not a routine diagnostic test in the standard hospital or university virus laboratory. Peripheral blood T-lymphocytes are separated from venous blood samples by Ficoll-Hypaque gradient centrifugation and stimulated with phytohemagglutinin for 3 days. The medium is removed and the lymphocytes are cultured in RPMI 1640 medium containing 10% fetal calf serum, 10% T-cell growth factor (interleukin-2), 2 µg/ml hexadimethrine bromide and 0.1% anti-human alpha-interferon sheep serum; this medium is changed twice weekly. Reverse transcriptase assays[3] are performed on cell-free supernatants twice weekly to monitor for virus replication. Usually virus is detected within 7–15 days of culture,[12,31] and these fresh isolates are propagated by inoculation of supernatants into lymphocyte cultures from normal human donors which have been stimulated by phytohemagglutinin during the preceding 3 days. Electron microscopic examination of thin sections, both of lymphocytes cultured from LAS patients and donor lymphocytes infected with the HIV isolate, show typical retrovirus particles,[31] with immature budding forms at cell surfaces and mature forms with eccentric electron-dense cores. Isolates are further characterized as HIV by immunofluorescence, ELISA and polyacrylamide gel electrophoresis.

Electron microscopic examination of thin sections of lymph node biopsies collected from 4 homosexual men in Perth, Western Australia, one of whom had AIDS and the other 3 had LAS, have revealed retrovirus particles with central or eccentric electron dense cores.[2] Both immature and mature retrovirus particles have been observed in biopsies from esophageal ulcers in 7 homosexual men in Vancouver, Canada[33] who presented with dysphagia in addition to LAS (Figure 22-1).

Antibodies to HIV are detected conveniently in patients' sera by several tests including: immunofluorescence assay for antibody to HIV p24 and gp41 antigens,[10] competitive radioimmunoassay[10] and ELISA[4,26] or radioimmune precipitation assay for antibodies to the p24 protein of HIV.[3,25] Tests such as immunofluorescence and ELISA are employed for routine screening purposes, and positive reactors are confirmed by western blot tests.

EPIDEMIOLOGY

Until June 1982 in USA, only 593 cases of AIDS were reported since the disease was first documented from health records in 1979.[7] Subsequent-

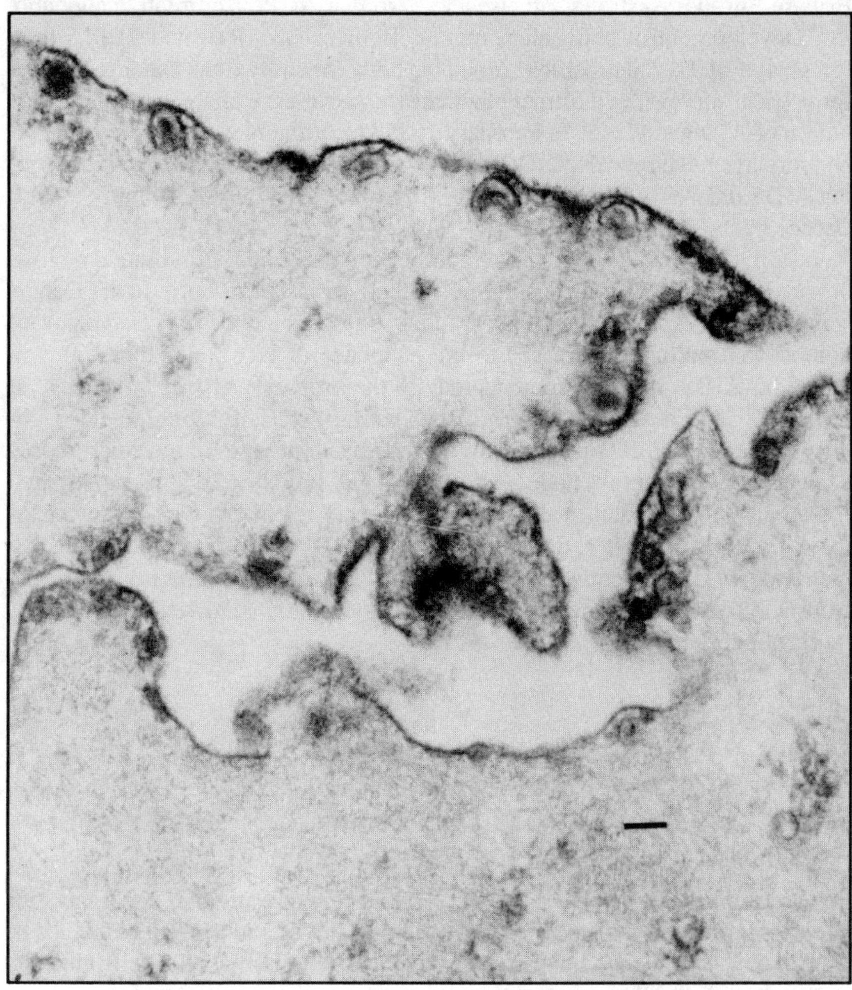

Figure 22-1: Retrovirus particles in thin sections of esophageal biopsy from a Vancouver man with lymphadenopathy syndrome and odynophagia (x59,400).[33]

ly the incidence of AIDS has increased dramatically, so that 2075 cases were reported in 1983 and 4386 throughout 1984.[9] By December 1989, a cumulative total of 112,240 cases with 66,493 deaths were reported in USA, with 25,781 new cases occurring in 1987, 29,157 new cases in 1988 and 18,298 new cases in 1989, which suggests that the epidemic wave is currently receding. Comparable escalation of reported AIDS cases has been observed in Great

Britain, Europe, Australia and elsewhere, so that AIDS is currently pandemic.

Development of convenient immunofluorescence, RIA and ELISA tests for assays of HIV antibodies routinely, both for individual patients and for serological surveys, will further elucidate the prevalence and geographic distribution of AIDS and LAS. In February 1985, these and more sophisticated antibody assays have revealed HIV infections in male homosexuals with or without AIDS or LAS in England (17–59%),[10] France (18–75%),[4] Denmark (9%),[20] Greece,[22] and West Germany (27–70%),[17] Switzerland (10–100%),[27] New York City (53–82%),[15] yet the antibody prevalence among volunteer blood donors in England,[10] France[4] and Switzerland[27] was virtually nil. In the Danish series, travel to the United States and increased number and frequency of homosexual partners, increased to the incidence of HIV antibodies.[20] Prevalence of AIDS is well documented in the tropical African countries of Rwanda[30] and Zaire,[23] and the Caribbean country of Haiti,[21] but it is not regularly associated with homosexuality in those countries. Electron microscopic examination of lymph node and esophageal biopsies in Australian[2] and Canadian[33] homosexual men with LAS revealed retrovirus particles morphologically typical of HIV. Seroconversions to HIV were found in 2 Canadian men and one subsequently died of AIDS. Isolations of HIV have been achieved from additional men with "mononucleosis syndrome" and retrovirus virions in esophageal biopsies.

PREVENTION

Protection of health-care personnel from risk of transmission of HIV, from known or suspected cases of AIDS or LAS, depends on strict observance of "universal precautions," including wearing of gloves and masks, avoidance of needlestick injuries and inadvertent contamination of abraded skin or mucous membranes with blood or secretions, plus adequate sterilization of all surgical and endoscopy equipment.[8] Dental personnel should also wear protective eyewear. Current American experience has shown that with good hospital isolation facilities, no nosocomial infections have occurred among 85 hospital workers with 28 of 29 serologically confirmed AIDS cases.[18] Infectivity of HIV was inactivated rapidly by sodium hypochlorite, 0.2% glutaraldehyde 0.1% or ethanol 25%,[29] all of which are suitable for routine sterilization of non-boilable instruments. It was also inactivated by heating at 56° C for 30 minutes, but not by 2×10^5 rad gamma radiation or 5×10^3 J/m^2 ultraviolet irradiation.[29]

REFERENCES

[1]Andreani T, Modigliani R, Le Charpentier Y, et al: Acquired immunodeficiency with intestinal cryptosporidiosis: possible transmission by Haitian whole blood. Lancet 1:1187, 1983.

[2]Armstrong JA, Horne R: Follicular dendritic cells and virus-like particles in AIDS-related lymphadenopathy. Lancet 2:370, 1984.

[3]Barré-Sinoussi F, Chermann JC, Rey F, et al: Isolation of a T-lymphotropic retrovirus from a patient at risk for acquired immune deficiency syndrome (AIDS). Science 220:868, 1983.

[4]Brun-Vezinet F, Rouzioux C, Barré-Sinoussi F, et al: Detection of IgG antibodies to lymphadenopathy-associated virus in patients with AIDS or lymphadenopathy syndrome. Lancet 1:1254, 1984.

[5]Centers for Disease Control: Persistent, generalized lymphadenopathy among homosexual males. MMWR 31:249, 1982.

[6]Centers for Disease Control: *Pneumocystis carinii* pneumonia among persons with hemophilia. MMWR 31:365, 1982.

[7]Centers for Disease Control: Update on Acquired Immune Deficiency Syndrome (AIDS): United States. MMWR 31:507, 1982.

[8]Centers for Disease Control: Acquired immunodeficiency syndrome (AIDS): precautions for health-care workers and allied professionals MMWR 32:450, 1983.

[9]Centers for Disease Control: Summary-cases of specified notifiable diseases, United States, 4 Jan. 1985. MMWR 33:720, 1985.

[10]Cheingsong-Popov R, Weiss RA, Dalgleish A, et al: Prevalence of antibody to human T-lymphotropic virus type III in AIDS and AIDS-risk patients in Britain. Lancet 2:477, 1984.

[11]Curran JW, Lawrence DN, Jaffe H, et al: Acquired immunodeficiency syndrome (AIDS) associated with transfusions. New Eng J Med 310:69, 1984.

[12]Ellrodt A, Barré-Sinoussi F, LeBras P, et al: Isolation of human T-lymphotropic retrovirus (LAV) from Zairian married couple, one with AIDS, one with prodromes. Lancet 1:1383, 1984.

[13]Gallo RC, Salahuddin SZ, Popovic M, et al: Human T-lymphotropic retrovirus, HTLV-III, isolated from AIDS patients and donors at risk for AIDS. Science 224:500, 1984.

[14]Gazzard BG, Shanson DC, Farthing C, et al: Clinical findings and serological evidence of HTLV-III infection in homosexual contacts of patients with AIDS and persistent generalized lymphadenopathy in London. Lancet 2:480, 1984.

[15]Goedert JJ, Sarngadharan MG, Biggar RJ, et al: Determinants of retrovirus (HTLV-III) antibody and immunodeficiency conditions in homosexual men. Lancet 2:711, 1984.

[16]Gottlieb MS, Schroff R, Schanker HM, et al: *Pneumocystis carinii* pneumonia and mucosal candidiasis in previously healthy homosexual men. Evidence of a new acquired cellular immunodeficiency. New Eng J Med 305:1425, 1981.

[17]Hehlmann R, Kreeb G, Erfle V, et al: Antibodies to HTLV-III in patients with acquired immunodeficiency or lymphadenopathy syndrome in West Germany. Lancet 2:1094, 1984.

[18]Hirsch MS, Worsmer GP, Schooley RT, et al: Risk of nosocomial infection with human T-cell lymphotropic virus III (HTLV-III). New Eng J Med 312:1, 1985.

[19]Laverdiere M, Tremblay J, Lavallee R, et al: AIDS in Haitian immigrants and in Caucasian women closely associated with Haitians. Can Med Ass J 129:1209, 1983.

[20]Melbye M, Biggar RJ, Ebbesen P, et al: Seroepidemiology of HTLV-III antibody in Danish homosexual men: prevalence, transmission and disease outcome. Brit Med J 289:573, 1984.

[21]Pape JW, Liautaud B, Thomas F, et al: Characteristics of the acquired immunodeficiency syndrome (AIDS) in Haiti. New Eng J Med 309, 945, 1983.

[22]Papevangelon G, Economidou J, Kallinikos J, et al: Lymphadenopathy associated virus in AIDS, lymphadenopathy syndrome, and classic Kaposi patients in Greece. Lancet 2:642, 1984.

[23]Piot P, Quinn TC, Taelman H, et al: Acquired immunodeficiency syndrome in a heterosexual population in Zaire. Lancet 2:65, 1984.

[24]Ragni MV, Urbach AH, Kierman S, et al: Acquired immunodeficiency syndrome in the child of a haemophiliac. Lancet 1:133, 1985.

[25]Safai B, Sarngadharan MG, Groopman JE, et al: Seroepidemiological studies of human T-lymphotropic retrovirus type III in acquired immunodeficiency syndrome. Lancet 1:1438, 1984.

[26]Salahuddin SZ, Groopman JE, Markham PD, et al: HTLV-III in symptom-free seronegative persons. Lancet 2:1418, 1984.

[27]Schupbach J, Haller O, Vogt M, et al: Antibodies to HTLV-III in Swiss patients with AIDS and pre-AIDS in groups at risk for AIDS. New Eng J Med 312:265, 1985.

[28]Scott GB, Buck BE, Leterman JG, et al: Acquired immunodeficiency syndrome in infants. New Eng J Med 310:76, 1984.

[29]Spire B, Barré-Sinoussi F, Montagnier L, Chermann JC: Inactivation of lymphadenopathy associated virus by chemical disinfectants. Lancet 2:899, 1984 and 1:188, 1985.

[30]Van de Perre P, Rouvroy D, Lepage P, et al: Acquired immunodeficiency syndrome in Rwanda. Lancet 2:62, 1984.

[31]Vilmer E, Barré-Sinoussi F, Rouzioux C, et al: Isolation of new lymphotropic retrovirus from two siblings with haemophilia B, one with AIDS: Lancet 1:753, 1984.

[32]Vilmer E, Fischer A, Griscelli C, et al: Possible transmission of a human lymphotropic retrovirus (LAV) from mother to infant with AIDS: Lancet 2:229, 1984.

[33]Wong KK, McLean DM, Rabeneck L: Retrovirus particles in esophageal biopsies in lymphadenopathy syndrome. Poster T-3, International Conference in Acquired Immunodeficiency Syndrome, Atlanta GA, 16 April 1985.

CHAPTER 23

CENTRAL NERVOUS SYSTEM VIRAL DISEASES

Viral infections of the central nervous system are classified clinically into aseptic meningitis, poliomyelitis and encephalitis (Table 23-1).

CLINICAL

ASEPTIC MENINGITIS

Aseptic meningitis is the syndrome arising from acute infection of the meninges with several serotypes of enterovirus, or mumps virus. Typical clinical features are sudden onset of headache accompanied by nausea and vomiting, fever with temperature elevation to 39° C, and stiffness of the neck.[31] This may cause patients to sit completely upright with the arms outstretched behind the trunk, giving the tripod sign. Characteristically the cerebrospinal fluid (CSF) shows an increased leukocyte count to between 50 and 5000 cells per μl (normal $<5/\mu l$, $<5/mm^3$), of which more than 50% (usually 90–100%) are lymphocytes, the levels of glucose (2.8–4.2 m mol/1, 50–75 mg/dl) protein (0.15–0.45 g/l, 15–45 mg/dl) and chloride (120–130 m mol/l, 120–130 m Eq/l)[21] remain normal. Occasionally during the first few hours of illness, the CSF cell count may show a higher proportion of polymorphonuclear cells than the leukocytes, but after 24 hours, lymphocytes usually predominate.

It is important to distinguish clinically between aseptic meningitis (viral) and purulent meningitis (bacterial) at the time of initial examination of the patient. In aseptic meningitis the patient usually shows a mild constitutional upset and is alert, but in purulent meningitis the patient is severely ill, with either pronounced irritability and drowsiness progressing to stupor, or excitable and difficult to control. The CSF in aseptic meningitis appears clear or slightly turbid, with lymphocytes predominating and normal chemistries, but CSF in purulent meningitis is turbid, virtually all cells are polymorphonuclears, the glucose is depressed below 2.8 m mol/l and the protein increased above 0.45 g/l. Gram staining of a smear of CSF reveals no microorganisms in aseptic meningitis, but bacteria such as *Neisseria meningitidis*

TABLE 23-1
TIME COURSE AND LABORATORY DIAGNOSIS OF CENTRAL NERVOUS SYSTEM VIRAL INFECTIONS

Syndrome	Virus species (family)	Incu-bation period	Duration of comm.	Duration of illness	specimen	Virus identification EM	Virus identification IF	virus isolation	Antibodies (paired sera) test	Antibodies (paired sera) initial detection	Antibodies (paired sera) persis-tence
Aseptic meningitis	Enterovirus (Picornaviridae)	4–8d	0 to 7d	3–5d	CSF feces	n/a	n/a	MK	NT	2–5d	20+ yr
	Mumps (Paramyxoviridae)	16–21d	–2 to +4d	2–4d	CSF throat	+	+	MK	HI S-CF	2–4d 2–4d	20+ yr 6 mo
Polio-myelitis	Poliovirus (Picornaviridae)	4–8d	0 to 14d	3–10d	feces	n/a	n/a	MK	NT	2–5d	20+ yr
Encephalitis	Togavirus (WEE) Bunyavirus (LAC)	4–14d	–3 to +1d (viremia)	3–20d	CSF, throat brain (fatal)	n/a	n/a	VERO, BHK,SM	HI NT ELISA CF	3–7d 10–14d	20+ yr 3 yr
	Rhabdovirus	2–26w	0 to 10d	5–10d	CSF, throat brain (fatal)	+ +	+ +	DH,VERO, SM	n/a		
	Herpesvirus	4–20d	0 to 5d	5–20d	CSF, throat brain (fatal)	+	+	DH,PH, CC	n/a		
	Measles	12–20d	–2 to +4d	3–20d	CSF, throat brain (fatal)	+	+	CC	HI IF NT ELISA	3–7d	20+ yr

Day 0:	day of onset of illness	BHK:	continuous baby hamster kidney cultures	NT:	neutralization	
–2:	two days before onset	MK:	primary monkey kidney cultures (rhesus)	ELISA:	enzyme-linked immunosorbent assay	
+4:	four days after onset	PH:	continuous polyploid human cells	DH:	continuous diploid human fibroblasts	
EM:	electron microscopy (negative stain)	VERO:	continuous monkey kidney cultures (grivet)	CC:	cocultivation of brain fragments	
		CF:	complement fixation	SM:	suckling mice	
IF:	immunofluorescence	HI:	hemagglutination inhibition			

or *Haemophilus influenzae* are usually observed in purulent meningitis. In tuberculous meningitis, the patient may exhibit board-like rigidity of the neck and spine. Although the CSF may show lymphocytosis, the glucose level is usually depressed, the protein level is elevated, and a web-like pellicle forms in the CSF on standing overnight at room temperature. This pellicle usually contains acid-fast *Mycobacterium tuberculosis* organisms. Leukemic infiltration of the central nervous system may be accompanied by the presence of primitive leukocytes in the CSF, but no microorganisms.

The incubation period of enteroviral (aseptic) meningitis is 4–8 days and mumps meningitis 14–21 days. Diagnosis of aseptic meningitis should be established by immediate microscopic examination of CSF obtained as soon as possible after onset of fever, headache and neck stiffness. Since meningeal symptoms arise from increased intracranial pressure, from outpouring of fluid and lymphocytes from the inflamed meninges into the subarachnoid space, removal of 5–10 ml CSF during lumbar puncture usually causes relief from these symptoms within 24 hours. However, if lumbar puncture is not performed, headache and neck stiffness may persist for 3–5 days. Clinical recovery is complete within 5–7 days. Although obvious sequelae are rare, 16% of virologically confirmed enteroviral meningitis in a group of Seattle children showed severe neurological disorders and others showed speech delay or behavioral problems,[48] whilst transient muscle weakness has been noted during epidemic spread of non-polio enteroviruses in California[40] and elsewhere.

Mumps meningitis may occur in 0.5–2.0% patients with mumps.[2,9,30,38] Meningitis without parotitis has occurred in 33–41% of laboratory cases of mumps meningitis. Male cases outnumber female cases by 2:1–3:1. Mumps meningitis is encountered more frequently during winter and spring; enteroviral meningitis occurs more commonly during the warmer months.[38] The incubation period of mumps meningitis ranges from 14 to 21 days. Meningeal symptoms usually persist no longer than 3 days, when lumbar puncture is performed during the initial 1–2 days after onset of headache and neck stiffness, but they may persist as long as 5–7 days, particularly when lumbar puncture is delayed or omitted.

Duration of communicability of enteroviruses by the feces is about 7 days following onset of meningitis. Mumps virus is communicable, by airborne droplets from mumps meningitis patients, from 2 days before to 4 days after onset of meningitis, but this period may be extended, particularly if parotid swelling appears several days after meningeal signs. Therefore it is important that cases of aseptic meningitis be nursed in appropriate isolation facilities within hospitals in order to prevent nosocomial infections.

POLIOMYELITIS

Flaccid paralysis of one or more groups of skeletal muscles, characteristically accompanied by intense pain and spasm, usually begins 1–2 days after onset of aseptic meningitis. Minor illness comprising mild fever, headache and nausea may affected patients 2 or more days before meningeal signs. Classically, poliomyelitis patients are alert and apprehensive during the meningeal phase of development of paralysis over a period of 2–3 days, when affected muscle groups are exquisitely tender and in spasm. Paralysis arises from selective destruction of motor neurons in the anterior horn of the spinal cord grey matter. Occasionally motor neurons of the brain stem may be affected alone, or with those of the spinal cord, causing central respiratory or cardiovascular failure or, more commonly a flaccid bulbar palsy affecting the facial and pharyngeal muscles, causing difficulty with swallowing.

Clinical distinction between poliomyelitis and the Guillain-Barré syndrome (acute ascending polyneuritis) is important. Poliovirus patients show flaccid paralysis of random groups of skeletal muscles, Guillain-Barré syndrome patients exhibit symmetrical flaccid paralysis of the lower extremities, often ascending to involve the upper extremities and diaphragmatic musculature. The CSF in poliomyelitis shows lymphocytosis and normal chemistries, but in the Guillain-Barré syndrome there are no cells and the protein concentration is raised beyond 2.0 g/l with normal glucose and chloride levels.

The etiology of the Guillain-Barré syndrome is obscure, because no virus has been isolated consistently from CSF or other specimens from patients. During widespread administration of inactivated swine influenza vaccine (A/New Jersey/76 $H_{sw_1} N_1$) to residents of the United States in 1976, the risk of development of the Guillain-Barré syndrome was 8–14 fold higher among recipients of this vaccine than among those who were unvaccinated.[8]

The incubation period of poliomyelitis is 4–8 days or possibly as long as 15 days. Although meningeal signs and apprehension usually have abated within 3–5 days, especially after performance of lumbar puncture, mild to severe degrees of flaccid paralysis may persist indefinitely in limb muscles. Progressively increasing degrees of active movement of the affected musculature, under careful daily supervision and encouragement by physiotherapists, may enable patients to regain a substantial degree of limb function through the substitutionary involvement of unaffected muscle groups adjacent to the paralyzed muscles. Involvement of the basal ganglia affecting the respiratory and cardiovascular centers may terminate fatally, especially during pregnancy.[50]

ENCEPHALITIS

Sudden onset of hyperpyrexia (40–43° C), together with severe headache and clouding of consciousness, progressing through stupor to coma, signifies the development of encephalitis. Frequently convulsions occur at the time of onset and persist intermittently for several days. Spastic weakness, frank hemiparesis and focal epilepsy may involve the limbs. The development of neck stiffness and lymphocytosis of CSF indicate concomitant meningitis. Although encephalitis is infrequently induced by poliovirus, and occasionally by a group B coxsackievirus[35] or echovirus-11[42] infections during the puerperium, it is found commonly in arbovirus infections and in rabies. Rarely encephalitis complicates infection with herpesvirus and measles (Table 23-1).

Symptoms arise from destruction of cerebral or cerebellar neurones as a direct result of viral multiplication in the central nervous system immediately after the viremic phase of infection, and thus appear within an incubation period of 1–3 weeks after exposure to the infectious arthropod bite as an arboviruses, or virus-shedding patients as in herpes or measles, or longer intervals following bites by rabid animals.

Measles virus may remain dormant in central nervous tissue for several years, eventually causing subacute sclerosing panencephalitis (SSPE). This syndrome appears 2–11 years after onset of measles in 5.2–9.7 per million reported cases[7] and comprises progressive dementia, myoclonic jerks, pyramidal and extrapyramidial signs, an electroencephalogram with regular periodic complexes, and measles antibody titers in both IgM and IgG components of CSF globulins, usually at 8- to 32-fold lower titers than in serum.[22]

Post-infectious encephalitis, which arises from perivascular demyelination within the central nervous system, may appear 1–3 weeks after onset of acute exanthematous infections[11] with the following rates per 100,000 cases in USA during 1978: measles 48.4, mumps 154.6, rubella 5.5, chickenpox 26.0. Average percentage case fatality rates were measles 14.0, mumps 1.3, rubella none, chickenpox 23.1, thus showing the severity of this complication.

LABORATORY DIAGNOSIS

ASEPTIC MENINGITIS (ENTEROVIRAL AND MUMPS)

The best single test for diagnosis of enteroviral or mumps meningitis is isolation of the causative agent from CSF, by inoculation of primary monkey kidney tissue cultures and incubation at 35–37° C, until cytopathic effects are observed 3–7 days later. Enteroviruses induce shrinkage of cells with pyknosis of nuclei, and the virus isolate within the supernatant fluid is serotyped by neutralization tests, according to techniques described in a textbook.[32] Mumps virus induced syncytia, and serotyping is accomplished with 2 hours by hemagglutination inhibition tests using the supernatant as antigen, or by indirect immunofluorescence.

Same-day techniques of electron microscopy will reveal the presence of paramyxovirus virions in CSF of patients within 15 minutes after submission of specimens to the laboratory, and these virions are serotyped as mumps virus 2 hours subsequently by indirect immunofluorescence.

Good supportive evidence of enteroviral or mumps infection as the cause of aseptic meningitis is obtained from isolation of these viruses from throat swabs or garglings collected within 4 days after onset, and enteroviruses may be isolated from feces or rectal swabs collected within 4–7 days after onset of meningitis.

Serological confirmation of a recent infection requires collection of two blood samples, the first within 1–2 days after onset and the second sample 1 or more days after defervescence i.e. usually 4–7 days after onset. Enteroviral antibodies are titrated in neutralization tests, mumps antibodies by hemagglutination inhibition or neutralization.

POLIOMYELITIS

Polivirus is isolated readily from feces of paralyzed patients 1–28 days after onset, and from their throats 1–4 days after onset, but rarely if ever from CSF, using tissue culture techniques identical to those for enteroviruses. Serological confirmation of infection requires neutralization tests on paired sera collected at similar time intervals to other enteroviruses.

ENCEPHALITIS

TOGAVIRUS AND BUNYAVIRUS (ARBOVIRUSES)

Brain provides the best material for attempts at isolation of arboviruses from fatal cases of encephalitis. Small portions are macerated and dispersed in maintenance medium, then inoculated: (a) intracerebrally into families of suckling mice aged less than 48 hours, which are observed for signs of encephalitis during the subsequent two weeks; (b) into tissue cultures of VERO cells (continuous rhesus kidney) and BHK cells (continuous baby hamster kidney) which are overlaid with agarose and examined for plaque formation after incubation for as long as 1 week. After suckling mice exhibit hunching, ruffled fur and convulsions i.e. encephalitis, usually within 2–6 days after inoculation, brains are removed: (a) portions are dispersed in maintenance medium and serotyped by neutralization tests in mice; (b) other portions are dispersed in sucrose, extracted with acetone and assayed for hemagglutinin using goose erythrocytes at several pH and temperature values, and if hemagglutinin is detected, serogrouping is performed by hemagglutination inhibition. Full details are described in a textbook on techniques.[32] When plaques are observed in tissue cultures, single plaques are removed aseptically, dispersed in maintenance medium and serotyped in plaque-reduction neutralization tests.[32]

Virus isolation should always be attempted from specimens obtained during the acute stage of illness, particularly CSF and throat secretions, by inoculation of suckling mice and tissue cultures, but success is achieved rarely.

Pairs of sera should always be sought from patients, during this initial 3 days after onset and again after a further 3 days or more, whenever the temperature has remained normal at least for 24 hours. Rising titers of hemagglutinin inhibiting antibody give evidence of the particular serogroup of arbovirus infecting the patient, and serotype specific-responses are obtained in neutralization and ELISA tests. Antibodies detected by these procedures persist at least 20 years. Antibodies are first detected by complement fixation 10–14 days after onset, and they persist no longer than about 3 years.

RHABDOVIRUS (RABIES)

Virus isolation should always be attempted from throat and CSF of patients during life, and from portions of brain post mortem, by procedures comparable to those for arboviruses. Immediate evidence of rabies virus infection in brain smears, especially from Ammon's horn of the hippocampus, is obtained by indirect immunofluorescence.

HERPESVIRUS AND MEASLES

Portions of brain obtained at biopsy or post mortem are minced into small fragments using scalpel blades, and these fragments are co-cultivated with susceptible tissue culture monolayers (diploid human fibroblasts or certain continuous polyploid lines such as HeLa). Both these agents promote fusion of brain cells to tissue culture cells, the incomplete virus genome within brain cells is transferred to the susceptible tissue culture cells, in which it multiplies to liberate complete virus into the supernatant, and induce characteristic cytopathic effects (grape-like clusters in herpesvirus, syncytia in measles). These fresh isolates are serotyped by immunofluorescence or neutralization.

These viruses may occasionally be isolated from CSF of patients within the initial 2–3 days after onset of encephalitis by inoculation of tissue cultures as above. Isolation of these viruses from throat specimens offers merely circumstantial evidence that encephalitis has been induced by them.

Serological tests are of considerable value in diagnosis of measles encephalitis where increases of antibody titer may be detected within the first week after onset by hemagglutination inhibition, immunofluorescence, neutralization or ELISA. In cases of subacute sclerosing panencephalitis, antibodies are found in the IgM as well as the IgG component of CSF, but usually at titers 8–32 fold lower than in serum. However antibody determinations are of no value in diagnosis of herpesvirus encephalitis.

EPIDEMIOLOGY

ASEPTIC MENINGITIS

Aseptic meningitis affected between 3197 and 11,740 persons annually in the United States (annual incidence rates per 100,000 were 1.5 to 5.1) between 1972 and 1984.[12,20] During the decade 1970–79, aseptic meningitis was associated with 61% of enterovirus isolates in USA[12] and encephalitis was associated with 17% enteroviral isolates. Monthly prevalence of aseptic meningitis closely paralleled the high prevalence of enteroviruses during the summer months of June through October (Figure 23-1), which was 6.5 times higher than during the remaining 7 cooler months.[12] Males were involved 1.5 times more commonly than females. Persons under 20 years of age comprised the majority (55%) of cases, with 35% cases aged less than 10 years. Virus isolations were achieved from CSF in about 30% of cases, the remaining isolations were obtained from throat or fecal samples. Echoviruses comprised 76% of virus isolations from aseptic meningitis, group B coxsackieviruses 21%, group A coxsackieviruses 4% and polioviruses 2%.

Enteroviruses commonly associated with aseptic meningitis in USA between 1970 and 1979 include the following serotypes: (a) Echovirus 9 (2238 isolates) showed 3 epidemic peaks in 1971, 1975 and 1979,[12] with epidemic spread maximum during August and 84% of isolates were associated with meningitis (60%) and encephalitis (24%); (b) Coxsackievirus B5 (1867 isolates) showed one epidemic peak in 1972, with epidemic spread maximum during August and 92% of isolates were associated with meningitis (77%) and encephalitis (15%). A further large outbreak of coxsackievirus B5 aseptic meningitis occurred throughout USA during 1983, particularly in Texas where the epidemic peaked in June.[16] Echovirus 11 (1509 isolates) peaked in 1979 and a smaller peak occurred in 1972, with 70% of isolates associated with meningitis (56%) and encephalitis (14%) and 55% of echovirus 11 infections involved children aged less than 1 year. Echovirus 4 (1448 isolates) peaked in 1971 and a smaller peak occurred in 1978, with 95% of isolates associated with meningitis (75%) and encephalitis (20%), and the highest proportion of cases (27%) children aged 5–9 years. Echovirus 6 (1150 isolates) peaked in 1972 and 1977, with 85% of isolates associated with meningitis

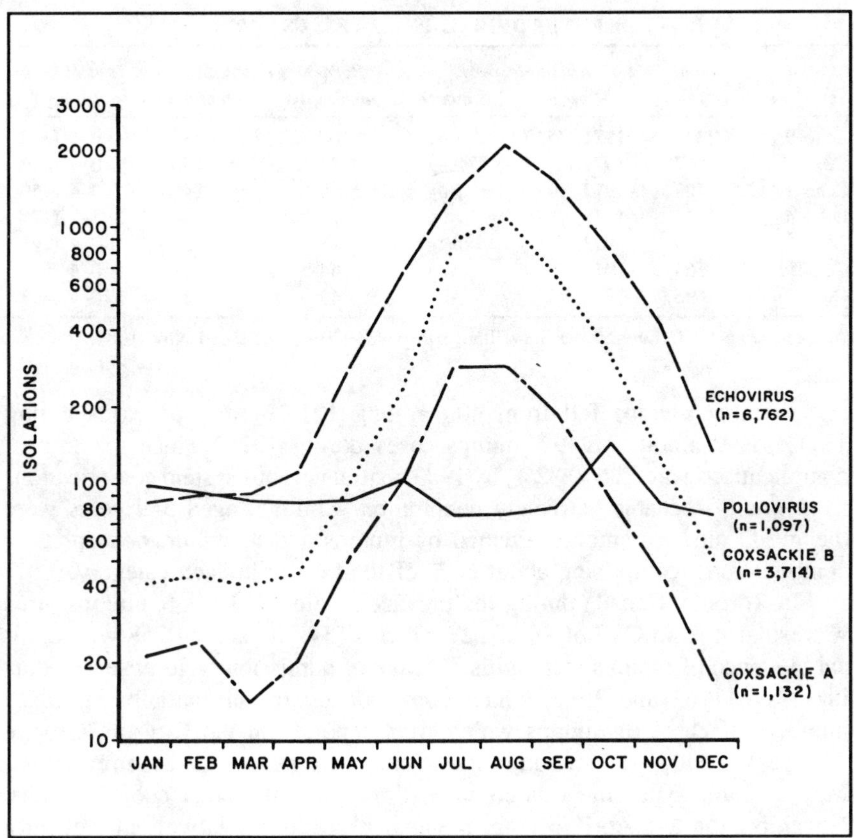

Figure 23-1: Enterovirus isolations, by etiologic agent and month of onset of illness, United States, 1970–1979

(75%) and encephalitis (10%), and the highest proportion of cases (30%) affected children aged less than 5 years, predominantly those under 1 year of age. Coxsackievirus B4 (764 isolations) and coxsackievirus A9 (696 isolations) were endemic throughout the 1970's with relatively small fluctuations in their annual incidence, but in each case August was the peak month of prevalence. (Table 23-2).

Mumps meningitis has comprised a steadily decreasing proportion of the total cases of aseptic meningitis in USA, corresponding with profound decline of total mumps cases from annual incidence rates per 100,000 of 90–180 before licensure of live mumps vaccine in 1967 to 1.4 representing 3355 cases during 1983.[18] (Figure 19-8). Total cases of aseptic meningitis and encephalitis

TABLE 23-2
MAJOR ENTEROVIRAL ISOLATES, USA 1970–1979

Serotype	Total isolates	Epidemic peaks year	month	Percentage isolates meningitis	encephalitis	Peak age group (yr)
Echo 9	2238	1971, 75, 79	Aug	60	24	0–4 (32%)
Cox B5	1867	1972	Aug	77	15	0–4 (44%)
Echo 11	1509	1972, 79	Aug	56	14	0–4 (55%)
Echo 4	1448	1971, 78	Aug	75	20	5–9 (27%)
Echo 6	1150	1972, 77	Aug	75	10	0–4 (29%)
Cox B4	764	1972, 76, 79	Aug	44	14	0–4 (50%)
Cox A9	696	1972, 73, 78	Aug	49	2	0–4 (42%)

Adapted from CDC Enterovirus Surveillance Report 1970–1979. Issued Nov. 1981.

complicating mumps fell from 400 among 121,924 mumps cases during 1971, to 99 among 38,492 mumps cases during 1976.[9] Since the rate of complications was 0.26–0.32%, by 1983 central nervous system complications from mumps became extremely uncommon. Children aged 5–9 years were the group most commonly affected by mumps and its meningoencephalitic complications, comprising about 60% of total cases in each category.

In Toronto, Canada during the prevaccine era 1959–1966, mumps virus was isolated from CSF of 78 of 227 patients (34.4%) among 258 with clinical evidence of mumps meningitis.[38] Peaks of admission were observed during 1960, 1963 and 1966, which corresponded to substantially increased numbers of cases of mumps which were reported in the City of Toronto. The peak monthly rate of admission with mumps meningitis occurred during May, but this syndrome was common throughout the other cooler months, November through April. Mumps meningitis occurred relatively infrequently during the warmer summer months July through October, with minimum incidence during September. However enteroviral meningitis occurred commonly during the warmer months June through October in Toronto[36] in common with the United States.[12] Substantially reduced mumps incidence in Canada during recent years, following routine use of mumps vaccine combined with measles and rubella vaccines, shortly after the first birthday, has rendered mumps meningitis extremely rare; the last case encountered by the author in Vancouver occurred in April 1981.

POLIOMYELITIS

Annual total of reported cases (with rates per 100,000 in parenthesis) of paralytic poliomyelitis in the United States[15] have fallen from a pre-vaccine peak of 21,269 (13.7) in 1952, to 2499 (1.5) in 1957, which was two years after licensure of inactivated poliovirus vaccine in 1955. This decline was continued to 1964 to 106 cases (0.09), two years after licensure of live oral poliovirus vaccine in 1962 to 20 cases (0.010) in 1971, 7 cases (0.003) in 1981 and 4 cases (0.002) in 1984[20] (Figure 23-2). Among the 167 paralytic

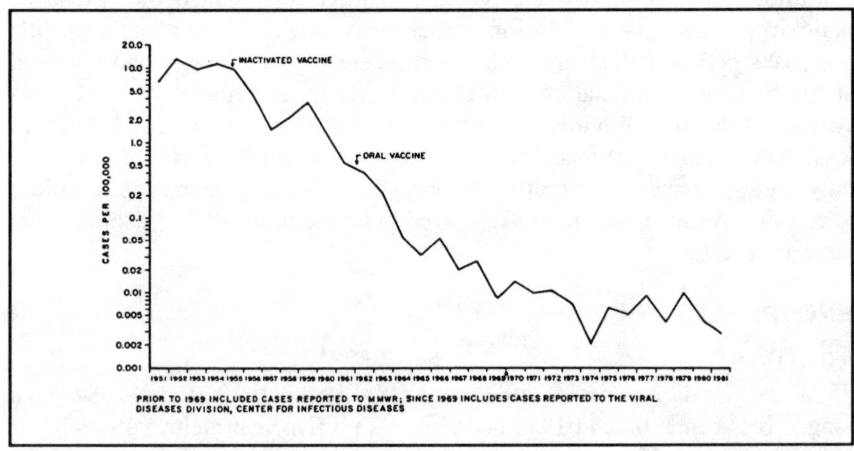

Figure 23-2: Reported paralytic poliomyelitis attack rates, United States, 1951–1981

cases investigated virologically between 1969 and 1981,[15] virtually all epidemic and imported cases were caused by poliovirus 1, most of which were mild-type strains. Most of the vaccine-associated cases were associated with poliovirus 2 or poliovirus 3 strains with vaccine-like characteristics. These were assayed by temperature-marker and modified Wecker tests before 1978, and by van Wezel tests or oligonucleotide mapping of (45 isolates) between 1978 and 1983.[29] Canadian incidence of paralytic poliomyelitis has paralled the US downward trend from 20 cases (1 per 100,000) in 1964, two years after licensure of live oral poliovirus vaccine, to between 0 and 3 cases per year between 1965 and 1984,[27] except during summer 1978 when 8 paralytic cases due to poliovirus 1 occurred among household contacts of visitors from an unvaccinated community in Holland, where poliovirus was epidemic.[26]

In most developed countries in Europe, Japan, Australia and New Zealand, vigorous pursuit of universal campaigns of poliovirus vaccination during the past two decades has virtually eliminated paralytic poliomyelitis, in common with United States and Canadian experience. However in Finland where no cases of poliovirus have been reported during the past 2 decades, following widespread immunization using 6 doses of inactivated poliovirus vaccine, 6 paralytic cases due to poliovirus 3 occurred between October and December 1984, 3 of whom had received 5 doses of inactivated vaccine.[45] These isolates were "not vaccine-like." Poliovirus 3 was also isolated from sewage from

Helsinki and other Finnish cities in 1984, for the first time since the period of 1971–1981 when regular sewage samples revealed no polioviruses. Oral poliovirus vaccine was distributed to the entire Finnish population of about 5 million, through a mass campaign, and effectively halted the spread of poliovirus. Similarly in Taiwan which was free of major poliomyelitis outbreaks between 1975 and 1981, and where 80% of infants had received at least 2 doses of trivalent live oral poliovaccine, an outbreak of 1031 paralytic cases due to poliovirus 1 occurred between May and October 1982.[30] At least 65% paralytic patients were unvaccinated and 19% received one dose only, but since the vaccine efficacy was 98% after 3 or more doses, failure to receive adequate vaccination appeared to be the most likely reason for this large outbreak.

ENCEPHALITIS

ARBOVIRUSES

Encephalitis reportings throughout USA between 1970 and 1984 have ranged between 1302 and 1950 per year, with a five year median 1979–83 of 1595, except in 1975 when reportings peaked at 4308[11,20] (Figure 23-3).

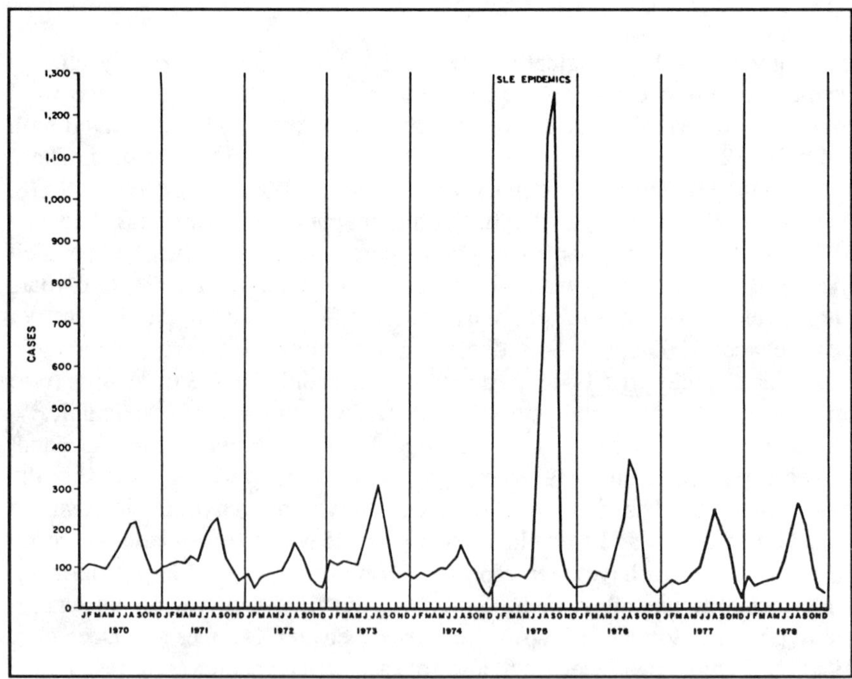

Figure 23-3: Encephalitis—reported cases by month of onset, United States, 1970–1978

Between 70 and 427 cases per year were attributed to arboviruses, approximately 200–600 cases were caused by other viruses, but causes of the remaining 900–1700 cases were indeterminate. Regularly each year, most cases occurred during the warm summer months June through October, with peaks of both arbovirus cases and those of indeterminate etiology occurring during August or September. Of 3451 confirmed arbovirus cases between 1970 and 1978, 73% were causes by St. Louis encephalitis (SLE) and 20% were due to California serogroup (CAL) viruses, whilst 6% were due to western equine encephalomyelitis (WEE), 0.8% to eastern equine encephalomyelitis (EEE), all of which were mosquito-borne, and 0.1% were due to tickborne Powassan (POW) virus. However 1815 of 2514 SLE cases, 133 of 207 WEE cases, and 160 of 679 CAL cases occurred during the major epidemic year 1975.

The geographic distribution of SLE and WEE extends largely from the Ohio-Mississippi Basin westward to California and Pacific Northwestern States.[11] During the 1975 epidemic, which recorded the highest ever annual incidence of SLE, particularly high attack rates were observed in Mississippi and in metropolitan Chicago where the disease had not been recognized previously.[6] North Dakota and adjacent Manitoba experienced high attack rates of WEE. Over 100 cases of SLE occurred in Canada along the north shore of Lake Erie,[44] in addition to 429 cases in Ohio. Southwards, these arboviruses are prevalent in Florida[43] and Texas, and northwards they extend through prairie grassland and parkland of the Canadian Province of Saskatchewan as far as 53° N,[4] where there is a sharp transition into boreal forest. These agents have repeatedly caused encephalitis principally in the San Joaquin and Sacramento valleys of California for many years, but during the summer of 1984, SLE cases were encountered for the first time in coastal suburban communities of Orange County and Los Angeles County.[19] Although both viruses may affect persons of all ages, characteristically SLE involves adults, particularly senior citizens[43] who experience case fatality rates 7–16%; typically WEE involves children and young people. In some outbreaks such as WEE in Manitoba during 1981[41] about 25% virologically confirmed cases of WEE infection exhibited aseptic meningitis without encephalitic manifestations.

Natural vectors of SLE and WEE viruses are culicine mosquitoes. In the Ohio-Mississippi Basin, mosquitoes of the *Culex pipiens* complex[24] are particularly important vectors of SLE both in small rural communities and in large urban centers where the mosquitoes breed periodomestically. In Western USA from the great plains to the Pacific Northwest and California, *Culex tarsalis*[46] is the most important mosquito vector species; it breeds in semipermanent collections of water particularly in irrigation areas. *Culex tarsalis* is also the principal natural vector of SLE and WEE viruses in the Canadian prairie provinces of Saskatchewan and Manitoba.[41] In Florida, the tropical mosquito *Culex nigripalpus* is an important vector.

Natural vertebrate reservoirs of infection are wild birds, particularly those which live near bodies of water or periodomestically. Young birds develop symptomless viremia 2 days after bites by infected mosquitoes, and they serve as sources of infection for mosquitoes which bite these birds during the succeeding 2–4 days. Virus replication occurs within the mosquito tissues, and salivary glands contain substantial virus titers after 2–3 weeks of extrinsic incubation at summertime temperatures, at which time the virus is transmitted by biting other birds. Humans become infected by mosquitoes tangential to this natural bird-mosquito cycle (Figure 23-4). Although this is

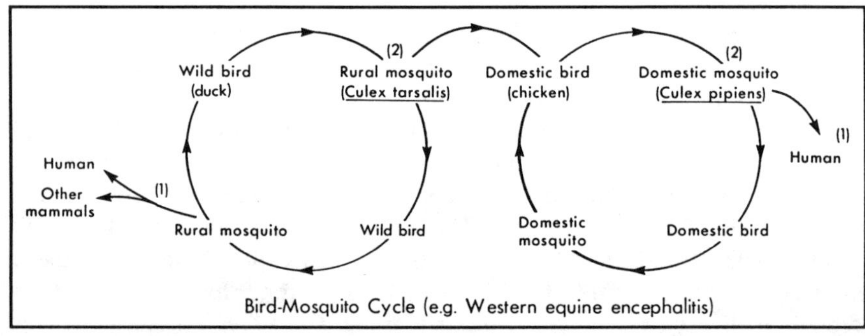

Figure 23-4: Bird-mosquito cycle of arbovirus transmission in nature eg. western equine encephalitis virus. Reproduced with permission from McLean DM 1980. Virology in Health Care, Williams and Wilkins, Baltimore, p. 171.

the normal mechanism of arbovirus transmission in nature, recent experimental evidence with SLE virus has demonstrated the possibility of transovarial transmission.[24]

California serogroup infections causing encephalitis or aseptic meningitis in North America have arisen from infections with 2 serovarieties of the La Crosse serotype. (a) The La Crosse (LAC) serovariety has caused serologically or virologically confirmed cases of central nervous system disease, frequently encephalitis, in 24 States from the Ohio-Mississippi Basin eastwards to the Atlantic Seaboard,[5] and virus isolations have been achieved from *Aedes sp.* mosquitoes collected in 13 of these States. The principal mosquito vector, *Aedes triseriatus,* breeds in tree holes and accumulations of water in used-tire yards adjacent to human habitations; the principal vertebrate reservoirs are squirrels and rabbits or hares. During summer, humans become infected tangentially to this natural cycle (Figure 23-5). In addition to this

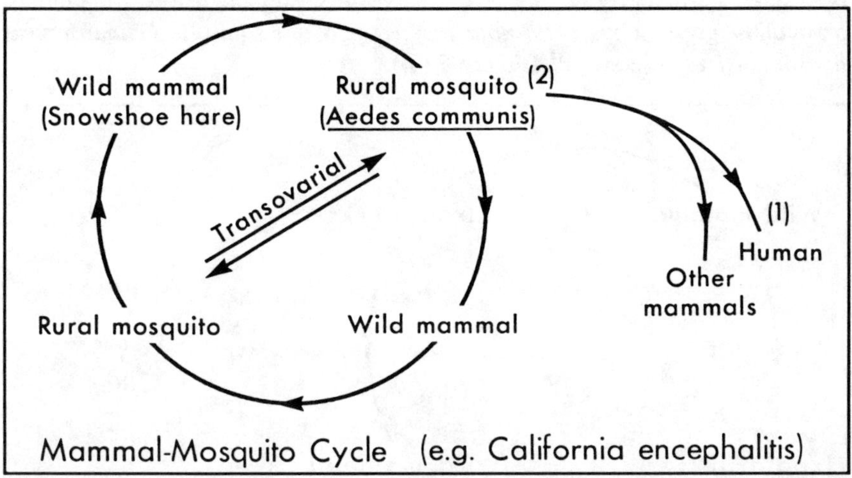

Figure 23-5: Mammal-mosquito cycle of arbovirus transmission in nature, including transovarial transfer eg. California serogroup viruses such as La Crosse and snowshoe hare serovarities. Reproduced with permission from McLean DM 1980. Virology in Health Care, Williams and Wilkins, Baltimore, p 172.

summertime cycle of transmission, transovarial transfer[3] provides an important overwintering mechanism for persistence of CAL serogroup viruses in localities between successive summers (b) The Snowshoe hare serovariety (SSH) has caused serologically confirmed cases of aseptic meningitis in woodland areas of eastern Canada[1] in Ontario and Quebec. Geographically, SSH prevalence extends from these regions, together with upstate New York and Montana, northwards through the boreal forest and open woodland of subartic Canada, including the Yukon Territory[39] and Alaska, with *Aedes communis* as an important vector and snowshoe hares plus ground squirrels as major vertebrate reservoirs.

Serological evidence of human infection has been obtained with two additional CAL serogroup agents: (a) Jamestown Canyon subtype has been associated with encephalitis in Indiana[25] and New York State,[49] and virus has been isolated from mosquitoes collected in these States and in Southwestern States;[5] (b) Trivittatus virus has caused inapparent infections,[49] and it has been isolated from mosquitoes collected in States bordering the Great Lakes from New York to Minnesota, but also in the Dakotas and Southeastern States.[5]

Powassan (POW) virus was first isolated from a fatal case of encephalitis in rural Ontario, Canada in 1958.[34] Scientific reports of an additional 18 cases from Ontario, Quebec, New York State and Pennsylvania have been published in 1983.[23] This virus is maintained in nature by a cycle involving hard ticks, particularly *Ixodes cookei* as vectors, and small forest mammals, particulary groundhogs *(Marmota monax)* and red squirrels *(Tamiasciurus hudsonicus)* as reservoirs[37] (Figure 23-6).

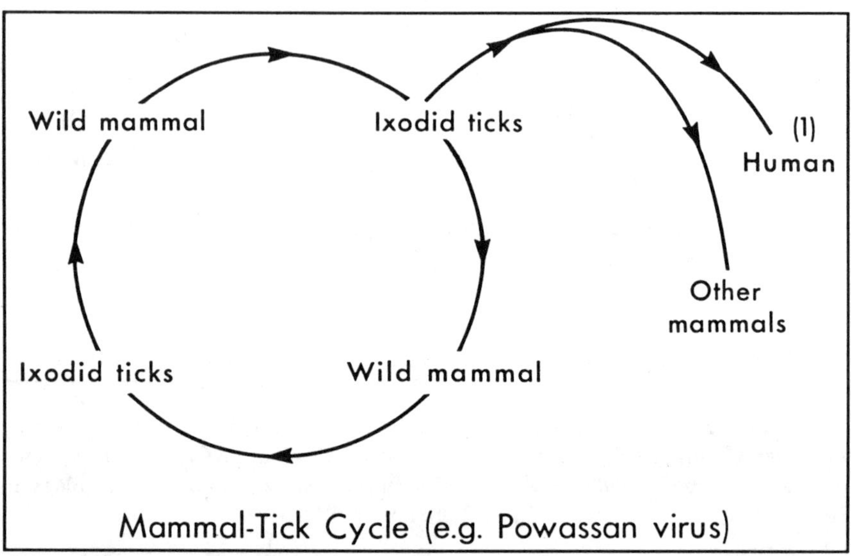

Figure 23-6: Mammal-tick cycle of arbovirus transmission in nature eg. Powassan virus. Reproduced with permission from McLean DM 1980. Virology in Health Care, Williams and Wilkins, Baltimore, p 174.

Arboviruses cause encephalitis in all six zoogeographic regions throughout the world, but a particular serotype is usually restricted to one region. Mosquito-borne flaviviruses are represented in North America by SLE virus, the Orient by Japanese B encephalitis virus, Australasia by Murray Valley encephalitis virus, South America by Rocio virus and Africa by West Nile virus. Tick-borne flaviviruses cause encephalitis in North America by POW virus, in Europe by tick-borne encephalitis virus and in Siberia by Russian spring-summer encephalitis virus. The epidemiology of these and other arboviruses is discussed in a textbook.[31]

RABIES

During the past decade, rabies has caused between 1 and 4 fatal cases each year in USA except 1980 and 1982 when no cases were recorded.[17,20] On the other hand, rabies has been identified in 2627 to 5896 wild or domestic animals annually between 1975 and 1984. Important reservoir animals, comprising about 85% of proved rabid infections, are skunks, foxes, raccoons and bats,[17] with cattle, dogs and cats comprising a minority of infected species. Rabies is endemic in wild animals in most parts of the world, except Australasia which is maintained free of rabies through enforcement of strict quarantine laws. Rabies is transmitted from animals to humans by salivary contamination of bite wounds. On two recent occasions however, rabies was transmitted by corneal grafts obtained from donors during the incubation period of rabies.[10,28]

PREVENTION

MUMPS MENINGITIS

Administration of one subcutaneous dose of live mumps virus vaccine containing 5000 TCD_{50} of the attenuated Jeryl Lynn strain,[14] usually as a trivalent combination with live measles and rubella vaccines (MMR), to all children as soon as possible after the first birthday, has induced immunity in a sufficiently high proportion of the US population that mumps and consequently mumps meningitis have been virtually eliminated since 1982. Con tinuing vaccination of infants will be required for several years in order to prevent attacks by importation of mumps, inadvertently by travellers from endemic areas, who arrive during the incubation period. The vaccine efficacy approaches 90%, and vaccine-induced immunity has persisted at least 15 years.[14]

POLIOMYELITIS

Paralytic poliomyelitis has been virtually eliminated from North America, most of Europe, some Asian countries and Australasia through prolonged programs of administration of 3 doses of trivalent oral poliovirus vaccine (Sabin) during the first year of life, followed by boosters upon school entry.[13,29] In addition to long duration of immunity, extending for 20 years or more, live poliovaccine inhibits colonization of the intestine by wild poliovirus strains, thus substantially reducing their circulation in the community. The risk of contracting a paralytic infection following administration of oral poliovaccine is less than 0.25 per million.[13] However Holland and the Scandinavian countries[45] have achieved profound reduction of incidence of paralytic disease through the subcutaneous injection of 4 doses of trivalent inactivated poliovaccine (Salk) during the initial 12 months of life followed by a booster upon school entry, similar to the US recommendations.[13] Although an additional booster of inactivated vaccine is recommended currently, future more potent inactivated vaccines may induce long-term immunity following two doses only.[47] Unfortunately, the intestinal carriage of wild-type poliovirus strains remains unaffected following inactivated vaccine. Although inactivated vaccines may be substituted for live oral vaccines during times of unavailability of the live product for routine immunization, they cannot be used for control of epidemic spread of poliovirus, for which live vaccine is essential, as in Finland during late 1984.[45]

RABIES

POSTEXPOSURE PROPHYLAXIS

Following bites by wild mammals such as skunks, bats, foxes or other carnivorous animals, administration of human diploid cell rabies vaccine (HDCV) should be commenced immediately, accompanied by one dose of rabies immune globulin, human (RIG).[17] HDCV is an inactivated virus vaccine prepared from fixed rabies virus propagated in human diploid cells WI-38 and inactivated with tri-n-butyl phosphate plus β-propiolactone in USA, or grown in MRC-5 diploid cells and inactivated with β-propiolactone in France, and distributed in vials as 1.0 ml doses. The first dose of HDCV should be administered intramuscularly as soon as possible after exposure and repeated on days 3, 7, 14 and 28. The dose of RIG is 20 international units per kg body weight intramuscularly.

Following bites by domestic dogs and cats which appear healthy, antirabies treatment is not normally prescribed unless the animal becomes rabid during the succeeding 10 days, or if the animal is sacrificed and rabies antigen is demonstrated in the brain.

All bite wounds and scratches require immediate and thorough washing with soap and water. Tetanus prophylaxis and measures to control bacterial infection should be given as indicated.

PREEXPOSURE IMMUNIZATION

Veterinarians, animal handlers and some laboratory technicians comprise risk groups who should be offered preexposure prophylaxis against rabies. Three doses of HDCV are administered intramuscularly on days 0, 7 and 28, and additional boosters to maintain adequate antirabies antibody titers should be offered at intervals of approximately 2 years.

REFERENCES

[1]Artsob H, Spence L, Surgeoner G, et al: Snowshoe hare virus activity in Southern Ontario. Can J Pub Health 73:345, 1982.

[2]Azimi PH, Cramblett HG, Haynes RE: Mumps meningoencephalitis in children. JAMA 207:509, 1969.

[3]Beaty BJ, Thompson WH: Delineation of La Crosse virus in developmental stages of transovarially infected *Aedes triseriatus*. Am J Trop Med Hyg 25:505, 1976.

[4]Burton AN, McLintock J: Further evidence of western encephalitis infection in Saskatchewan mammals and birds and in reindeer in Northern Canada. Can Vet J 11:232, 1970.

[5]Calisher CH, Thompson WH eds: California Serogroup Viruses. Alan R Liss Inc, New York, 1983.

[6]Centers for Disease Control: Encephalitis Surveillance Summary 1975, issued May 1977.

[7]Centers for Disease Control: Measles Surveillance Report No. 10, 1973–1976, issued July 1977.

[8]Center for Disease Control: Follow-up on Guillain-Barré syndrome - United States. MMWR 26:7, 1977.

[9]Centers for Disease Control: Mumps Surveillance, July 1974–December 1976, Issued July 1978.

[10]Centers for Disease Control: Human-to-human transmission of rabies via corneal transplant. MMWR 29:25, 1980.

[11]Centers for Disease Control: Encephalitis Surveillance. Annual Summary 1978, issued May 1981.

[12]Centers for Disease Control: Enterovirus Surveillance Report, 1970–1979, Issued Nov. 1981.

[13]Centers for Disease Control: Poliomyelitis prevention. MMWR 31:22, 1982.

[14]Centers for Disease Control: Mumps vaccine. MMWR 31:617, 1982.

[15]Centers for Disease Control: Poliomyelitis Surveillance Summary 1980–1981, issued Dec. 1982.

[16]Centers for Disease Control: Coxsackievirus B5 meningitis - Texas, 1983. MMWR 33:281, 1984.

[17]Centers for Disease Control: Rabies prevention - United States, 1984. MMWR 33:393, 1984.

[18]Centers for Disease Control: Mumps - United States, 1983–84. MMWR 33:533, 1984.

[19]Centers for Disease Control: St. Louis encephalitis - California, MMWR 33:649, 1984.

[20]Centers for Disease Control: Summary-cases of specified notifiable disease United States. MMWR 33:720, 1985.

[21]Conn RB ed: Current Diagnosis 7. W. B. Saunders Co, Philadelphia 1984 p. 1317.

[22]Connolly J, Haire M, Hadden DSM: Measles immunoglobulins in subacute sclerosing panencephalitis. Brit Med J 1:23, 1971.

[23]Embil JA, Camfield P, Artsob H, Chase DP: Powassan encephalitis resembling herpes simplex encephalitis. Arch Int Med 143:341, 1983.

[24]Francy DB, Rush WA, Montoya M, et al: Transovarial transmission of St. Louis encephalitis virus by *Culex pipiens* complex mosquitoes. Am J Trop Med Hyg 30:699, 1981.

[25]Grimstad PR, Shabino CL, Calisher CH, Waldman RJ: A case of encephalitis in a human associated with a serological rise to Jamestown Canyon Virus. Am J Trop Med Hyg 31:1238, 1982.

[26]Health and Welfare Canada: Poliomyelitis in contacts of Netherlands Travellers - Ontario, Alberta and British Columbia. Can Dis Wkly Rep 4:157, 1978.

[27]Health and Welfare Canada: A Guide to Immunization for Canadians, 2nd ed 1984.

[28]Houff SA, Burton RC, Wilson RW, et al: Human-to-human transmission of rabies virus by corneal transplant. New Eng J Med 300:603, 1979.

[29]Kim-Farley RJ, Bart KJ, Schonberger LB, et al: Poliomyelitis in the USA: virtual elimination of disease caused by wild virus. Lancet 2:1315, 1984.

[30]Kim-Farley RJ, Rutherford G, Lechfield P, et al: Outbreak of paralytic poliomyelitis, Taiwan. Lancet 2:1322, 1984.

[31]McLean DM: Virology in Health Care. Williams and Wilkins, Baltimore 1980.

[32]McLean DM: Immunological Investigation of Human Virus Disease. Churchill Livingstone, Edinburgh 1982 pp 47–51.

[33]McLean DM, Wong KK: Same-day Diagnosis of Human Virus Infections. CRC Press, Boca Raton FL, 1984 pp 66–67.

[34]McLean DM, Donohue WL: Powassan virus: isolation of virus from a fatal case of encephalitis. Can Med Ass J 80:708, 1959.

[35]McLean DM, Donohue WL, Snelling CE, Wyllie JC: Coxsackie B5 virus as a cause of neonatal encephalitis and myocarditis. Can Med Ass J 85:1046, 1961.

[36]McLean DM: Coxsackieviruses and echoviruses. Am J Med Sc 251:351, 1966.

[37]McLean DM, Cobb C, Gooderham SE, et al: Powassan virus: persistence of virus activity during 1966. Can Med Ass J 96:660, 1967.

[38]McLean DM, Larke RPB, Cobb C, Griffis ED, Hackett SMR: Mumps and enteroviral meningitis in Toronto, 1966. Can Med Ass J 96:1355, 1967.

[39]McLean DM, Lester SA: Isolations of snowshoe have virus from Yukon mosquitoes, 1983. Mosq News 44:200, 1984.

[40]Magoffin RL, Lennette EH, Hollister AC, Schmidt NJ: An etiological study of clinical paralytic poliomyelitis JAMA 175:269, 1961.

[41]Manitoba Ministry of Health: Western Equine Encephalitis in Manitoba. Dec 1982.

[42]Nagington J, Wreghitt TG, Gandy G, Roberton NRC, Berry PJ: Fatal echovirus-11 infections in outbreak in special-care baby unit. Lancet 2:725, 1978.

[43]Nelson DB, Kappus KD, Janowski HT, et al: St. Louis encephalitis - Florida 1977. Patterns of a widespread outbreak. Am J Trop Med Hyg 32:412, 1983.

[44]Ontario Ministry of Health: Arboviral Encephalitides in Ontario with special reference to St. Louis Encephalitis 1979.

[45]Public Health Laboratory Service: Communicable Disease Report 85/06 p 3. 1985.

[46]Reeves WC, Hammon W Mc D: Epidemiology of the Arthropod-borne Viral Encephalitides in Kern County, California 1943–52. University of California Publications in Public Health, Vol 4, 1962.

[47]Salk D, VanWezel AL, Salk J: Induction of long-term immunity to paralytic poliomyelitis by use of non-infectious vaccine. Lancet 2:1317, 1984.

[48]Sells CJ, Carpenter RL, Ray CG: Sequelae of central nervous system Enterovirus infections. New Eng J Med 293:1, 1975.

[49]Srihongses, Grayson MA, Deibel R: California serogroup viruses in New York State: the role of subtypes in human infections. Am J Trop Med Hyg 33:1218, 1984.

[50]Wingate MB, Meller HK, Ormiston G: Acute bulbar poliomyelitis in late pregnancy. Brit Med J 1:407, 1961.

CHAPTER 24

IMPORTED TROPICAL VIRAL INFECTIONS

Viruses exotic to North America (Table 24-1) are causing illnesses among steadily increasing numbers of travellers, upon their return to the Temperature Zone, after visits to tropical regions where these viruses are endemic.[26] These include arboviruses and certain non-arthropod-borne agents in similar ecological niches.

CLINICAL

Travel history is the most important single component of the clinical assessment of patients who develop fevers of unexplained origin within 2 weeks after their arrival in North America from the Tropics. Following appropriate bacteriological tests to exclude salmonellosis or shigellosis, and parasitological tests to eliminate amoebiasis, malaria or schistosomiasis, clues as to the identity of the possible causative virus are derived from a knowledge of the geographical distribution of arboviruses and certain non-arthropod-borne viruses customarily investigated by arbovirologists. Since arbovirus foci are frequently localized within a particular bioclimatic or vegetation zone within a country, the travel history should include details of urban or rural locations visited by the patient. It is also important to eliminate common virological syndromes such as measles or chickenpox, using a combination of same-day tests by electron microscopy and immunofluorescence, or enteroviral disease, by attempts at virus isolation plus serological procedures.

Clinical manifestations of tropical arbovirus infections include: yellow fever (hepatic involvement), dengue and other febrile infections with or without rashes or hemorrhagic phenomena (Table 24-1); encephalitis or aseptic meningitis (Chapter 23) may also arise from viruses endemic in some countries. Non-arthropod-borne agents, Lassa and Marburg viruses, induce hemorrhagic fevers, whilst rabies induces fatal central nervous system disease (Chapter 23).

YELLOW FEVER

Patients suddenly develop headache and fever, accompanied by generalized myalgia, nausea, vomiting, apprehension and injected conjunctivae.[31,43]

TABLE 24-1

TIME COURSE AND LABORATORY DIAGNOSIS OF TROPICAL VIRAL INFECTIONS IMPORTED INTO NORTH AMERICA

		Incu-	Duration of		Virus antigen (serum)				Antibodies (paired sera)		
	Virus species	*bation*						*virus*		*initial*	*persis-*
Syndrome	*(genus)*	*period*	*comm.*	*illness*	*specimen*	*EM*	*IF*	*isolation*	*test*	*detection*	*tence*
Yellow fever	yellow fever (Flavivirus)	3–6d	–1 to +4d (viremia)	3–10d	blood liver (fatal)	n/a	+ (liver)	VERO BHK SM MOS	HI NT CF	3–7d 10–14d	20+ yr 3 yr
Dengue	dengue 1–4 (Flavivirus)	4–14d	–1 to +2d (viremia)	3–10d	blood	n/a	n/a	VERO BHK SM MOS	HI NT ELISA	3–7d	20+ yr
Tropical fevers	Arthropod-borne: Ross River (Alphavirus), Oropouche (Bunyavirus), Rift Valley Fever (Phlebovirus) Non-arthropod-borne: Lassa (Arenavirus), Marburg (Filovirus) Incubation periods and laboratory identification resemble those for dengue and yellow fever										

BHK:	continuous baby hamster kidney cultures	CF:	complement fixation
VERO:	continuous monkey kidney cultures (grivet)	ELISA:	enzyme-linked immunosorbent assay
SM:	suckling mice (intracerebrally)	HI:	hemagglutination inhibition
MOS:	mosquitoes inoculated intrathoracically	NT:	neutralization

Convulsions may herald the onset of yellow fever in children. Jaundice may appear on the third day of illness, and hematemesis and melena, epistaxis and bleeding gums may also occur. Albuminuria and oliguria may also begin suddenly during the first week of illness.

The incubation period is 3–6 days. Illness usually persists 3–10 days. In severe cases, death may occur 3 days or more after onset of illness; midzonal necrosis is observed in the liver. The overall case-fatality rate is 5–10%. Mild cases may develop fever, headache and myalgia only; it is important to distinguish these cases of yellow fever from dengue or other tropical arboviruses, by isolation of virus from the blood, or appropriate serological tests. Care must be taken to distinguish yellow fever from hepatitis A or hepatitis B, from bacterial infections including leptospirosis and borreliosis, and from protozoan infections such as malaria, by appropriate laboratory tests.

DENGUE

Patients suddenly develop fever and severe frontal headache, accompanied by retro-ocular pain, myalgia, pain in the back and limbs ("break-bone fever"), perversions of taste, and lymphadenopathy, in the absence of persisting respiratory symptoms.[8,37] A maculopapular rash lasting 2–7 days may affect two-thirds of the patients and pruritus about half the patients.

The incubation period is 4–14 days. Fever may persist 3–5 days and it may show a remission followed by a relapse ("saddleback fever") in about half the patients. Leukopenia with relative lymphocytosis is a constant finding. Complete recovery is the rule after typical dengue.

Although clinically typical dengue usually arises from infection with one of 4 serotypes of dengue virus (Flavivirus), chikungunya (Alphavirus) has induced symptoms closely resembling dengue.[12]

HEMORRHAGIC FEVERS

In southeast Asia since 1958, and in islands of the Southwest Pacific since 1971, hemorrhagic manifestations including purpura, epistasis, hematuria and gastrointestinal hemorrhage, which are accompanied by varying degrees of shock, have been observed in association with the typical symptoms of dengue.[20,29] Both children and adults are affected, but in Southeast Asia the incidence of severe and fatal cases is highest among children aged 3–7 years. Thrombocytopenia with platelet counts below 100,000 per µl is found in about two-thirds of cases, persisting 1–2 weeks, but counts have been as low at 10,000–16,000 per µ l 4–6 days after onset. The case fatality rate from hemorrhagic dengue is 4–12%.

Similar hemorrhagic states have also been caused by chikungunya virus (Alphavirus)[38] and Kyasanur Forest disease virus (Flavivirus)[47] in eastern and western India respectively, but Congo-Crimean hemorrhagic fever virus (Nairovirus) in South Africa[34] and Korean hemorrhagic fever (also termed hemorrhagic fever with renal syndrome) due to Hantaan virus (Bunyaviridae) in Korea,[24] Greece,[2] Scotland[45] and elsewhere in Europe.

UNDIFFERENTIATED TROPICAL FEVERS

Febrile illnesses in the tropics may arise from infection with a wide range of arbovirus serotypes. Some infections resemble dengue with intense pain in the bones and muscles, others may be accompanied by polyarthritis. Mayaro (Alphavirus) caused fever, arthralgia and exanthema in Para State, Brazil during 1978,[33] comparable to earlier outbreaks of this syndrome in Trinidad 1954 and Para, Brazil in 1955. The bunyavirus Oropouche has caused 7 outbreaks of fever, rash and polyarthritis in Para, Brazil between 1961 and 1978.[32] Ross River (Alphavirus) caused an outbreak of fever and polyarthritis in Raratonga (Cook Islands) in 1980,[36] following earlier epidemic activity of this virus in Australia, New Guinea, the Solomon Islands, Fiji[1] and New Caledonia.[16] The phlebovirus Rift Valley fever (RVF) (Bunyaviridae) has caused extensive outbreaks of fever in Egypt in 1977 and 1978 with a case fatality rate about 0.3%[6] and in Central African Republic since 1974[18] following its introduction from sub-Saharan Africa. A serious, but well recognized complication of RVF, exudative lesions and retinal hemorrhages in both eyes, affected a Canadian visitor upon her return to Canada, 5 weeks after she developed fever, sweating, myalgia, fatigue, severe headache and neck stiffness, which began 3 days after visiting a nature reserve in Kenya during January 1979.[21] The nairovirus Congo-Crimean hemorrhagic fever (Bunyaviridae) caused fever with hemorrhages and jaundice clinically resembling yellow fever in the Upper Volta[39] and in Mauritania[40] during 1983, in addition to causing fatal hemorrhagic fever in a visitor to a nature reserve in Transvaal Province, South Africa in 1981,[34] but it caused fever and joint pains in patients near Stanleyville, Congo in 1956.[46]

NON-ARTHROPOD-BORNE AGENTS INVESTIGATED BY ARBOVIROLOGISTS (ROBOVIRUSES)

Lassa (Arenaviridae) and Marburg plus Ebola (Filoviridae) are important human pathogens in equatorial Africa which are not transmitted by arthropods. They are transmitted by: (a) contamination of abraded skin and mucous membranes with virus-containing urine from infected rodent reservoirs as in Lassa virus; (b) parenteral inoculation using instruments contaminated by monkey tissues (Marburg), or syringes contaminated by human blood (Ebola). These agents are now termed Roboviruses.

Lassa virus has induced severe generalized infections with high fever, headache, anorexia, nausea, vomiting, myalgia, pharyngitis with petechiae or ulcers, abdominal pain and hypotension during outbreaks near Jos, Nigeria in 1969[17] and Zorzor, Liberia in 1972,[28] with a case fatality rate of 40% or higher. Lassa hemorrhagic fever developed in a patient in London, England in January 1982, following her arrival 6 days earlier from Jos, Nigeria, and the patient recovered after several months of illness.[15]

Marburg and Ebola viruses both induce severe hemorrhagic fevers with case fatality rates 20–80%. Initial cases of Marburg virus infections occurred largely among workers in Marburg, West Germany with tissues from African green monkeys received recently from their natural habitat in Uganda.[41] During 1980, two human residents of Kenya contracted Marburg disease, one of whom died.[42] Many Ebola infections have occurred among patients and health workers in Zaire who routinely used inadequately sterilized syringes and needles,[30] thus permitting transmission of infected blood between individuals.

LABORATORY DIAGNOSIS

Whenever possible attempts should be made to isolate virus from samples of whole blood (preferably), or triturated blood clot or plasma, which are obtained by venepuncture 1–3 days after onset of fever. Suspensions should be inoculated: (a) intracerebrally into suckling mice aged less than 48 hours which are supervised daily for development of encephalitis during the succeeding 14 days; (b) monolayer cultures of continuous lines of baby hamster kidney (BHK) or African green monkey kidney (VERO) which are incubated under agarose overlay and observed for plaque formation during the succeeding week or more; intrathoracically into colonized *Aedes aegypti* or *Ae. albopictus*[19] or *Toxorhynchites amboinensis*[35] mosquitoes, which are incubated for 14 days or more at 32° C, and the salivary glands and mosquito brains are examined for presence of arbovirus antigen by direct immunofluorescence. Tissue cultures from the C6/36 clone of *Ae. albopictus* mosquito cells have revealed immunofluorescent foci 24 hours after inoculation with Ross River virus. Mosquitoes frequently are 10–100 times more susceptible to infection by small amounts of virus than suckling mice or tissue cultures.[27,35] Final serological identification of the fresh arbovirus isolates is conducted by hemagglutination inhibition tests and by neutralization tests either in suckling mice or in tissue cultures by plaque reduction (Chapters 10, 23). Precision of identification of dengue serotypes is enhanced using monoclonal antibodies.[22]

Serological methods are of vital diagnostic significance in the absence of virus isolation. Rising antibody titres in paired sera are observed by hemagglutination inhibition (HI), plaque reduction neutralization tests (PRNT) and IgM capture ELISA tests within one week after onset of illness, whilst complement fixing antibodies are not detected until 3–4 weeks after onset. With some flaviviruses such as dengue, especially where more than one serotype is prevalent, results of HI and PRNT tests may not indicate clearly the infecting serotype due to antigenic overlap. Indirect immunofluorescence tests are used extensively for detection of antibodies to Lassa and Marburg viruses,[23] but these procedures must be conducted in specially constructed isolation units due to the hazardous nature of these viruses.

EPIDEMIOLOGY

Yellow fever is endemic in tropical South America and the Caribbean. It is maintained in nature principally by a sylvan or jungle cycle in the forest canopy involving tree-dwelling monkeys as reservoirs and tree-hole breeding *Haemogogus* mosquitoes as vectors. Humans become infected by bites of forest mosquitoes, often during forest clearing operations. Yellow fever is also endemic in tropical Africa between latitudes 15° N and 15° S, extending northwards into Ethiopia and the Sudan. Principal sylvan vertebrate reservoirs are monkeys of the genera *Cercopithecus* (African green) and *Colobus*. Vectors are *Aedes africanus* in the forest, *Ae. simpsoni* in the forest fringe and plantation areas, and *Ae. aegypti* in urban areas. In equatorial Africa, Rift Valley fever and Congo-Crimean hemorrhagic fever viruses sometimes coexist in the same regions.[40,41]

Dengue is endemic in tropical portions of Central and South America and the Caribbean. Dengue epidemiology before 1980 has been summarized in a textbook.[25] Following the initial dengue-2 virus isolation in Trinidad in 1953, dengue-3 virus was first recognized in Puerto Rico in 1963, dengue-1 virus activity was initially identified in Puerto Rico in 1977 and 1978, and dengue 4 prevalence was confirmed serologically in Chicago resident who returned 4 days earlier by air from St. Barthelemy in 1981.[7] Dengue types 1, 2 and 4 viruses were isolated from humans in Mexico during 1983[10] where dengue was prevalent in all regions except desert and mountains. During 1982, dengue viruses were isolated from 6 persons with imported dengue after returning to the United States: dengue-1 virus in returnees from Mexico and New Delhi, India; dengue-2 from individuals exposed in Jamaica and Sri Lanka; dengue 4 from visitors to Puerto Rico and Martinique.[9] Serological confirmation of imported dengue was also obtained in travellers from other Caribbean islands, Central America, Southeast Asia, the Pacific

Islands, India and Africa. Hemorrhagic manifestations were observed in 2 cases of imported dengue.

Dengue virus is maintained in nature by a cycle involving humans both as reservoirs and target hosts for the disease, together with domestic mosquitoes *(Aedes aegypti)* or peridomestic mosquitoes (*Ae. albopictus* or *Ae. polynesiensis*) as vectors (Figure 24-1). Dengue virus is transmitted mainly

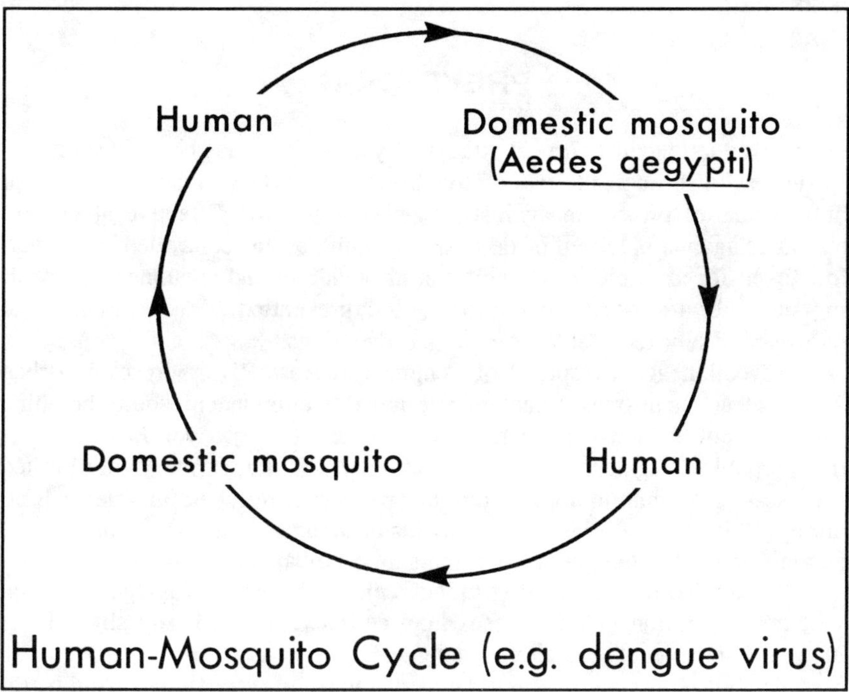

Figure 24-1: Human-mosquito cycle of arbovirus transmission (domestic cycle) eg. dengue virus. Reproduced with permission from McLean DM 1980. Virology in Health Care, Williams and Wilkins, Baltimore, p 170.

in urban areas where houses are unscreened against mosquitoes which breed readily in rainwater accumulations in tins, motor tires, or treeholes adjacent to human habitation.

Ross River virus has caused febrile illnesses, sometimes accompanied by maculopapular rash and arthralgia in humans residing in coastal areas of Australia, extending northwards from Newcastle, New South Wales (32° S, 152° E)[11] into tropical Queensland.[13] Epidemics of polyarthritis due to Ross River virus affected Fiji in 1979[1] and the Cook Islands in 1980[36] where virus was also isolated from *Ae. polynesiensis* mosquitoes. Serological evidence of Ross River virus infection was obtained in 6 subjects who developed fever, rash and polyarthritis upon return to U.S.A. from visits to Fiji, American Samoa or Australia during 1979.[4,5] The principal mosquito vector in the Pacific islands appears to be *Ae. polynesiensis*, and on the Australian mainland *Ae. vigilax*, and humans are both reservoirs and target hosts.

PREVENTION

Prevention against clinical attacks of yellow fever has been outstandingly successful through the use of live attenuated 17D vaccine.[44] This is the only means of protection against jungle yellow fever. Effective abatement measures against breed-up of domestic mosquitoes has controlled urban yellow fever, for example by screening of all windows and containers for holding of water for domestic purposes, and prevention of accumulation of rainwater in any receptacle near human dwellings.

Prevention against spread of dengue and Ross River viruses in urban areas is feasible through procedures designed to eliminate mosquito breeding sites adjacent to human habitations, comparable to urban yellow fever. Active prophylaxis against dengue-3 infection was first attempted, with limited success due to immunological overlap between serotypes, in Puerto Rico during 1966, through the use of attenuated dengue-1 mouse brain vaccine administered subcutaneously.[3] A promising candidate dengue-4 strain, attenuated by passage in primary dog kidney cells followed by passage and final vaccine preparation in fetal rhesus lung cells induced rash and slight fever in 2 of 8 recipients, but altered dengue-4 virus was recovered from these persons, thus rendering this candidate strain unsuitable for further administration to humans.[14] Attempts are in progress to prepare live attenuated dengue vaccines which immunize humans but which remain attenuated after growth in recipients.

REFERENCES

[1]Aaskov JG, Matiaka JU, Lawrence GW, et al: An epidemic of Ross River virus infections in Fiji 1979. Am J Trop Med Hyg 30:1053, 1981.

[2]Antoniadis A, Pyrpasopoulos M, Sion M, et al: Two cases of hemorrhagic fever with renal syndrome in Northern Greece. J Infect Dis 149:1011, 1984.

[3]Bellanti JA, Bourke ATC, Buescher EL, et al: Report of dengue vaccine field trial in the Caribbean, 1963: a collaborative study. Bull WHO 35:93, 1966.

[4]Centers for Disease Control: Ross River virus outbreak - Fiji. MMWR 28:323, 1979.

[5]Centers for Disease Control: Ross River virus infection - American Samoa. MMWR 29:50, 1980.

[6]Centers for Disease Control: Rift Valley fever - Egypt. MMWR 20:178, 1980.

[7]Centers for Disease Control: Dengue 4 infections in U.S. travellers to the Caribbean. MMWR 30:249, 1981.

[8]Centers for Disease Control: Imported dengue type 4 - Florida. MMWR 30:622, 1982.

[9]Centers for Disease Control: Imported dengue fever - United States, 1982. MMWR 32:145, 1983.

[10]Centers for Disease Control: Dengue - Mexico, 1983. MMWR 33:203, 1984.

[11]Clarke JA, Marshall ID, Gard G: Annually recurrent epidemic polyarthritis and Ross River virus activity in a coastal area of New South Wales. I. Occurrence of the disease. Am J Trop Med Hyg 22:543, 1973.

[12]Deller JJ, Russell PK: Chikungunya disease. Am J Trop Med Hyg 17:107, 1968.

[13]Doherty RL, Carley JG, Best JC: Isolation of Ross River virus from man. Med J Austral 1:1083, 1972.

[14]Eckels KH, Scott RMcN, Bancroft WH, et al: Selection of attenuated dengue 4 viruses by serial passage in primary kidney cells. V Human response to immunization with a candidate vaccine prepared in fetal rhesus lung cells. Am J Trop Med Hyg 33:684, 1984.

[15]Emond RTD, Bannister B, Lloyd G, et al: A case of Lassa fever: clinical and virological findings. Brit Med J 285:1001, 1982.

[16]Fauran P, Donaldson M, Harper J, et al: Characterization of Ross River viruses isolated from patients with polyarthritis in New Caledonia and Wallis and Futura Islands. Am J Trop Med Hyg 33:1228, 1984.

[17]Frame JD, Baldwin JM, Gocke DJ, Troup JM: Lassa fever, a virus disease of man from West Africa. I. Clinical description and pathological findings. Am J Trop Med Hyg 19:670, 1970.

[18]Georges AJ, Wahid SA, Meurier DYM, et al: Serological equivalence of endemic Zinga virus and Rift Valley fever virus in Central African Republic. Lancet 1:1338, 1983.

[19]Gubler DJ, Suharyono W, Lubis I, et al: Epidemic dengue 3 in Central Java associated with low viremia in man. Am J Trop Med Hyg 30:1094, 1981.

[20]Halstead SB, Voulgoropoulos E, Tien NH, Udomsadki S: Dengue hemorrhagic fever in South Vietnam: report of the 1963 outbreak. Am J Trop Med Hyg 14:819, 1965.

[21]Health and Welfare Canada: A case of Rift Valley fever with retinopathy. Canada Diseases Weekly Report 5:189, 1979.

[22]Henchal EA, McCown JM, Seguin MC, et al: Rapid identification of dengue virus isolates by using monoclonal antibodies in an indirect immunofluorescence assay. Am J Trop Med Hyg 32:164, 1983.

[23]Johnson KM, Taylor P, Elliott LH, Tomari O: Recovery of a Lassa-related arenavirus in Zimbabwe. Am J Trop Med Hyg 30:1291, 1981.

[24]Lee HW, Lee PW, Johnson KM: Isolation of the etiologic agent of Korean hemorrhagic fever. J Infect Dis 137:298, 1978.

[25]McLean DM: Virology in Health Care. Williams and Wilkins, Baltimore 1980.

[26]McLean DM: Imported arbovirus infections. in Recent Advances in Clinical Virology 3. ed AP Waterson, Churchill Livingstone 1983, p 237.

[27]McLean DM, Grass PN, Judd BD, et al: Bunyavirus isolations from mosquitoes in the western Canadian arctic. J Hyg 79:61, 1977.

[28]Mertens PE, Patton R, Baum JJ, Monath TP: Clinical presentation of Lassa fever cases during the hospital epidemic at Zorzor, Liberia, March-April 1972. Am J Trop Med Hyg 22:780, 1973.

[29]Moreau JP, Rosen L, Saugrain J, Lagraulet J: An epidemic of dengue on Tahiti associated with hemorrhagic manifestations. Am J Trop Med Hyg 22:237, 1973.

[30]Pattyn S, Jacob W, van der Groen G, et al: Isolation of Marburg-like virus from a case of hemorrhagic fever in Zaire. Lancet 1:573, 1977.

[31]Pinheiro FP, Travassos da Rosa APA, Travassos da Rosa JFS, et al: An epidemic of yellow fever in Central Brazil 1972–1973. I. Epidemiological studies. Am J Trop Med Hyg 27:125, 1978.

[32]Pinheiro FP, Travassos da Rosa APA, Travassos da Rosa JFS, et al: Oropouche virus. I. A review of clinical, epidemiological and ecological findings. Am J Trop Med Hyg 30:149, 1981.

[33]Pinheiro FP, Freitas RB, Travassos da Rosa JF, et al: An outbreak of Mayaro virus disease in Belterra, Brazil. I. Clinical and virological findings. Am J Trop Med Hyg 30:674, 1981.

[34]Public Health Laboratory Service; a case of Congo/Crimean hemorrhagic fever in South Africa. Communicable Disease Report 81/19, p 3.

[35]Rosen L: The use of *Toxorhynchites* mosquitoes to detect and propagate dengue and other arboviruses. Am J Trop Med Hyg 30:177, 1981.

[36]Rosen L, Gubler DJ, Bennett PH: Epidemic polyarthritis (Ross River) virus infection in the Cook Islands. Am J Trop Med Hyg 30:1294, 1981.

[37]Russell PK, Buescher EL, McCown JM, Ordonez J: Recovery of dengue viruses from patients during epidemics in Puerto Rico and East Pakistan. Am J Trop Med Hyg 15:573, 1966.

[38]Sarkar JK, Pavri KM, Chaterjee SN, et al: Virological and serological studies in cases of hemorrhagic fever in Calcutta. Material collected by the Calcutta School of Tropical Medicine. Indian J Med Res 52:684, 1964.

[39]Saluzzo JF, Digoutte JP, Cornet M, et al: Isolation of Crimean-Congo hemorrhagic fever and Rift Valley fever viruses in Upper Volta. Lancet 1:1179, 1984.

[40]Saluzzo JF, Digoutte JP, Camicas JL, Chauvancy G: Crimean-Congo hemorrhagic fever and Rift Valley fever in south-eastern Mauritania. Lancet 1:116, 1985.

[41]Siegert R, Shu HL, Slenczka W, et al: Zur Atiologic einer unbekanten, von Affen ausgegangenen, menschlichen Infektionskrankheit. Deutsch Med Wochenschr 92:2341, 1967.

[42]Smith DH, Johnson BK, Isaacson M, et al: Marburg-virus disease in Kenya. Lancet 1:816, 1982.

[43]Spence L, Downs WG, Boyd C, Aitken THG: Description of human yellow fever cases seen in Trinidad in 1959. West Indian Med J 9:273, 1960.

[44]Strode GK: Yellow fever. McGraw Hill, New York 1951.

[45]Walker E, Pinkerton IW, Lloyd G: Scottish case of hemorrhagic fever with renal syndrome. Lancet 2:982, 1984.

[46]Woodall JP, Williams MC, Simpson DIH: Congo virus: a hitherto undescribed virus occurring in Africa. II. Identification studies. East African Med J 44:93, 1967.

[47]Work TH: Russian spring-summer virus in India. Kyasanur Forest disease. Progr Med Virol 1:248, 1958.

PART IV

CHAPTER 25

LABORATORY DIAGNOSIS OF VIRUS INFECTIONS

Knowledge of the proper time and procedure is the central issue in laboratory diagnosis of virus infections. Allied health professionals play a vital role in achieving rapid and accurate results of diagnostic tests through: (a) collection of the appropriate samples from their patients at the correct moment of time during the patient's illness; (b) accurate labelling of specimens; (c) placing specimens in appropriate transport medium and ensuring adequate refrigeration during transit to the laboratory; (d) arranging transit of specimens by the most expeditious mode. Upon receipt of results of virological tests, allied health professionals should comprehend their relevance to the manner in which each category of professional works with the patient: (a) to promote expeditious recovery from illness; (b) to prevent spread of infection to other patients, staff or visitors.

SPECIMENS

SAME-DAY TESTS (VIRUS IDENTIFICATION—PRESUMPTIVE)

VESICLES are punctured with a scalpel or #26 gauge hypodermic needle; the fluid, or scraping from the base of the vesicle, is applied directly to: (a) a carbon-coated 300-mesh electron microscope grid; (b) several wells on a teflon-coated immunofluorescence slide. Slides are air-dried, then fixed immediately by immersion in chilled acetone for 10 minutes, followed by drying.

THROAT garglings, or nasopharyngeal secretions or throat swabs, are suspended in 2 ml transport medium in snap-cap or screw-cap vials and conveyed to the laboratory without refrigeration, if transit time is less than 30 minutes, or in a suitable container with ice at 4° C, if transit times are longer than 30 minutes but not more than 24 hours. In the laboratory, the specimen is centrifuged at 2000 x g for 10 minutes to deposit epithelial cells and bacteria. Cellular deposit is applied to: (a) electron microscope grids; (b) wells on immunofluorescence slides which are then fixed in acetone as above.

CSF is applied directly to: (a) electron microscope grids; (b) immunofluorescence slides which are fixed in acetone as above.

FECES is conveyed directly to the laboratory in snap-cap or screw-cap vials. Portions about 1 gram are dispersed with 2 ml water and suspensions are: (a) placed directly on electron microscope grids; (b) centrifuged at 2000 x g for 10 minutes to deposit coarse particles and the supernatant is used in ELISA tests.

MODE OF TRANSIT

Specimens are conveyed to the laboratory on the day of collection, or as soon as possible thereafter, by any convenient mode. Prompt transit ensures prompt results. Refrigeration is not required.

VIRUS ISOLATION TESTS (VIRUS IDENTIFICATION—DEFINITIVE)

VESICLES are punctured with a scalpel or #26 gauge needle and the fluid, or scrapings from the base of the vesicle on the puncturing instrument, are dispersed in 2 ml transport medium in snap-cap or screw-cap vials. Transport medium is usually tissue culture minimal essential medium containing at least 5% fetal bovine serum or 0.75% bovalbumin fraction V; the added protein stabilizes the virus infectivity during transport to the laboratory and is mandatory in order to achieve good results from attempts at virus isolation.

THROAT garglings or nasopharyngeal secretions or throat swabs are suspended immediately in 2 ml transport medium.

CSF is collected directly into snap-cap or screw-cap vials.

FECES is conveyed directly to the laboratory in snap-cap or screw-cap vials; rectal swabs which show obvious fecal staining are immersed in 2 ml transport medium in snap-cap or screw-cap vials.

OTHER FLUID SPECIMENS such as urine, joint aspirate, pericardial aspirate are transported expeditiously to the laboratory without transport medium. However biopsy fragments should always be immersed in transport medium.

MODE OF TRANSIT
Virus Laboratory in Same Institution as Patient. Convey the specimen by personal messenger so as to reach the virus laboratory within 30 minutes after their collection from the patient. Refrigeration is not required during transit. At the laboratory, the specimens require holding refrigerated at 4° C until inoculation into appropriate tissue cultures.

Transit Time Less Than 24 Hours. Pack the specimens in a styrofoam or comparable insulated shipping container with ice cubes or pre-frozen refrigerant packs. Ship to the laboratory by the most expeditious mode e.g. taxi within urban areas, parcels courier or air express from rural areas.

Ship only on Mondays through Thursdays, never ship on Fridays or one day before a statutory holiday.

Transit Time Longer Than 24 Hours. Pack the specimens in a styrofoam or comparable insulated shipping container with a sufficient quantity of Dry Ice to maintain the specimens frozen at $-70°$ C for at least 72 hours. Specimens should be flame-sealed in glass ampoules if at all possible; this prevents possible viral inactivation by seepage of CO_2 through teflon or rubber seals of snap-cap or screw-cap vials at ultra-low temperatures. Immediately after collection from patients, whilst specimens are awaiting shipment, the specimens should be stored frozen at $-70°$ C in an electric ultra-low temperature cabinet. Similarly, upon arrival at the testing laboratory, specimens should be transferred promptly to an ultra-low temperature cabinet to await virus isolation attempts.

Alternatively, where facilities for holding and transporting of specimens frozen at $-190°$ C in liquid nitrogen are available, this offers an equally satisfactory means of preservation of virus viability in specimens until tested.

Plan the transportation schedule so that specimens are estimated to arrive at the testing laboratory on Mondays through Thursdays, or at least one day before a statutory holiday.

SEROLOGICAL TESTS (CONFIRMATORY AND EPIDEMIOLOGICAL)

DIAGNOSIS OF ILL PERSONS. Collect 2–5 ml clotted blood by venepuncture using a sterile syringe and # 21 or 22 gauge needle, or vacutainer with a similar needles: (a) immediately upon obtaining the history and conducting the initial physical examination as soon as possible after onset of illness; *plus* (b) one day or more after the temperature returns to normal accompanied by obvious clinical improvement of the patient (frequently the interval between collection of this pair of blood samples is 3–7 days). Do not collect the second blood sample until the temperature has remained normal, at least 24 hours. Send these clotted blood samples to the laboratory as promptly as possible, without refrigeration if the estimated transit time is less than 48 hours. For transit times exceeding 48 hours, or if the samples are likely to freeze during winter, or to become excessively heated during summer, separate the serum from the clot within 2 hours of collection of the sample, and dispatch the serum only. Good practice suggests holding the first blood sample in a refrigerator on the ward where the patient is located in hospital, until the second sample is collected several days later; sera are pipetted away from clots into sterile vials, and the serum pair is shipped together.

EPIDEMIOLOGICAL SURVEYS. These are employed to determine the prevalence of a virus serotype in a population at a particular point in time. On a stated day, 2–5 ml samples of clotted blood are collected by vene-puncture from representative members of each age range e.g. 20 persons aged 5–9 years, another 20 aged 15–19 years and so on. Sera are conveyed unrefrigerated by the epidemiological team from the collection site to the laboratory on the day of collection, then held refrigerated overnight and sera are separated from clots on the following morning. Less satisfactory alterna-tive arrangements are the collection of blood from residents of a district whenever these residents can be located during the course of a week, separat-ing sera from clots after holding the blood samples overnight in refrigerators, and shipping the sera piecemeal to the laboratory.

LABELLING OF SPECIMENS

All specimens must be labelled with self-adhesive stickers containing essential details such as patient's full name, address, sex, date of birth, hos-pital or other serial number, attending physician's name, date of collection. Accompanying requisitions (one per sample) should state, in addition to the above demographic data, the disease syndrome or system affected and the date of onset of present illness.

Upon receipt by the testing laboratory, all the above data are entered in an accession book or fed into a computer and a sequential accession number is assigned to each specimen.

PRINCIPLES OF TESTS

SAME-DAY TESTS

ELECTRON MICROSCOPY. After adding phosphotungstic acid as a negative stain to the specimen on an electron microscope grid, the specimen is examined in an electron microscope at magnifications up to 200,000 x or more. In our laboratory, this is accomplished with a Philips EM300 electron microscope. Virus particles with morphology typical of a family e.g. Para-myxoviridae, will be observed in virus-positive specimens within 10 minutes. The report "paramyxovirus particles seen" is telephoned immediately to the hospital ward or the attending physician, and represents a presumptive virological diagnosis of immediate clinical relevance to the future treatment and prognosis of the patient.

IMMUNOFLUORESCENCE. With the virus family established by electron microscopy, preliminary serotyping of the infecting virus is undertaken by indirect immunofluorescence. For paramyxovirus particles in a patient with an acute respiratory infection, three common serotypes are parainfluenza types 1 and 3 and respiratory syncytial (RS) virus. Antisera to the viruses are added to wells on teflon-coated multispot slides containing centrifuged deposit from throat samples, incubated, washed, fluorescein-labelled anti-species antiserum is added, incubated, washed, counterstained with naphthalene black, washed and the slides are examined by incident ultraviolet light. Apple-green fluorescent points in cells treated with parainfluenza-1 antiserum indicate that the infecting serotype was parainfluenza-1. This result is telephoned or faxed to the hospital ward within 3 hours of collection of the specimen.

VIRUS ISOLATION TESTS

All specimens suspended in transport medium are centrifuged at 2000 x g for at least 10 minutes to deposit bacteria. Supernatants in 0.1 ml aliquots are inoculated into plate or tube tissue cultures of primary rhesus monkey kidney, continuous human diploid fibroblasts and sometimes continuous human polyploid epithelial cells. Plates are incubated stationary in humidified CO_2 incubators, tubes are rolled at 1 revolution every 5–10 minutes in incubators, and examined for cytopathic effects each day for 7–14 days according to the virus. Some arboviruses may require continuous African green monkey (VERO) cells to exhibit cytopathic effects, and often virus isolation is enhanced by overlay with agarose, when plaque formation is observed after several days incubation. Virus liberated into the tissue culture supernatant at the time of cytopathic effect is typed by neutralization (enteroviruses) or hemagglutination inhibition (mumps). Influenza and parainfluenza viruses are not usually cytopathic but the tissue culture supernatant contains hemagglutinin, which is serotyped by hemagglutination inhibition. Herpes-viruses cause clumping of tissue culture cells which appear as grape-like clusters—these cells are dislodged by forceful pipetting, they are placed on teflon-coated multispot slides and serotyped by immunofluorescence.

These results definitively establish the freshly isolated virus as the particular serotype which infected the patient at the time of illness. Usually 4–10 days are required to achieve the final result. It is entered into the patient's health record after transmittal to the hospital ward by computer or intramural messenger, or to the attending physician by mail or fax. Although essential for epidemiological purposes, these results usually come through too late to influence the course of clinical management of the patient, but they are useful in prognosis.

SEROLOGICAL TESTS

Paired sera from patients are always tested together. It is important to defer testing until receipt of the second specimen. Evidence that a patient's illness was caused by a particular serotype is demonstrated either by a conversion of the patient's antibody status from negative to positive, or by at least a fourfold of antibody titer between collection of sera.

Hemagglutination inhibition tests are preferred for antibody titrations whenever the virus is a hemagglutinating agent e.g. influenza, parainfluenza, rubella, because they are technically straightforward and they are completed within 2 hours. In some systems, these tests are being superseded by enzyme immunoassay (ELISA) tests which, although they may require 3–4 hours for performance, are completed by a printout from a spectrophotometer. Neutralization tests in tissue culture (cytopathic inhibition in tube cultures or plaque reduction in plate cultures) are required for enterovirus antibody determinations—these require 3–4 days for completion. All the above tests detect antibodies which appear shortly after defervescence.

Immunofluorescence (indirect) tests are used routinely for determination of antibodies to Epstein-Barr virus (mononucleosis) and they may be adapted to any virus system, provided that multispot slides are seeded with virus-infected tissue culture cells. Antibodies in the IgM (initial 4–6 weeks after onset) or IgG (long term persistence) components of serum proteins are determined using fluorecein-labelled antibodies to human IgM or IgG respectively.

Radioimmunoassays are used routinely for detection of antibodies to hepatitis A and hepatitis B. Particularly with hepatitis A, determination of antibodies in the IgM component indicates current infection. This provides the only convenient means for diagnosis of hepatitis A infection, because the virus is difficult to detect routinely in patients' feces. Enzyme immunoassays may soon supersede radioimmunoassays in hepatitis diagnosis.

LABORATORY ASSISTANCE IN WORK OF ALLIED HEALTH PROFESSIONALS (WITH NOTES ON COST EFFECTIVENESS)

Close observation of patients by allied health professionals, especially nurses and physiotherapists, often alerts the health team to an emergent viral infection. Several examples illustrate the role of these members of the health team in prevention of nosocomial infections.[3]

MEASLES. Rash involving the face and trunk, together with a runny nose and watery eyes, may be noticed by an admitting nurse in a child who was referred to hospital for elective surgery. Performance of an electron microscopic-examination of throat secretions may reveal paramyxovirus particles suggestive of measles within 1/2 hour of specimen collection, whilst the patient is held in an isolation cubicle. This is confirmed as measles within 3 hours by immunofluorescence. The patient is returned home until the rash and fever have remitted completely after one week. This immediate presumptive test, at an insured cost about $28, has prevented the admission of a case of measles who, almost certainly, would have transmitted measles nosocomially to other nearby hospitalized patients at a cost exceeding $300 per day for each additional day of hospitalization. This represents a benefit:cost ratio about 10:1.

CHICKENPOX. Development of vesicles over the face and trunk, and fever in a child already hospitalized with an orthopedic condition, is usually observed first by a physiotherapist or nurse. Prompt identification of the infecting agent as varicella virus by immunofluorescence, with or without electron microscopy, during the succeeding 3 hours, provides adequate scientific justification for transfer of this patient to isolation facilities, thus preventing nosocomial spread of chicken pox which causes particularly severe disease in immunocompromized patients. The cost saving ratio 10:1 is similar to early recognition of measles.

GASTROENTERITIS. Increase in the frequency of passing stools in a subject with chronic diarrhea may first be observed by the attending dietician or the nurse who then recommends the collection of feces for virological examination. Identification of rotavirus within 1/2 hour by electron microscopy, or 3–4 hours by ELISA, indicates the virological cause of the acute-on-chronic gastroenteritis, and necessitates isolation of the patient to prevent nosocomial transmission of rotavirus. The cost saving ratio again is about 10:1.

VACCINATION PROGRAMS (COST EFFECTIVENESS AND WORKING OF PROFESSIONALS)

The Commonwealth of Massachusetts Department of Public Health in 1981 found that, from commencement of a public immunization program against measles in 1966, the annual reported cases of measles fell by 19% from 19,152 cases in 1965 to 59 cases in 1980, an estimated decrease of 237,953 cases of measles.[1] The cost of vaccination of more than 3 million persons was $3,713,029. Without this measles vaccination program, the cost of caring for patients with measles and complications was estimated at $12,048,905, instead of the actual $448,361. This represented a saving of $7,887,515. Cost savings for a 99% reduction in the annual incidence of mumps through vaccination programs from 1969 to 1980 were $1,816,558. For a 95% reduction in rubella incidence through vaccination between 1970 and 1980, cost savings were $6,427,110. Additional cost savings throughout USA are likely to be achieved from 1985 onwards through the virtual elimination of congenital rubella syndrome by universal vaccination of infants after their first birthdays.[2]

Rubella affected 47 of 2983 health care personnel at a Massachusetts tertiary-care facility during spring 1979.[4] The index case worked in the dietary department, and infection spread in two waves to health workers in most departments, of whom 12% were devoid of rubella antibodies. As a result, 475 employee workdays were lost and one pregnancy was terminated. The total cost of the outbreak was estimated at $50,000 for extra staff, lost worktime and additional laboratory tests. An additional cost was provision of rubella vaccine to 1974 of 2983 (66%) employees in attempts to prevent further spread of rubella.

REFERENCES

[1]Fiumara NJ. Cost-benefit effectiveness for vaccination programs. Presented at a Symposium on Immunization; the Means to Eradicating Infectious Diseases, Montreal, Canada. 9 March 1981.

[2]Hinman AR, Bart KJ, Orenstein WA, Preblud SR: Rational strategy for rubella vaccination. Lancet 1:39, 1983.

[3]McLean DM, Wong KK: Same-day diagnosis of human virus infections. CRC Press, Boca Raton, FL, 1984.

[4]Polk BF, White JA, DeGirolami PC, Modlin JF: An outbreak of rubella among hospital personnel. New Eng J Med 303:541, 1980.

GLOSSARY OF VIROLOGICAL TERMS

Antigen: organic substance (usually protein, MW >12,000) which stimulates the reticuloendothelial system to make antibodies and/or to show increased reactivity towards the antigen.

Antibody: serum protein (globulin MW >70,000) produced by reticuloendothelial system in response stimulation by an antigen, which reacts specifically with that antigen.

Attenuated: virus infects a person and induces immunity without causing illness.

B-cells (lymphocytes): lymphocytes which produce antiviral antibodies.

Capsid: anatomical arrangement of protein subunits (and nucleic acid) within the virion. Some fully infectious virions are naked capsids (eg. adenovirus), others require an outer proteinaceous envelope (eg. influenza virus).

Capsomere: fundamental virus structural protein subunit.

Cytopathic effect: microscopically visible change in the cell following virus growth within it.

Deoxyribonucleic acid (DNA): nucleic acid containing purine or pyrimidine bases and deoxyribose (a sugar with 5 carbon atoms).

Electron microscope: machine for magnifying objects to x300,000 using the substantially shorter wavelength of a beam of electrons than a beam of visible light. Objects as small as 0.3 to 1.0 nm can be visualized.

Endemic: cases occur infrequently during each year.

Envelope: lipoprotein coat surrounding the virus capsid. The protein is usually derived from host cells under stimulation by the virus.

Epidemic: small or large clusters of cases occurring over a narrow time frame.

Exotic: imported from another country or region.

Genome: virus-specific nucleic acid (RNA or DNA). Viruses do not contain both RNA and DNA.

Host: human or other living creature (may be as small as an individual cell) which a virus may infect.

Immunity: ability of a person to remain without illness following a further encounter with the same virus serotype.

Incidence rate: frequency or risk of occurrence of a virus infection during some specified interval of time eg. number of cases per 100,000 per year.

Indigenous: present within a community from year to year.

Infect: ability of a virus to invade a host (or an individual cell) an multiply inside it.

Nanometer: 10^{-9} meter. Virus sizes range from 20 to 300 nm (1 nm = 1 mμ).

Nucleocapsid: combination of nucleic acid and protein, often appearing as strands as in influenza virus.

Pandemic: world-wide occurrence of cases over an extensive duration.

Pathogen: ability of a virus to infect and cause disease (mild to severe).

Prevalence rate: frequency or risk of occurrence of a virus infection at some point in time eg. number of cases per 100,000 on 22 March 1985.

Prophylaxis: prevention of infection by vaccine or antiserum administration.

Rate: ratio of number of persons with disease as the numerator and number of the total population at risk as the denominator.

Ribonucleic acid (RNA): nucleic acid containing purine or pyrimidine bases and ribose (a sugar with 5 carbon atoms).

Sign: clinical features which are found on examination of the patient eg. enlarged spleen, elevated temperature.

Sporadic: single case, or cases of infection scattered randomly through a community.

Susceptible: able to support virus multiplication ie. able to be infected by a virus.

Symptom: clinical features which the patient describes eg. pain, nausea.

Syndrome: cluster of symptoms and signs of characteristic of a particular disease.

T-cells (lymphocytes): lymphocytes which induce cell-mediated immunity.

Titer: reciprocal of the highest dilution (ie. lowest concentration) of a virus preparation to induce infection, or of a serum sample which contains detectable antibody activity.

Vaccine: living attenuated virus, or killed virus which induces immunity against subsequent infection by the same virus serotype.

Virion: virus particle

Virulent: ability of a virus to infect and cause illness (mild to severe).

Virus: microorganism <300 nm diameter containing only RNA or DNA (but not both), which multiplies only inside living cells of susceptible hosts.

INDEX

Virus distinction from bacteria 4

W
Western Equine Encephalitis (WEE) 7, 167,
        171, 349
Weil-Felix test 230

Y
Yellow fever
    clinical 175, 347
    epidemiology 7, 167, 352
    HI 171
    mice 7, 167, 351
    vaccine (17D) 92, 354